Collaborating for Student Success

A Guide for School-Based Occupational Therapy

Edited by Barbara Hanft, MA, OTR, FAOTA,
and Jayne Shepherd, MS, OTR, FAOTA

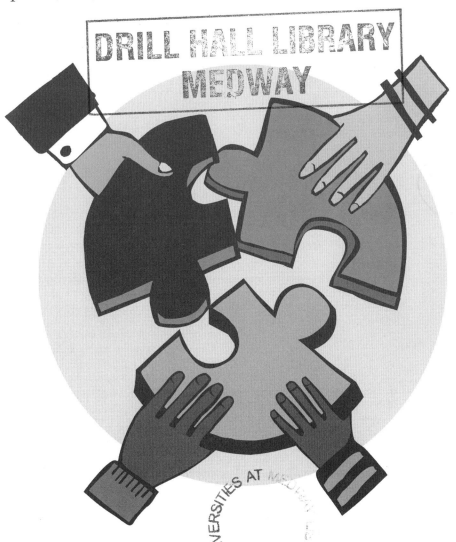

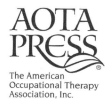

AOTA PRESS®
The American
Occupational Therapy
Association, Inc.

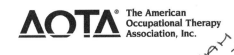

AOTA® The American
Occupational Therapy
Association, Inc.

Centennial Vision

We envision that occupational therapy is a powerful, widely recognized, science-driven, and evidence-based profession with a globally connected and diverse workforce meeting society's occupational needs.

Vision Statement

The American Occupational Therapy Association advances occupational therapy as the pre-eminent profession in promoting the health, productivity, and quality of life of individuals and society through the therapeutic application of occupation.

Mission Statement

The American Occupational Therapy Association advances the quality, availability, use, and support of occupational therapy through standard-setting, advocacy, education, and research on behalf of its members and the public.

AOTA Staff

Frederick P. Somers, *Executive Director*
Christopher M. Bluhm, *Chief Operating Officer*
Maureen Freda Peterson, *Chief Professional Affairs Officer*

Chris Davis, *Director, AOTA Press*
Sarah D. Hertfelder, *Continuing Education Program Manager*
Caroline Polk, *Project Manager*
Michael Melletz, *Book Production Manager*
Linda Weidemann, Wolf Creek Press, *Compositor*
Carrie Mercadante, *Production Editor*

The American Occupational Therapy Association, Inc.
4720 Montgomery Lane
Bethesda, MD 20814
Phone: 301-652-AOTA (2682)
TDD: 800-377-8555
Fax: 301-652-7711
www.aota.org

To order: 877-404-AOTA (2682)

Disclaimers

This publication is designed to provide accurate and authoritative information in regard to the subject matter covered. It is sold or distributed with the understanding that the publisher is not engaged in rendering legal, accounting, or other professional service. If legal advice or other expert assistance is required, the services of a competent professional person should be sought.

*—From the Declaration of Principles jointly adopted by the American Bar Association
and a Committee of Publishers and Associations*

It is the objective of the American Occupational Therapy Association to be a forum for free expression and interchange of ideas. The opinions expressed by the contributors to this work are their own and not necessarily those of the American Occupational Therapy Association.

ISBN-13: 978-1-56900-247-6
ISBN-10: 1-56900-247-9

Library of Congress Cataloging-in-Publication Data
Collaborating for student success : a guide for school-based occupational therapy/edited by Barbara Hanft and Jayne Shepherd. p. ; cm.
  Includes bibliographical references and indexes.
  ISBN-13: 978-1-56900-247-6
  ISBN-10: 1-56900-247-9
  1. Occupational therapy for children. 2. Children with disabilities—Education
3. Children with disabilities—Rehabilitation.
I. Hanft, Barbara E. II. Shepherd, Jayne. III. American Occupational Therapy Association.
  [DNLM: 1. Occupational Therapy—methods. 2. Child. 3. Disabled Children—education. 4. Disabled Children—rehabilitation. 5. Faculty. 6. Group Processes. WS 368 C697 2008]

RJ53.O25C65 2008
362.17'8083--dc22

2008010416

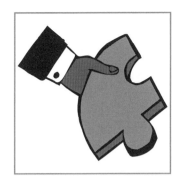

Contents

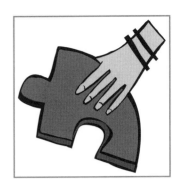

Dedication

In honor of our ASPIIRE colleagues who inspire us to
collaborate,
communicate,
coordinate, and
cogitate.

And our family partners who support us every day:
Roland and Fred.

Acknowledgments

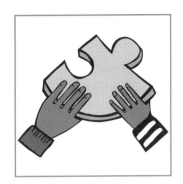

We could not possibly have written a book about collaborating without seeking the wisdom of a select group of therapists, educators, families, and administrators who live and breathe teamwork in their daily interactions in the schools. In honor of their unique perspectives and experiences, we identify these individuals at the end of each chapter.

Two extraordinary groups of reviewers critiqued our manuscript at two critical stages: our first draft and the extended rewrite. The following occupational therapy students at the University of Southern California, led by their faculty, Diane Kellegrew and Jean Pacifica-Banta, in a course on school-based practice poured over our first draft and sent us more than 100 pages of commentary.

Kelly Bloom
Sara Cassone
Courtney Daniels
Inbal Fraiman
Kory Fukuwa
Anthony Gallegos

Samana Khan
Rebecca Kim
Sophia Lin
Christine Nakamura
Denver Nino
Melissa Schofield

Karen Smikahl
Britt Sorensen
Sarah Tompkins
Maritza Villegas
Rebecca Zino

Three expert clinicians, Chris Knippenberg, Jean Polichino, and Judie Sage, completed an in-depth review with astonishing speed and critiqued our final manuscript from the perspective of providing "helpful help" for building the collaborative skills of occupational therapists who are currently working or desire to work in education settings.

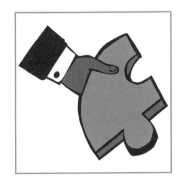

About the Authors

Barbara Hanft, MA, OTR, FAOTA, co-editor of this volume, has 35 years of experience as a clinician, lecturer, and lobbyist. An occupational therapist with a graduate degree in counseling psychology, she has managed a rural early intervention program, directed therapeutic services in an urban special education setting, and developed a private practice as a developmental consultant. Hanft has designed a broad range of professional development programs, including a nationally recognized model in-service to promote family-centered care in early intervention programs. Recognized as a Fellow by the American Occupational Therapy Association (AOTA) in 1989 for her leadership and advocacy in pediatrics, Hanft lobbied Congress in 1986 on behalf of AOTA to amend the Individuals With Disabilities Education Act (IDEA) to create preschool and early intervention programs. In 1995, she was awarded a Presidential Citation by AOTA for developing Promoting Partnerships, a leadership project focused on bringing education and early intervention administrators together with occupational therapy practitioners and educators to enhance services and supports to children and their families.

Hanft teaches, writes, and consults nationwide with schools, early intervention programs, and related community agencies regarding family-centered care in natural environments, child development, and special education and related services in the public schools. With more than 25 publications in early childhood and team collaboration, Hanft was awarded the Jeannette Bair Writer's Award by AOTA for co-authoring "School-Based Practice: Moving Beyond 1:1 Service Delivery," published in *OT Practice* in 2002. She has also co-authored two best-selling books: *The Consulting Therapist: A Guide for Occupational and Physical Therapists in Schools* and *Coaching Families and Colleagues in Early Childhood*.

Jayne Shepherd, MS, OTR, FAOTA, co-editor of this volume, has worked for more than 26 years as a therapist and occupational therapy educator. A former special education teacher, she understands the unique needs of teachers working with related services personnel. Before coming to academia, Shepherd worked as a clinician, fieldwork coordinator, and supervisor in acute care, rehabilitation, and inpatient and outpatient settings for children and adults. She teaches at Virginia Commonwealth University (VCU) and consults with varied pediatric and special education programs in Virginia.

Shepherd has taught in multiple interdisciplinary grants for infant intervention, early childhood education, and Maternal and Child Health. From 1994 to 1999 she directed a 5-year pre-service and in-service grant, Interdisciplinary School-Based Training for Occupational and Physical Therapists. This grant was highlighted during AOTA's Promoting Partnerships project as an example of how to work with a state's Department of Education to develop and fund education for therapists. As the School System co-liaison for the Virginia Occupational Therapy Association and as an AOTA Associations of Service Providers Implementing IDEA Reforms in Education (ASPIIRE) Partnership Cadre member, Shepherd has organized and presented at numerous conferences related to school-based practice.

Shepherd is the assistant chair and director for postprofessional education at VCU. She coordinates Fieldwork I and teaches content related to pediatrics, school-based practice, assistive technology, therapeutic activities, and clinical reasoning. Her research interests and publications are in school-based therapy, adolescent transition services from school to community, assistive technology in pediatrics, activities of daily living and instrumental activities of daily living, and play.

Gloria Frolek Clark, MS, OTR/L, BCP, FAOTA, is a 1977 graduate of the University of North Dakota's occupational therapy program. She has an MS in early childhood special education from Iowa State University and is a doctoral student. During the past 30 years, Frolek Clark has specialized in occupational therapy services for pediatric clients in home, community, and school settings. She was cofounder and chair of the AOTA School System Special Interest Section (SSSIS) and is a member of the current SSSIS. While on the AOTA Commission on Practice, she contributed to the development of the *Occupational Therapy Practice Framework* and many other official AOTA documents. Frolek Clark has presented nationally on early intervention services and school-based practice; has authored several book chapters and articles on practice; and was appointed to the AOTA Specialty Board, Pediatric Panel. She is AOTA's representative to the National Association of State Directors of Special Education's IDEA Partnership Projects funded through the U.S. Department of Education, Office of Special Education Programs. Frolek Clark works for the Heartland Area Education Agency in the Adel office providing occupational therapy services in early intervention, preschool, school-age, and community programs and is a consultant for the Iowa Department of Education in Des Moines.

Yvonne Swinth, PhD, OTR/L, FAOTA, is professor at the University of Puget Sound and continues to work one day a week at the University Place School District in Tacoma, Washington. She has more than 20 years of experience in school-based practice and has presented locally, nationally, and internationally on topics related to services for children. She is the editor of the current AOTA Online Course for school-based therapists, *Occupational Therapy in School-Based Practice: Contemporary Issues and Trends.* Swinth is a past chairperson of AOTA's SSSIS and has served as the education and research liaison to the SSSIS prior to that. She is also an AOTA representative on the National IDEA Resource Cadre of the federally funded IDEA Partnership Projects, U.S. Department of Education, Office of Special Education Programs, and is co-chair of

Occupational Therapists in Schools, a standing committee for the Washington Occupational Therapy Association. Swinth has presented internationally and nationally on topics related to school-based practice and has authored more than 10 book chapters and articles specific to service delivery in the schools. She is analyzing data from a national research project that is addressing efficacy and efficiency in school-based occupational therapy.

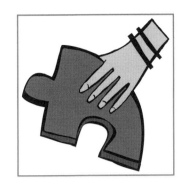

List of Reflections, Resources, Tables, and Figures

Chapter 4

Chapter 5

Chapter 6

Chapter 7

Appendix: Exhibits and Worksheets

Introduction

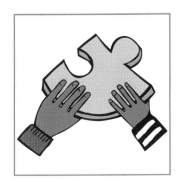

Barbara Hanft, MA, OTR, FAOTA, and
Jayne Shepherd, MS, OTR, FAOTA

Collaborating for Student Success: A Guide for School-Based Occupational Therapy is designed as both a textbook and an American Occupational Therapy Association (AOTA) Self-Paced Clinical Course (the continuing education instructions and exam are in a separate packet) to engage school-based occupational therapists in collaborative practice with education teams. The ultimate goal of team collaboration for occupational therapists is to ensure that students engage in educationally relevant occupations as part of their typical school routines, or *paces*, within a variety of school *places* and *spaces*, such as the classroom, cafeteria, gymnasium, and community work sites.

Why This Topic Now?

It is widely accepted by occupational therapists working in diverse settings that collaboration is great to engage in and is a valuable part of teamwork. But what it actually looks like in education—and how to do it effectively to promote student performance—is akin to the tale of the blind men touching an elephant's tusk, ear, tail, or foot and deciding that the particular part touched describes all there is to know about an elephant.

Throughout our teaching, conversations, and visits with school-based practitioners over the years, we have heard *collaboration* described as team meetings, informal discussions, working in the classroom, helping teachers and aides, and general getting along with one's teammates. Few therapists connected collaboration to how effectively a student engaged in typical school occupations. Collaboration was essentially regarded as another service model, an intervention, a new name for consultation, and the latest education trend. Although acknowledged as a good thing to do with teachers and families, collaboration with team members was separate from what occupational therapists did with students to help them develop the skills and behaviors they needed to be successful in school. We rarely heard collaboration described as an *interactive team process* focused on student performance and influenced by critical personal and contextual variables.

We decided to write a practical guide highlighting *how* occupational therapists collaborate effectively with family and education partners in the schools and connecting collaboration to the mandate in the Individuals With Disabilities Education Act (IDEA) and No Child Left Behind Act to help all students participate in the general curriculum. Collaboration does not "happen" just because an occupational therapist and teacher work together in the same classroom or because a parent and therapist talk to one another.

To accomplish our goal, we reflected on our experiences teaching in university and continuing education programs and working in the schools as occupational therapists (as well as Jayne's experience as a special educator and Barbara's experience as an elementary school guidance counselor). We knew that we could not possibly write about collaboration without collaborating ourselves with a score of experienced and articulate parents, public school students, therapists, occupational therapy students, teachers, and administrators. We enlisted two experts in school-based practice, Gloria Frolek Clark and Yvonne Swinth, to share their school expertise and describe the successes and challenges practitioners encounter daily when providing collaborative services and supports to students, teams, and school systems. Finally, we poured through the occupational therapy, school psychology, and education literature (both print and online) on collaboration and teamwork in school-based practice.

Objectives for the Target Audience

The key to effective collaboration in education settings is learning to use one's professional knowledge and interpersonal skills to blend hands-on services for students with team and system supports for families, educators, and the school system at large. Seven chapters discuss the essential topics that shape collaborative practice (see table).

We targeted our content for *experienced* school-based occupational therapists who already know how to provide pediatric occupational therapy evaluations, assessments, and intervention and who understand the federal and state laws, regulations, and policies that govern public education (or at least know who to talk to about their impact on school-based practice). Our content is appropriate for occupational therapy therapists and occupational therapy assistants; however, our intent is not to address their role delineation in education settings. Note that the terms *occupational therapist* and *therapist* are used throughout AOTA publications and Self-Paced Clinical Courses. That choice does not exclude the important role the occupational therapy assistant has in meeting the needs of people who need occupational therapy. The occupational therapist is responsible for all aspects of occupational therapy service delivery and is accountable for the safety and effectiveness of the occupational therapy delivery process. The occupational therapy assistant delivers occupational therapy services under the supervision of and in partnership with the occupational therapist in accordance with (1) state regulations; (2) the AOTA *Standards of Practice for Occupational Therapy* (AOTA, 2005c); (3) the *Occupational Therapy Code of Ethics (2005)* (AOTA, 2005a); (4) the *Guidelines for Supervision, Roles, and Responsibilities During the Delivery of Occupational Therapy Services* (AOTA, 2004a); and (5) the *Standards for Continuing Competence* (AOTA, 2005b) and the *Scope of Practice* (AOTA, 2004b).

Eight general objectives guided our selection of content for the seven chapters in this combination textbook and Self-Paced Clinical Course:

1. Identify the characteristics and challenges of providing collaborative occupational therapy services and supports within a historical perspective of working in inclusive schools.

2. Illustrate the collaborative roles occupational therapists engage in to support students with disabilities in multiple school contexts within the context of a general education curriculum.

3. Analyze the contextual variables that influence how students, families, and education personnel collaborate in an interactive team process.

4. Describe strategies and approaches for building team partnerships, including mentoring and coaching other school-based therapists.

5. Review the evidence for providing in-context team supports to ensure students' participation in inclusive environments.

6. Consider practical strategies for resolving challenges related to participating on collaborative teams to provide occupational therapy services and supports.

7. Recognize the communication and teaming skills needed to effectively engage in collaboration to support student learning within different environments in a school.

8. Identify the process of initiating and sustaining changes in practice and influencing families/education personnel to engage in collaboration with occupational therapists.

Key Topics Covered in This Volume

Chapter	Topics
1	Definition of *collaboration* Hands-on services with team supports Team and system supports Benefits and challenges of collaboration
2	*Faces:* Core and extended school teams *Places and spaces:* School environments *Paces:* Routines, schedules, classroom culture Contextual influences on collaboration
3	Characteristics of collaborative teams Collective decision making Team operations and communication Mentoring and coaching
4	School-based occupational therapy Applying the *Occupational Therapy Practice Framework: Domain and Process** (AOTA, 2002) in education settings Early intervening services (EISs) Collaboration during evaluation, assessment, and intervention
5	Communicating about occupational therapy Managing workload Administrative support for flexible services Documenting collaborative services and supports
6	Stages of team development Problem-solving strategies Principles of negotiation Conflict resolution
7	Encouraging reluctant collaborators Family perspectives Change process in schools Initiating systemwide collaboration

*Revisions to the *Framework* were pending at the time this publication went to press; where possible, the authors have tried to be mindful of those changes.

What Readers Will Find in Each Chapter

Our guide for school-based collaboration categorizes and organizes information in a user-friendly manner; we hope you will adapt our information and strategies to your own school setting. Each chapter includes these special features:

- *Learning objectives* focus therapists on what they can expect to learn to build on their knowledge of school-based practice.
- Quotes presented as *Voices* share the perspectives of students, parents, educators, administrators, occupational therapy students, and experienced school-based therapists.
- *Collaboration in Action* vignettes illustrate key concepts about the collaborative process and demonstrate how occupational therapists provide collaborative hands-on services and team and system supports.
- *"Remember this"* selections emphasize key points for occupational therapists to keep in mind about collaboration in education settings.
- *Resources* suggest online, video, and print resources for extended reading on a particular subject.
- *Reflections* present questions and points to assist occupational therapists with applying the chapter contents to specific situations frequently encountered in school settings.
- *Tables, figures,* and *exhibits* organize information in a visual format for easy referral; a special feature is the pie charts that illustrate the percentage of hands-on services and team and system supports provided by an occupational therapist in selected vignettes (see sample at left). The vignettes about students and accompanying pie charts are summarized in Exhibit A in the Appendix.
- *Worksheets* present topical information in a format that can be put into immediate use.
- The *Appendix* includes reference material from IDEA and blank, reproducible copies (some of which are included on the enclosed CD-ROM) of all worksheets described in each chapter.

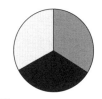

KEY:
- ☐ Hands-on services (HO)
- ■ Team supports (TS)
- ▨ System supports (SS)

What We Hope Readers Will Do With This Information

Research on effective professional development indicates that practitioners must find ways to apply the material from a workshop presentation or print resource in their own settings as soon as possible. The literature on system change also emphasizes that one cannot change everything at once and often must "go slow to go fast." Below are suggestions for enlisting colleagues to help readers consider and implement the content presented:

- Review the worksheets with a colleague and consider how you each might use it in your schools to promote team collaboration.
- Talk with occupational therapists (and other professionals) in school districts in your state and contrast their school-based practice with the collaborative teaming illustrated in the Collaboration in Action vignettes.
- Ask another occupational therapist who uses collaborative practices effectively to coach or mentor you.

- Form a reading group or an online discussion group to explore your district's hot topics addressed in the book.
- Share Chapter 5 with your supervisor and ask for a meeting with other occupational therapists to review how your workload is defined and documented.
- Choose one new collaborative strategy and invite a team member whom you think would be open and willing to try it with you.
- Share your collaborative success stories (toot your horn and inspire others) within your teams and school system, your state networks, and the School System Special Interest Section of AOTA.

A Challenge for School-Based Therapists

Occupational therapists have much to offer students, teams, and school districts; however, their services and supports are often underutilized in the education system. We challenge readers to let go of old models of providing school-based therapy, search out evidence-based practices, and develop the interpersonal skills to collaborate with team members within the complex context of public education. Reflect on your current practice and identify the "missed opportunities" for sharing your expertise and knowledge to promote student success at school. Are occupational therapists involved in your school's response to intervention teams or early intervening services? Can you join the playground renewal committee or the assistive technology or behavioral supports teams? Reframe how you use your expertise by blending hands-on student services, as needed, with team and system supports. Build on your interpersonal and communication skills to assume a leadership role within your team or school system to ensure that students acquire the skills and behaviors they need to participate in school, and ultimately, contribute to their community!

NOW . . . as we describe in the following chapters, pick up the *pace* and collaborate with different *faces* in a variety of school *places* to support teams to achieve student success!

References

American Occupational Therapy Association. (2002). Occupational therapy practice framework: Domain and process. *American Journal of Occupational Therapy, 56,* 609–639.

American Occupational Therapy Association. (2004a). Guidelines for supervision, roles, and responsibilities during the delivery of occupational therapy services. *American Journal of Occupational Therapy, 58,* 663–667.

American Occupational Therapy Association. (2004b). Scope of practice. *American Journal of Occupational Therapy, 58,* 673–677.

American Occupational Therapy Association. (2005a). Occupational therapy code of ethics (2005). *American Journal of Occupational Therapy, 59,* 639–642.

American Occupational Therapy Association. (2005b). Standards for continuing competence. *American Journal of Occupational Therapy, 59,* 661–662.

American Occupational Therapy Association. (2005c). Standards of practice for occupational therapy. *American Journal of Occupational Therapy, 59,* 663–665.

CHAPTER 1

2 . . . 4 . . . 6 . . . 8 . . .
How Do You Collaborate?

Barbara Hanft, MA, OTR, FAOTA, and
Jayne Shepherd, MS, OTR, FAOTA

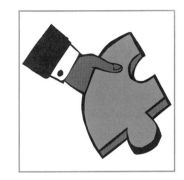

You can't beat it [collaboration]. When you're working with each other and you're trying to get the same results, there's nothing like it.

—Teacher describing her collaboration with an occupational therapist
(as quoted in field notes, Dillon, Flexman, & Probeck, 1996)

Chapter 1 lays the foundation for understanding school-based collaboration as an interactive team process focused on helping *all* students participate in school lessons and activities. For occupational therapists, the ultimate goal of team collaboration is to ensure that students engage in educationally relevant occupations as part of their typical school routines or *paces* within a variety of *places* and *spaces* such as the classroom, cafeteria, gymnasium, and community work sites. The key to effective collaboration in education settings is learning to use one's professional knowledge and interpersonal skills to blend hands-on services for students with team and system supports for families, educators, and the school system at large. Chapter 1 introduces the essential topics that shape collaborative practice:

- Hands-on and team supports in school lessons and activities
- System supports
- Benefits and challenges of collaboration.

After reading this material, readers will be able to

- Identify how legal mandates and professional guidelines for providing special education and related services in the least restrictive environment in public schools influence collaboration among therapists, families, and education staff;
- Recognize that occupational therapists collaborate with team members by blending hands-on services for students, if needed, with team supports, system supports, or both;
- Recognize the benefits of providing services and supports within the context of students' typical school lessons and activities; and
- Identify the personal, interpersonal, and system challenges to effective school-based collaboration.

Key Topics

- Definition of *collaboration*
- Hands-on services with team supports
- Team and system supports
- Benefits and challenges of collaboration

1

Part 1: Collaboration in Education Settings

Collaboration in Action: Three scenarios

Reflection 1.1

Vignettes of Ricardo, Shelley, and Lorinda

• With whom do these therapists collaborate?

• How do they use their occupational therapy expertise to promote the performance and participation of Michele, Rohinton, and incoming kindergartners in school lessons and activities?

Ricardo, a registered occupational therapist, uses collaborative consultation to assist a physical education (PE) teacher to adapt his curriculum for Michele, a second-grade student with Asperger syndrome. Michele is easily excited, and Ricardo helps the teacher modify physical activities and games so Michele can participate in PE with her classmates. Ricardo also talks with Michele's parents about appropriate extracurricular activities for her.

Shelley, a certified occupational therapy assistant, shares responsibility with Rohinton's special education teacher to implement his individualized education program (IEP) goals to develop functional work skills for future employment. Shelley reinforces the functional literacy and math skills Rohinton has learned in class and teaches him to ride on a city bus (e.g., recognize signs, count change, signal where to stop).

Lorinda, a registered occupational therapist, volunteered to serve on a district task force to design and implement a program to screen all incoming kindergarten students for basic school "survival" skills (e.g., sit and listen, follow directions, identify colors, put on a hat and coat, color with a crayon).

Occupational therapists across the country, like Ricardo, Shelley, and Lorinda, are finding effective and creative ways to collaborate with educators, families, and other school personnel (see Reflection 1.1). Their stories illustrate three key roles that occupational therapy practitioners blend to promote collaboration in education settings: team supports, system supports, and hands-on with team supports. Hands-on services, when needed by a student or students, should always be combined with team supports, system supports, or both, preferably within the context of typical school lessons and daily activities. For example, Shelley combined hands-on services to Rohinton with team supports for his special education teacher. Ricardo provided team supports by collaborating with Michele's PE teacher and parents, and Lorinda supported her school system by contributing to a districtwide screening initiative.

Team supports involve assisting families, as desired, and education colleagues in their efforts to promote their children's learning and participation in school. As observed by one mother,

Family Voices: Occupational therapy support

My son, Jake, was born with a birth defect in his forearms that does not allow him to rotate his hands palms up. He is also sensitive in his palms and the front side of his body and does not have a lot of upper-body tone. My favorite part of OT is when the therapist shows *me* how to work with Jake. It is good when his school therapist can work with him, but she can't be there all the time—so it is much better when she helps me know the steps to take in teaching him things he needs to learn such as how to button or tie his shoes. It seems crazy to a 9-year-old if you make him button and rebutton a shirt during his school day. However, if he does it as he dresses in the morning, it makes much more sense.

—Melanie Cashion, parent of fourth-grade student Jake, North Carolina

Jake's occupational therapist provided knowledge and support to help his mother understand his needs and practice emerging skills in a context that is meaningful to him. As illustrated here and in the introductory vignettes with Ricardo, Shelley, and Lorinda, occupational therapy in an education setting is a related service designed to help students with disabilities benefit from specially designed instruction so that they can access and participate in the general curriculum with their "typical" peers. Resource 1.1 identifies the definition of *special education* in the Individuals With Disabilities Education Improvement Act of 2004 (IDEA).

Description of *Collaboration*

What is *collaboration,* and how does it influence the interaction among team members?

> **School-based collaboration is an interactive team process that focuses student, family, education, and related services partners on enhancing the academic achievement and functional performance of *all* students in school.**

The essence of collaboration is reflected in three words that describe how collaboration works: *interactive team process.* Teamwork drives the engine for collaborative

---

Resource 1.1. Definition of *Special Education* in the Individuals With Disabilities Education Improvement Act of 2004 (34 CFR § 300.39)
(Note that key words influencing collaboration are in boldface.)

Special education.

(a) *General.*

   (1) *Special education* means **specially designed instruction**, at no cost to the parents, **to meet the unique needs of a child with a disability**, including—

   (i) Instruction conducted in the classroom, in the home, in hospitals and institutions, and in other settings; and

   (ii) Instruction in physical education.

   (2) The term includes each of the following, if it meets the requirements of paragraph (a)(1) of this section:

   (i) Speech-language pathology services, or any other related service, if the service is considered special education rather than a related service under State standards;

   (ii) Travel training; and

   (iii) Vocational education.

(b) *Individual terms defined.* The terms in this definition are defined as follows:

   (3) *Specially-designed instruction* means **adapting**, as appropriate to the needs of an eligible child under this part, **the content, methodology, or delivery of instruction—**

   (i) To address the unique needs of the child that result from the child's disability; and

   (ii) To **ensure access of the child to the general curriculum,** so that the child can meet the educational standards within the jurisdiction of the public agency that apply to all children.

(Authority: 20 U.S.C. § 1401(29))

**Resource 1.2. Definitions of School-Based
Collaboration and Related Terms**

- *Collaboration:* formal and informal interactive processes among teachers and related services personnel for planning, development, and monitoring of interdisciplinary interventions (Barnes & Turner, 2000, p. 83); working together for a common end using three basic approaches—consulting, coaching, and teaming (Fishbaugh, 2000, p. 3); a system of planned cooperative activities where general educators and special educators share roles and responsibilities (Wiggins & Damore, 2006, p. 49); an interactive process in which individuals with varied life perspectives and experiences join together in a spirit of willingness to share resources, responsibility, and rewards in creating inclusive and effective educational programs and environments for students with unique learning capacities and needs (Rainforth & York-Barr, 1997)

- *Collaborative teaming:* two or more people working toward a common goal (Rainforth & York-Barr, 1997)

- *Collaborative team:* a group of people with a common goal and a shared belief system who work with parity and distributed functions in a collaborative teaming process (Thousand & Villa, 2000)

- *Collaborative teamwork:* a group of educators, related service providers, and family members who work together to pursue shared goals and share skills for implementing specific educational strategies or programs to support children with disabilities to learn in general education classes (Giangreco, Prelock, Reid, Dennis, & Edelman, 2000)

- *Interpersonal collaboration:* Conveys how an activity occurs, not what individuals are doing; collaboration is more than cooperation, coordination, and compromise; it yields shared meaning, decision making, and accountability (Friend & Cook, 2007)

- *Collaborative consultation:* an interactive process that enables teams of people with diverse expertise to generate creative solutions to mutually defined problems (Idol, Nevin, & Paolucci-Whitcomb, 1987, p. 1)

- *Collaborative school consultation:* interaction in which school personnel and families confer, consult, and collaborate as a team to identify learning and behavioral needs and to plan, implement, evaluate, and revise as needed the educational programs for serving those needs (Dettmer, Dyck, & Thurston, 1999, p. 6).

Remember this . . .
Hands-on services, team supports, and *system supports* are descriptors of collaborative practice, not service models.**

relationships among individuals with different personalities, areas of expertise, and responsibilities. *Education partners* include teachers, administrators, paraprofessionals, and school staff such as custodians and secretaries. *Related services partners* include occupational and physical therapists, assistive technology specialists, nurses, psychologists, social workers, and speech–language pathologists.

Team membership varies as a student moves from grade to grade and from school to school because a student and his or her family partners, not a teacher or a principal, are the heart of any team (Hanft, Shepherd, & Read, in press). Team members bring diverse educational backgrounds, lifestyles, and professional and family experiences, as well as expectations, values, and beliefs about working on teams, educating children, and addressing disability (see Chapter 2, "Team Faces and Spaces," and Chapter 3, "Teamwork vs. the Lone Ranger," for further discussion of influences on collaborative teaming). Resource 1.2 identifies how collaboration, collaborative teaming, and related terms are described in the education literature; note how the terms overlap and complement one another, forming a foundation for general and special educators and therapists to work together to achieve common goals.

Collaboration, as an interactive team process, is both an art and a science (Idol, 1990). The science of collaboration focuses on team operations and management and also on applying the evidence of the benefits of collaboration to facilitate student participation and achievement throughout a school environment. The art of collaboration is a function of how seamlessly occupational therapists interact with team members to select and blend their hands-on services for students with team and system supports. Figure 1.1 illustrates the three roles that occupational therapists blend when collaborating with team members: hands-on services for students, team supports and system supports. When occupational therapists integrate hands-on services with team and system supports, they draw on their expertise to help achieve specific outcomes for students, teams, and the school system. Students improve their academic achievement and functional performance, team members increase their competency, and school systems offer proficient education programs.

A simplified version of the collaboration graphic (Figure 1.1) accompanies the extended practice vignettes throughout the book. Consider how the proportions of hands-on services and team/system supports provided by each occupational therapist vary by each student's goals and progress; team faces; and school places, spaces, and paces.

Figure 1.2 identifies typical hands-on services and team and system supports provided by occupational therapists in an education setting. Obviously, the propor-

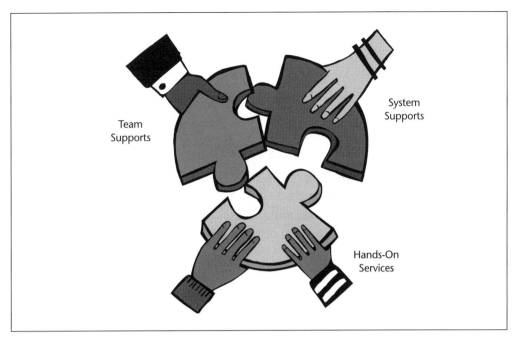

Figure 1.1. The art of collaboration.

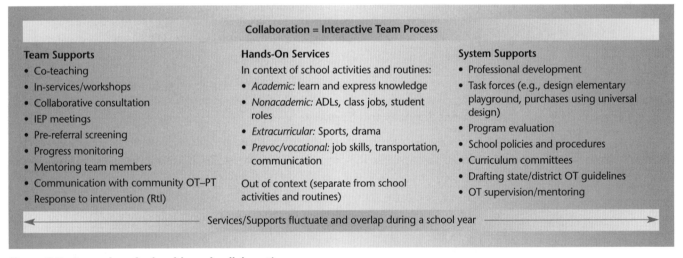

Figure 1.2. Examples of school-based collaboration.

Note. IEP = individualized education program; OT–PT = occupational therapist–physical therapist; ADLs = activities of daily living; Prevoc = prevocational.

tion of supports and services provided for each student and team will change depending on a student's projected outcomes and progress toward achieving stated goals. Other key variables that affect the proportion of occupational therapy supports and services provided to each student (and school) include

- *Faces,* key team members and their knowledge and experience related to addressing students' educational needs;
- *Places* and *spaces,* the education environments in which students learn and interact with their peers and teachers; and
- *Paces,* the structure, routine, and culture of school activities and interactions with peers and adults.

We selected the terms *hands-on services, team supports,* and *system supports* as descriptors of collaborative practice in the schools. Neither collaboration nor these descriptive terms are service models; rather, they refer to a *process* that families, education personnel, and therapists engage in to share their knowledge and experience to ensure that all children participate successfully in the general education curriculum, to the extent possible.

Hands-On Services With Team Supports

Hands-on services with team supports are interventions provided by occupational therapists to promote the academic achievement and functional performance of individual students as well as selected groups. Hands-on services should *always* be paired with team supports, system supports, or both, preferably in the context of typical school lessons, activities, and routines (Case-Smith & Cable, 1996; King et al., 1999). The intended outcome of hands-on/team supports is to collaborate with teachers and other team members to ensure that students learn and participate, with their peers, in academic instruction and lessons, nonacademic activities such as lunch and PE, and prevocational and vocational education. As expressed succinctly by one fourth-grade student,

> My OT also helped me in gym. We shot bows and arrows in archery. My bow was too tight, so they got my teacher to make it looser for me. I couldn't pull it back before. My friends made fun of me, so the OT helped me get the teacher to make it easier. Now I like archery.

> —Jake Cashion, fourth-grade student, North Carolina

In-Context Services and Supports

A student's daily routines and contexts should provide the primary setting for all occupational therapy services and supports. Professional guidelines also emphasize the importance of working with students in the context of their daily school activities (AOTA, 2002; Dunn, 2000; Jackson, 2007; Polichino, 2004; Swinth, Spencer, & Jackson, 2007). In the vignettes included at the beginning of this chapter, Shelley provides hands-on services and team supports to Rohinton by planning with his special education teacher and then teaching him to travel on his community's bus system. In this instance, her individualized intervention is provided in a community context (i.e., a city bus) in which Rohinton will practice his emerging literacy and math skills when he uses public transportation.

Therapist Voices: Practicing skills in context

Interventions provided in natural settings during daily routines are most likely to be applied consistently. Intervention methodologies using curriculum content and classroom materials are most likely to achieve maximum contextual integration and replication. (Clark, Polichino, & Jackson, 2004, p. 684)

A major decision when providing in-context intervention is for occupational therapists and their teammates to consider what materials and resources are available to promote student learning and how specific activities, lessons, and environments can be modified so that a student can participate as independently as possible with the least amount of adult assistance. The following vignette illustrates how an occupational therapy student and her clinical instructor provided hands-on services with team supports (i.e., collaborative consultation and in-class modeling) for a general educator to successfully integrate sensory strategies for one student in a classroom activity that benefits all students.

Therapist Voices: Including all students

We are using activities and images from the SticKids program to help establish sensory breaks for my student with a disability. The other students benefit as well. I go into the class and teach four new activities a week. Each time I go, the class shows good return demonstration, we review the activities from previous weeks, and choose a student to pick and lead an activity for that day. I also review the parameters of using the activities in class with the students such as which ones are OK to do anytime, which are appropriate for particular times in the day, classroom rules, etc. I visit the class on a weekly basis and meet with the teacher to see how things are going; if it is working; if the exercises are helpful and manageable; how my student is doing with the exercises and is functioning in class; and any other concerns, questions, or ideas the teacher may have. I always make sure to run the new exercises by the teacher before I introduce them to the students to ensure they meet her needs and will fit in her classroom.

—Maritza Villegas, occupational therapy student,
University of Southern California

All students, especially those with disabilities, benefit from accessing school materials and the general curriculum through materials and instruction that is based on universal design of learning rather than specialized equipment or separate instruction (Goodrich, 2004). Figure 1.3 applies the principles of universal design and identifies adaptation strategies for facilitating students' participation in school lessons and activities. The in-context strategies (e.g., "adapt materials, equipment and toys") allow a child to participate as independently as possible without adult assistance and are considered less restrictive than out-of-context strategies. Occupational therapists should first consider using in-context strategies, or a combination of them, before initiating out-of-context strategies (e.g., "student works with adult in separate space from peers").

By providing in-context supports and services, occupational therapists follow the least restrictive environment (LRE) mandate in IDEA to educate children with disabilities with their typical peers (see Exhibit 1.1A in the Appendix for the IDEA definition of LRE).

Therapist Voices: Adapting the context

Modifying the environment in some way that allows a child to participate or providing a child with specific types of equipment are the least intrusive types of adaptation strategies. Removing a child from the typical environment so that the child is doing something different with an adult, generally in a one-

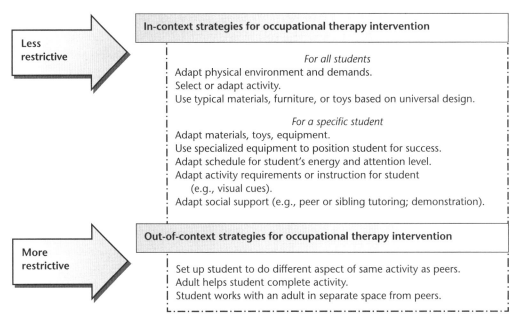

Figure 1.3. Providing occupational therapy in the least restrictive environment.

From Campbell, P. H. (2000). Promoting participation in natural environments by accommodating motor disabilities. In M. Snell & F. Brown (Eds.), *Instruction of students with severe disabilities* (5th ed., pp. 291–329 [p. 325]). Upper Saddle River, NJ: Prentice Hall. Copyright © 2000 by Prentice Hall. Adapted with permission.

on-one situation, is the most restrictive. The framework [Figure 1.3] is not meant to suggest that more restrictive options are never needed in particular situations or with certain children but rather that restrictive interventions should not be tried as a first solution. They should only be used when other categories of adaptation have been tried with no success. (Campbell & Milbourne, 2006, p. 6)

Out-of-Context Services and Supports

The courts have determined that the critical issue in special education is the provision of a free appropriate public education (FAPE; see Exhibit 1.1A in the Appendix for the IDEA definition). Students with disabilities may not be excluded from a general education classroom simply because it is easier to educate them in segregated settings. Moreover, schools must show a good-faith effort to include a student in the general education classroom with appropriate services and aids before deciding that the student cannot benefit from such instruction. In 1989, the Fifth Circuit Court of Appeals established the following two-part test for determining when a school district has met its obligation to include students with disabilities in regular education classes (*Daniel R.R. v. State Board of Education,* 1989).

1. *Can education in the general environment, with supplementary services and aids, be achieved satisfactorily?* Therapeutic services, including modifications for the classroom recommended by therapists, would qualify as supplemental services and aids if needed by the student to function *satisfactorily* in the school (note that optimum function is not required for FAPE).

2. *When special education is necessary, has the student been included to the maximum extent possible?* This question also applies to how, and where, occupational therapy and other related services are provided. Therapy that is isolated from a student's daily routine and schedule could be considered more restrictive than therapy provided within typical school settings and student routines.

Occupational therapists should work with students outside the context of regular school activities and routines only when needed to assist students to begin to acquire specific skills and behaviors necessary to achieve their IEP goals or for student privacy. Consider these student and teacher perspectives regarding working with an occupational therapist in and out of context:

Student Voices: Out-of-context intervention

When my OT helps me with buttoning my pants it is OK to do it by myself. I don't want to do it with other people around. My OT also helps me learn to type, and sometimes my teacher helps me write stuff because my hands get tired. That is OK to do in class with my friends.

—Jake Cashion, fourth-grade student, North Carolina

Teacher Voices: In-context intervention

The highly specialized training and expertise of an occupational therapist is essential in teaching a student to perform such tasks. However, we have found that students do not necessarily transfer or generalize skills when these skills are taught in isolation, even by the most talented occupational therapist. It is crucial that the expertise of the occupational therapist be used in the context or environment in which the targeted task will be naturally performed in the day-to-day routine of the student.

—Beverly Cipollone, special educator, and Janet Harris, first-grade teacher (Cipollone & Harris, 1999, p. 3)

If hands-on services with team supports must be provided out of context to a student's daily school lessons and activities, IDEA requires that a justification be included on the student's IEP indicating why and specifying the duration of the separate intervention (34 CFR § 300.320 (a)(5); see Exhibit 1.1A in the Appendix).

Occupational therapy services must be provided in the environment that has the fewest restrictions while still meeting the student's needs as they relate to the ability to benefit from education. Removal from the general education classroom is a very restrictive option and should be carefully considered in the context of the child's primary needs; less restrictive options usually are available, and legally they must be used if they meet these needs. (Polichino, Clark, & Chandler, 2005)

Hands-on services for students provided out of context to their daily school activities should still be combined with team supports, system supports, or both to

Remember this . . .
Hands-on services for students provided out of context to their daily school activities should still be combined with team supports, system supports, or both.

ensure that the student generalizes the skills and behaviors acquired in isolated places or spaces to daily school lessons and activities. Skills needed for personal care activities (even those that require privacy) can be practiced in the classroom with creative planning, as suggested below.

Therapist Voices: Meaningful practice

Rehearsing skills such as dressing and undressing for toileting with students with limited cognition is not meaningful when practiced separate from their daily routines. They do not understand why they are undressing, then pulling their pants right up without using the toilet! Instead, I ask their mothers to send snack to school in something that snaps, unbuttons, or zips. Guess what? Undoing fasteners to get snack out is far more engaging and doesn't require weekly OT sessions in the therapy room.

Another strategy I've used for a child working on an IEP goal of shoe tying (but who doesn't wear tie shoes!) is to talk with her teacher about incorporating tying a bow as part of her behavior plan. Whenever the child accomplishes a task in class, she ties a bow on a special dowel rather than put a sticker on a chart.

—Judith Schoonover, occupational therapist and
assistive technology specialist, Virginia

The following scenario presents an opportunity to consider how to provide in-context hands-on services with team supports using the adaptation strategies outlined in Figure 1.3. Derrick, an occupational therapist, provides out-of-context hands-on services to Julio, a preschooler. Julio plays well with his peers and understands what he hears but has significant problems with expressive language as well as with eating his lunch and snack in the allotted time.

What could be...

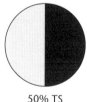

50% TS
50% HO

Collaboration in Action: Planning team supports

Derrick routinely provides hands-on services to his students in their classrooms. He decides to prompt Julio's oral–motor skills in a quiet area of his preschool classroom before lunch to work on his IEP goal of eating lunch within 20 minutes. (Note that Derrick's approach is the most restrictive out-of-context strategy identified in Figure 1.3.) Derrick never considers whether he is providing occupational therapy in the least restrictive environment for Julio and assumes that working with him in the back of the classroom makes his intervention educationally relevant. Derrick always makes a point to tell Marianne, Julio's teacher, what he worked on before he leaves the classroom to see his next student. However, he does not solicit observations or concerns from Marianne or suggest how she might promote Julio's emerging skill during other classroom activities.

In the scenario above, Derrick's missed opportunity for providing team supports is assuming that because the teacher can watch what he does with Julio, she will be able to follow through on her own. One teacher describes this as "swoop in, do

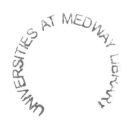

something and swoop out" intervention (Crystal Mallory, personal communication, November 8, 2007). Reflection 1.2 solicits ideas for translating Derrick's isolated intervention with Julio to hands-on service with team supports for Marianne, to enhance her effectiveness as Julio's teacher. Resource 1.3 suggests possible team supports Julio could provide.

When education partners collaborate effectively, hands-on services and team supports naturally flow together throughout the school year. The following sections describe the many different ways in which occupational therapists provide team and system supports and blend them with hands-on services to students.

> **Resource 1.3. Team Supports for Julio (based on adaptation strategies in Figure 1.3)**
>
> Select or adapt an activity for all students:
> - Help teacher schedule a transition activity from story time to lunch for all students (e.g., singing, humming, blowing on instruments, or playing "Simon Says" with mouth and tongue actions).
>
> Adapt activity requirements for a specific student:
> - Problem solve with Julio's mother to send food that he likes (Julio will try harder to chew favorite food)
> - Cut his lunch into bite-size pieces (all students eat different lunches).
>
> Adapt materials, toys, tools for a specific student:
> - Use a straw instead of a cup for Julio to drink liquids
> - Drink and eat smaller amounts at lunch to allow sufficient time for Julio to chew and swallow; follow up with snack later.

Team Supports

Team supports are the strategies and interactions that one team member uses to enhance the competency of another to facilitate students' academic achievement and participation in school. The immediate outcome is to enhance team members' mastery of new information and strategies to realize the long-term outcome of student achievement and participation in typical school activities and lessons.

Therapist Voices: Impact of team supports

Teachers find support through their collaborative efforts with the occupational therapist [who] provides resources to assist the teacher in the design of instruction, can assist in the classroom management of diverse learners, and can suggest additional strategies to be tried in the classroom. (Shasby & Schneck, 2005, p. 2)

Effective team supports increase the knowledge and skills of the key adults responsible for helping a student learn and interact with peers and adults (i.e., core team members). Occupational therapists should also consider assisting school staff such as custodians, bus drivers, and administrative assistants to reinforce students' targeted behavior when they interact with them, as reflected in the vignette below about modifying a student's social behavior.

Collaboration in Action: Supporting all school personnel

Adamo, an 8-year-old boy in second grade, was effusive when greeting and initiating contact with his peers and teachers. Adamo's core team (i.e., parents, second-grade teacher, special educator, speech–language pathologist, and occupational therapist) decided to help him learn more socially appropriate behaviors such as shaking hands when greeting others at school instead of hugging and kissing. Linda, an occupational therapist, recalled watching Adamo envelope Mr. Sylvester, a custodian, with his hearty embrace and suggested that the team be alert to observing Adamo's interactions with all school

Reflection 1.2

In-Context Intervention for Julio?

Consider how Derrick could combine hands-on and team supports for Julio and his teacher by suggesting in-context strategies. What could Marianne incorporate during lunch to help Julio finish on time? To guide your reflection, review Figure 1.3. (See Resource 1.3 for suggestions when you finish.)

75% TS
25% HO

personnel and share strategies with them to promote age-appropriate social interactions between Adamo, his peers, and other adults.

Other supports that occupational therapists provide team members include

- Helping to identify a student's ability profile of strengths, interests, and challenges and then developing a targeted intervention plan;
- Recommending strategies for educators to try in the classroom before referring students to special education (defined in IDEA as early intervening strategies and discussed in Chapter 4, "Getting Into a Collaborative School Routine");
- Participating on IEP teams to assess and develop students' IEPs;
- Jointly implementing intervention with educators, for example, co-teaching or zone instruction (setting up and facilitating centers for specific activities);
- Collecting data and conducting observations with family members and educators to assess the effectiveness of an intervention for a particular student; and
- Mentoring and coaching team members to acquire and refine their knowledge and skills (discussed in Chapter 3).

Although hands-on services should always be paired with team support, occupational therapists have found that team supports alone can be effective in assisting students to reach their goals (Dreiling & Bundy, 2003; Dunn, 1991; Kemmis & Dunn, 1996; VandenBerg, 2001). Team supports do not preclude short-term interaction with students to identify the source of student learning and behavior challenges, conduct trials of possible interventions, model selected strategies, and monitor student progress. Thus, team supports are not limited only to talking with teachers and other team members. In the opening vignettes of this chapter, Ricardo provided team supports through collaborative consultation with Michele's PE teacher to adapt the curriculum as well as with her parents to suggest extracurricular activities for Michele. It is very likely that Ricardo would also spend time observing Michele to find out what kind of sensory input focuses her before she engages in movement activities. He would then model effective strategies for the PE teacher and parents to use to help her calm down when she becomes too excited.

Occupational therapists should suggest strategies, activities, and interactions that team members can implement as appropriate to their knowledge, experience, and relationship with specific students. Judging what suggestions to give a particular team member, and how to share this information in a helpful manner, is an essential part of the art of collaboration (Hanft & Place, 1996). Applying the principles of adult learning studies (Donovan, Bransford, & Pellegrino, 1999) is dependent on one's communication and interpersonal skills (see Chapter 3 for further discussion).

Therapist Voices: Listening to learn what works

Martha [the occupational therapist] meets with José's teacher and explains the evidence she found on pencil grasp. She and the teacher discuss possible ways to motivate José to improve his legibility as well as to introduce adaptive

Remember this . . .
Team supports include short-term interaction with students and are not limited to talking with teachers and other team members.

strategies in the classroom, such as dark-lined paper and a spacing aid to support José's IEP goal. Martha is sensitive to the teacher's, parent's, and students' acceptance of the various strategies discussed and discards those that would make anyone uncomfortable. The strategies chosen will be ones that are acceptable to everyone involved; can be integrated into José's daily school routine with minimal time, training, and expense; and carry little or no risk to him. Martha then works with José's teacher to plan a data collection program so that José's progress while using the strategies can be measured and evaluated objectively. (Collins, 2006, p. 3)

In the scenario below, note how the occupational therapist and her teammates have worked out a plan to provide team supports through collaborative consultation with classroom teachers and build from the teachers' areas of strength to suggest new strategies and equipment.

Therapist Voices: Building on teacher strengths

I volunteered to participate on the assistive technology [AT] team for my district and then was offered further training to augment my OT expertise. Our team works collaboratively—for example, we read and share all referrals and then discuss who has the experience to address a student's learning issues, or who knows a particular student. We have established a precedent to provide AT consultation in pairs in order to blend our expertise. We do a classroom observation and look for what is going right in the classroom for the referred student, and then try some ideas and equipment to see how they can further support student learning and participation. We write up our observations and suggestions in a way that says, "Thank you for inviting us to your classroom, you are using such great AT already—here are some more ideas." Then we talk with the teacher to figure out the best way to help her and her assistants implement them.

—Judith Schoonover, occupational therapist and
assistive technology specialist, Virginia

Exhibit 1.2A in the Appendix includes a sample of the assistive technology team's recommendations for the classroom.

System Supports

System supports are the formal and informal initiatives, programs, and communications that occupational therapists and other team members engage in to ensure that a school district meets federal, state, and local requirements to educate all children. In the opening vignettes, Lorinda contributes her knowledge of child development to a school committee charged with designing and implementing a screening program for all incoming kindergartners in her school district. Examples of other system supports include

- Participating on task forces focused on playground design, transition to work, curriculum development, or assessment accommodations;

- Joining districtwide teams to provide specialized programs such as assistive technology or serve specific populations of students (e.g., autism spectrum disorder, low-incidence disability);
- Educating parents (e.g., alerting parents at a PTA meeting to the benefits of setting up homework routines for distractible students);
- Contributing to the development of state and local guidelines for occupational therapy services; and
- Providing continuing education to education team members and assisting other therapists in keeping abreast of current research and practices in occupational therapy and special education.

Occupational therapists often involve themselves in their school districts at the system level when they observe that students in various classrooms in different buildings need similar services to promote their learning and address behavior problems. As described in the vignettes below, occupational therapists take the initiative to develop school programs for specific students or groups.

Therapist Voices: System support for transition to community

I provided system support to my rural school district by suggesting that the transition coordinator and I talk with classroom teachers before school started to decide which classes (e.g., work study, home economics, or career exploration) would be most helpful for each student in the transition-to-work program. I thought if we visited students at their community job sites, it would help us consider what skills need to be taught in these classes to prepare them for their jobs. I also helped the transition coordinator set up an advisory board for the program, composed of business owners, family members, students, teachers, vocational rehabilitation staff, and myself.

—Judy Davis, occupational therapist, Colorado

Being involved at the system level gives occupational therapists an opportunity to apply their professional wisdom and experience to develop programs and policies to enhance the competency of education teams. Proficient school districts recognize when alternative programs must be developed to educate children with unique learning needs (e.g., preschoolers with autism spectrum disorder) and then ensure all members of the education team have the necessary skills and resources to do so.

Therapist Voices: System support for students with autism

I have received advanced training in using the TEACCH (Treatment and Education of Autistic and Related Communication Handicapped Children) methodology with individuals with autism along with some friends and colleagues—a speech–language pathologist, special educator, and parent. We serve as program consultants in the TEACCH approach across the state. Over the past year, we have been working with the State Department of Education to develop a training with multiple learning activities, three pilot sites, two general information meetings, and monthly interactive TV seminars in a "take and make" style to expand staff skills in using the specifics of the TEACCH approach.

Collaboration is a crucial part of our training and includes teaming to present the training, modeling the benefits for all staff, and most critical, partnering with parents. For the pilot programs across the state, local teams must be willing to commit their OT's time to the project for training and then assign the OTs to local school teams to provide program services, design the classroom environments, etc.

—Chris Knippenberg, occupational therapist, Vermont

As illustrated in these vignettes, occupational therapists who involve themselves in system supports help change attitudes about what therapists can do to support comprehensive school and community programs for students with different learning styles and needs. Collaboration among team members facilitates how information is shared and understood and provides a firm foundation for encouraging creative contributions from different professional and personal perspectives. Such a philosophy provides the foundation for occupational therapists to offer team and system supports in school settings and to decide whether and how to provide hands-on services for students, always blending them with supports to key team members.

Remember this . . .
- Hands-on services, when needed, should *always* be combined with team and system supports.
- Team supports include *interactions* with students as well as families and education partners.
- System supports are the programs and initiatives that ensure that a school district meets requirements to educate *all* children.

Part 2: From Service Models to Team Collaboration

Before 1975 (when IDEA was first enacted), therapeutic services for children with disabilities were most often provided in county health departments providing Crippled Children's Services under the Maternal and Child Health Act (illustrated in Table 1.1). Children with the most severe disabilities typically did not receive special education or school therapy services because they were not expected, or sometimes allowed, to attend public school (Turnbull, Stowe, & Huerta, 2007). In response to federal education laws and judicial decisions throughout the 1970s, public schools offered special

Table 1.1. Historical Perspective on Occupational Therapy in Schools

Time Span	Where Occupational Therapy Is Provided	Evolution of IDEA	How Occupational Therapists (OTs) Interact With Education Teams
1940–1974	Students receive occupational therapy in community health clinics, segregated schools, or private practices.	Education for children with disabilities is governed by state laws and regulations.	OTs direct parents and educators to carry out home and school programs as an adjunct to therapy.
1975–1990	Students receive occupational therapy in school spaces and places that are frequently separate from their daily education activities and lessons.	Education for the Handicapped Act (EHA) is enacted in 1975, mandating that a free appropriate public education for all children (kindergarten through 12th grade) be provided in all states by 1980.	OTs use three distinct models of service delivery: direct, consultation, and monitoring. Direct service in separate therapy spaces and places is typically provided two times per week (AOTA, 1989; Dunn, 1991).
1991–present	Occupational therapy continues to be provided in therapy sessions, although hands-on services with team supports is increasing within the context of typical school activities.	Reauthorization of the EHA in 1991 retitles it as the Individuals With Disabilities Education Act; the 1997 and 2004 reauthorizations highlight that children with disabilities who need special education should participate in the general school curriculum, to the extent possible.	OTs collaborate with educators, families, psychologists, and other therapists to help students achieve and participate in school by blending hands-on services with team and system supports.

education and related services to students with all levels of disabilities; however, these classrooms and therapy services were usually separate from the mainstream of what typical peers were learning and doing in each grade.

During the 1980s and 1990s, occupational therapists and other related service providers most often provided direct intervention by pulling students out of their classroom for one-on-one sessions in separate therapy rooms and spaces (Dunn, 1988; Sandler, 1997; Westling & Fox, 1995). The quote below vividly describes an occupational therapist's solo practice in the schools before she learned to collaborate with colleagues and family members.

Therapist Voices: My solo practice

In 1982, I drove a 45-foot Winnebago complete with a therapy room inside. I would go to the classroom to collect the student, provide treatment in the Winnebago, and return him or her to class. I rarely spoke with the teacher, other than the usual pleasantries. I communicated with the parents by phone or in person and contributed to the plan with clinically based occupational therapy goals that never seemed to overlap with academic issues. (Bowen-Irish, 2006, p. 23)

Remember this . . .
Choosing one service model for an entire school year is outdated and creates barriers to collaboration.

Occupational therapy during the 1980s and early 1990s was defined by three service models: direct, consult, and monitoring (Dunn, 1985, 1988). Therapists typically tried (and may still be required by administrative policy in some school districts) to select one model as the vehicle for providing their services for an entire school year. Choosing one service model for an entire school year is outdated and creates barriers to collaboration (Hanft & Place, 1996; Jirikowic et al., 2001). In recognition of these barriers, the Texas Board of Occupational Therapy Examiners has eliminated the service model terminology in lieu of using the *Occupational Therapy Practice Framework* language (Jean Polichino, personal communication, November 9, 2007).

From the 1990s to the present, the movement for inclusion has emphasized that children with disabilities have a right to participate in school activities and instruction with their peers (see Exhibit 1.1A in the Appendix for the definition of least restrictive environment). This concept was fully incorporated in the amendments to the IDEA in 1997 and 2004 as "ensuring access of the child to the general curriculum" (see the definition of special education and specially designed instruction in Resource 1.1). Therapists and educators who historically worked independently in self-contained classrooms and separate therapy spaces currently have collaborative teaming responsibilities mandated by professional guidelines (Clark, Polichino, & Jackson, 2004; Jackson, 2007) and federal legislation (IDEA, 2004). Deboer and Fister (1994) illustrated the evolving perspectives of therapists and special educators regarding their services for students with disabilities in school settings:

- *Self-contained class:* "I do special ed/therapy by myself."

- *Resource or pull-out:* "I do the special ed/therapy *part* myself."

- *Collaborative teaming:* "Together, *we* educate children."

Blending Supports and Services

One artful decision that teams must make about collaboration is how to provide special education and related services to maximize students' learning and participation in typical school activities. Collaboration needs to occur on a regular basis and "involve coworking with children as well as time for mutual knowledge exchange" (Priest & Waters, 2007, p. 146). Collaborative services and supports should not be left only to formal team meetings, which are difficult to hold because of therapists' travel time, workloads, and conflicting schedules (Barnes & Turner, 2000). Nor should occupational therapy be provided only through hands-on services for students, particularly in sessions out of context from their typical school lessons and activities (Dunn, 2000; Jackson, 2007; Knippenberg & Hanft, 2004; Swinth, Chandler, Hanft, Jackson, & Shepherd, 2003). Special and regular educators have also been encouraged to engage in dialogue with related service providers to figure out how to "push in" supports and services to the general education classroom and other school contexts rather than "pull out" students to separate special education classes and therapy spaces (Snell & Janney, 2005; Thousand & Villa, 2000).

Remember this . . .
As school-based therapists, we must educate ourselves, parents, and team members and focus on desired outcomes rather than service delivery models. (Shepherd, 1999)

Forcing a choice between hands-on services or team supports (e.g., collaborative consultation) drastically narrows the options for team members to work together to promote students' academic achievement and functional performance in school-related occupations. It also reduces the opportunities for therapists to observe a student's in-context performance and incorporate specific strategies for team members to implement with students. Table 1.2 contrasts blended occupational therapy services and supports with a traditional therapy model for elementary, middle and high school students.

A collaborative model blends hands-on services with team and system supports and provides flexibility in figuring out *how* to achieve students' goals to ensure their learning and participation in school. Parents, teachers, and occupational therapists should focus on how to blend services and supports to achieve education outcomes for students. Too often, the discussion at IEP meetings focuses narrowly on selecting service models and therapy goals. Consider the following comments about common goals and flexible intervention, hallmarks of collaborative teaming.

Family Voices: Shared goals

Flexibility means being open to new learning and sometimes learning to let go of what has been taught or practiced in the past. Flexibility means replacing "that's how I do things" with "whatever it takes, in partnership with others, for this particular child to be successful." It is the shift from "my occupational therapy goals" to "our goals together." (Gretz, 1999, p. 3)

Remember this . . .
The model of service delivery (e.g., direct or consultative) need not be and should not be an "either–or" proposition but rather a "both–and" consideration. (Gretz, 1999, p. 3)

Teacher Voices: Learning from therapists

By using an integrated therapy service model, regular and special educational teachers and instructional assistants are able to observe and learn teaching techniques used by occupational therapy practitioners for even greater carryover and long-term benefits for the student. (Cipollone & Harris, 1999, p. 3)

Table 1.2. Examples of In-Context vs. Out-of-Context Occupational Therapy Services and Supports

Results of Occupational Therapy Evaluation	Desired Learning or Participation Outcomes	Therapy Room Model (Out of Context)	Natural Context Model (In Context)
A third-grade student with autism has problems with sensory processing, contributing to poor modulation of nervous system (NS) arousal and result-ng in problems with transitions.	Independently transition between activities and environments, meeting timelines for daily routines.	Pull from instruction to segregated therapy room using a sensory integration frame of reference (30- to 60-minute sessions, two times per week)	*Hands-on/team supports:* Work with student to identify calming and alerting strategies to effect appropriate modulation for daily routine. *Team supports:* Provide in-service to instructional personnel and family on strategies for helping student anticipate and manage change, including Social Stories, picture schedule, and auditory cues. *Systems supports:* Develop a "bank" of visual symbols and post on the district Intranet to share with all school personnel (one 60-minute in-service; 2 hours first 6 weeks, then 30 minutes per 6 weeks)
A middle school student with spina bifida at T1 is not participating in physical education; the student does not attend class or sit on the sidelines.	Participate in grade-level physical education.	No occupational therapy intervention. IEP team places student in adaptive physical education (special class for children with disabilities)	*Hands-on/team supports:* Work with student to identify adaptations needed to change into physical education uniform and teach sequence for donning and doffing uniform in locker room area with other students during changing time. Work with student and physical education teacher to adapt activities to allow participation in fitness and leisure activities. Recommend needed accommodations and curriculum modifications to IEP team. (30 minutes weekly for first 6 weeks, then 30 minutes per semester)
A senior high student with a traumatic brain injury has poor motor skills and impulsive behavior and wants to continue taking photos for the yearbook (a pre-accident role).	Interact with peers without touching, interrupting, or yelling.	Pull from elective activity for motor and social re-training (60 minutes per week)	*Team supports:* Collaborate on behavior intervention plan for peer interactions; meet regularly with team to problem solve unanticipated occurrences. *Hands-on/team supports:* Collaborate with instructional team and family to target level of yearbook photo activities for adapting or retraining; model how to grade motor challenges during yearbook class. Include peers in activities with student (3 hours first 6 weeks, then 1 hour next 6 weeks).

From Polichino, J. (2004). Moving out of the "therapy room." In Y. Swinth (Ed.), *Occupational therapy in school-based practice: Contemporary issues and trends* [AOTA Online Course, Lesson 7]. Bethesda, MD: American Occupational Therapy Association. Copyright © 2004 by the American Occupational Therapy Association. Adapted with permission.

IEP = Individualized education program.

Therapist Voices: Blending roles

Choosing the best intervention strategy for a student can be accomplished only if flexible models of service are available. Occupational therapists must consider meeting educational needs in the natural environment, such as the classroom, playground, library, or lunch room. (Polcyn & Bissell, 2005, p. 1)

Benefits and Challenges of Collaboration

The daunting task of keeping up with new developments in one's profession and community has led to an increasing reliance on collaboration in diverse work settings from education to industry to information technology. Findings from 133 studies indicate that cooperative work relationships among adults have promoted higher achievement, greater support, and higher self-esteem (Johnson & Johnson, 1987). Some of the most significant innovations of the 20th century (e.g., personal computer, aviation technology, feature-length animated films) resulted from the extended collaboration of a team of dedicated and talented people (Bennis & Biederman, 1997).

Teacher Voices: Collaboration in the 21st century

We live in a fast-paced time that demands multitasking and a growing sensitivity to world issues. Communication, collaboration, and cooperation are factors that can contribute to effective performance in this age, regardless of whether one is referring to business deals, political campaigns, the protection of the environment, or the education of children. (Wiggins & Damore, 2006, p. 49)

Why collaborate in education settings? The short answer is that collaboration in public school settings is mandated in the IDEA, and research supports its effectiveness. Collaboration among team members is mandated by IDEA for educating students with disabilities in the following areas:

- Assessment and implementation of a student's IEP

- IEP development

- Education in the least restrictive environment

- Discipline and behavior support plans

- Mediation to resolve disagreements regarding special education and related services

- Transition to work.

Collaboration among general educators to enhance instruction for all students is an accepted practice for teaching core academic areas, particularly in middle schools, across the nation (Fishbaugh, 2000; Friend & Cook, 2007). *Colleague-to-colleague* collaboration, also referred to as *peer coaching,* reduces the isolation many educators and therapists encounter when providing itinerant services or being the only teacher in a classroom (Gersten, Morvant, & Brengelman, 1995; Hasbrouck & Christen, 1997; see Chapter 3 for additional information about coaching). Students themselves have functioned as peer tutors for students with disabilities, helping them learn academic lessons and acquire social and communication skills for future employment (Samaha & DeLisi, 2000; Van Meter & Stevens, 2000).

Another form of collaboration common in education settings is partnerships among universities, public schools, and community agencies to prepare teachers and related services personnel to address current trends and needs in the field. Examples of collaboration between occupational therapy faculty and students with public school personnel are as follows:

- Entry-level graduate occupational therapy students at Virginia Commonwealth University, in collaboration with an alternative high school administrator and the teachers working in Education for Employment classes, co-developed a transition portfolio for students.

- Occupational therapy students at Concordia University in Wisconsin worked with a case manager for students with learning disabilities to develop a 15-week life skills course for a local high school. Activities were developed and distributed to the teachers and students in a hard copy and an electronic copy for future use (personal communication, Christine Moser, April 20, 2007).

- After meeting with school-based occupational therapists and educators, occupational therapy students at Virginia Commonwealth University designed, fabricated, and evaluated adaptive projects for students with disabilities (e.g., Social Stories, schedule boards, communication boards, lap trays, slant boards, talking books, assistive technology positioners, adapted games and puzzles).

- Occupational therapy students at the University of Mary in Bismarck, North Dakota, partnered with community agencies and groups affiliated with schools in several projects. They have implemented indirect fine motor skills development, sensory, and social skills programs at a local Head Start; have implemented social skills groups; and have developed booklets describing developmentally appropriate and adaptable ideas for after-school programs. Students also worked with the Parks and Recreation Department to address accessibility issues to promote student participation in leisure activities (personal communication, Carol Olson, April 20, 2007).

The benefits of collaboration in general and special education are supported by evidence from both research and practice, from preschool through high school (Idol, Nevin, & Paolucci-Whitcomb, 1996; Villa, Thousand, Nevin, & Malgeri, 1996; Walther-Thomas, Korinek, McLaughlin, & Williams, 2002). Occupational therapists and other education team members can improve student and team outcomes by blending hands-on services, when needed, with team and system supports to enhance students' education outcomes. Table 1.3 summarizes 11 studies that assessed the impact of hands-on occupational therapy services with team supports (or team supports alone) on student outcomes and teacher–family satisfaction. It is noteworthy that in the studies that contrasted direct therapy with consultation, the direct services included team supports (Case-Smith, 2002) and the teacher consultation included hands-on services to students (Bayona, McDougall, Tucker, Nichols, & Mandich, 2006). Blending hands-on services with team supports was evident in both conditions in many of the studies.

When therapy, education, and family partners collaborate on school teams, they form partnerships that sustain all team members in their efforts to provide meaningful caregiving and effective intervention to ensure that children and youths participate fully in school, family, and community life (Hanft et al., in press). Rather than viewing collaboration solely as a helpful instructional tool, collaboration "is the foundation on which successful contemporary public schools are based, as well as the most effective means by which to provide services to students with disabilities and other special needs" (Friend & Cook, 2007, p. xix).

Table 1.3. Evidence for Improved Student Outcomes With Collaborative Occupational Therapy Services and Supports in Education Settings (1989–2006)

Source	Student Population	Intervention (Using Authors' Terms)	Occupational Therapist (OT) Roles	Student Outcomes
Bayona, McDougall, Tucker, Nichols, & Mandich (2006)	23 Canadian children, 5 to 8 years old, with no neurological disorder but problems with writing and using school materials	5 to 10 consultative visits to teachers and parents in school settings, based on student assessment data (duration of intervention: average 5.5 months)	Hands-on with team supports (86% of therapists report providing direct service during classroom consultations)	Improvement in written and fine motor skills of students was statistically significant and practically meaningful; teachers increased child individualized strategies from 26% to 70%; teachers reported moderate level of satisfaction with consultation, and parents reported moderate to high level of satisfaction.
Dreiling & Bundy (2003)	22 children, 3 to 5 years old, in special education preschool with gross motor, fine motor, or visual–motor delays	*Consultation group:* 1 day/week in class observing students and planning with teachers; 1 day/month in team meeting; meet with parents as needed. *Direct–indirect group:* 1.5 hours/week every 3 weeks in classroom + half-day team meeting/week (duration of intervention: 1 school year)	Team supports Hands-on with team supports	Both groups were equally effective in addressing goals related to mild motor performance.
Case-Smith (2002)	29 children, second to fourth grade, in special education and occupational therapy for problems with handwriting	*Direct therapy:* 30 minutes/week of individualized sessions; high levels of collaboration with teachers reported for students in intervention group (duration of intervention: 7 months)	Hands-on (out of context) with team supports	Students in intervention group increased an average of 14% in letter legibility and 15 of 29 students improved legibility greater than 90%; no improvement in numeral legibility or speed was noted.
King et al. (1999)	50 Canadian children, 4 to 12 years old, with various diagnoses, who also received physical therapy, occupational therapy, or speech–language therapy	Direct therapy, monitoring, and collaborative consultation between therapists, teachers, and parents were provided in school visits from speech–language, occupational, and physical therapists (duration of occupational therapy: 3 months, 2 times/week for 45 minutes)	Hands-on with team supports	98% of children made progress in their education goals (e.g., copying from the board, holding a pencil correctly, and keyboarding), with many gains maintained over the 6-month follow-up. Improvement on standardized measures was clinically significant in the targeted area of school productivity. Parents and teachers reported a high degree of satisfaction with the combined collaborative consultation and direct intervention.
VandenBerg (2001)	4 children, 5.9 to 10 years old, who received school-based occupational therapy for hyperactivity and sensory modulation problems	OT guides teachers to give children weighted vests to wear for 20 to 30 minutes during table-top classroom activities, e.g., drawing, counting, coloring, writing, pasting, cutting, or organizing materials (duration of intervention: 6 sessions over 15 days)	Team supports	Increased on-task behavior (17% to 25%) in all 4 children; teachers report more cooperation and decreased hyperactivity; children request to wear the vests for longer intervals.
Fertel-Daly, Bedell, & Hinojosa (2001)	5 children, 2 to 4 years old, with pervasive developmental disorder and sensory modulation difficulties	OT and teacher used weighted vest for each child for 2 hours on arrival at preschool in self-contained classroom; each child continued daily school program working 1:1 with aide in the classroom (duration of intervention: 15 sessions over 6 weeks)	Hands-on with team supports	Increased attention to task (e.g., building with blocks, scribbling, and snipping with scissors) and decreased self-stimulatory behaviors (e.g., rocking, spinning objects, hand biting, and squinting)
Kemmis & Dunn (1996)	10 children, 5.9 to 9.7 years old, with diagnoses of learning disorder, behavior disorder, or developmental delay	Collaborative consultation: 10 OT–teacher pairs plan strategies for teacher to carry out during weekly 60-minute meetings to target performance deficits in learning, socialization, and communication or sensory processing (duration of intervention: 1 school year)	Team supports	In-context intervention strategies, remedial and compensatory, were equally successful (63% of criterion for student performance met)

(continued)

Table 1.3. Evidence for Improved Student Outcomes With Collaborative Occupational Therapy Services and Supports in Education Settings (1989–2006) *(continued)*

Source	Student Population	Intervention (Using Authors' Terms)	Occupational Therapist (OT) Roles	Student Outcomes
Davies & Gavin (1994)	18 children, 3 to 5 years old, diagnosed as developmentally delayed with moderate to severe gross or fine motor delays	*Individual–direct group:* two 30-minute sessions each of occupational therapy and physical therapy per week in therapy clinic. *Group–consultation group:* one 30-minute occupational therapy group/ week in classroom; one 30-minute physical therapy group/week in clinic; in-services, resources, answering questions, integrating therapeutic activities in daily activities. (Duration of intervention: 7 months)	Hands-on (out of context) Hands-on with team supports	Students in both groups demonstrated significant increases in fine and gross motor skills in clinic, home, and academic potential testing.
Oliver (1990)	24 children, 5 to 7 years old, in regular education with resource room or self-contained special education; all had delayed writing readiness and learning difficulties	*Direct therapy:* One time/week for 30 minutes focused on multisensory stimulation, large movement patterns, and writing readiness skills *Supplementary program:* additional programming designed by the OT for teacher, aide, or parent to implement a minimum of 10 minutes 3 times/week. (Duration of intervention: 1 school year)	Hands-on with team supports	Results demonstrated an improvement of 17 months in writing readiness for Group 2 ($n = 6$); Group 3 ($n = 6$) gained 12 months. Parents and teachers report satisfaction with and usefulness of supplementary materials.
Dunn (1990)	14 students, 2.9 to 6 years old, in special education, experiencing a minimum 1 year delay in gross, fine, or self-help skills	*Direct service group:* out of classroom, 60 minutes per week; only neutral or supportive comments shared with teachers. *Collaborative consultation group:* 60 minutes/week for observation, planning, recommendations, and demonstrations. (Duration: 24 hours over 1 school year)	Hands-on with team supports	Children in both groups achieved 75% of Individualized education program (IEP) goals; 60% of teachers in the consultation group reported larger OT contributions and more positive attitudes compared with 34% of teachers in direct service group.
Palisano (1989)	34 elementary students, 6 to 9 years old, with learning disabilities	*Direct service group:* small–large group occupational therapy two times/week + small group PT one time/week *Consultation group:* large-group occupational therapy one time/week and in-class consultation one time/week + follow-up by teacher three times/week (Duration of intervention: 6 months, 75 to 105 minutes/week)	Hands-on (out of context) Hands-on with team supports	Students were compared on three motor and visual–motor tests; therapist-directed group improved more in visual–perceptual skills (clinically but not statistically significant); consultation group improved significantly in motor skills.

Specifically, school-based collaboration among related service, education, and family partners can produce the following benefits for students, teams, and school districts:

- Inclusion of children with disabilities in the general education curriculum
- Shared accountability to reach desired outcomes for students
- Enhanced team competency by sharing knowledge and resources
- Support for individualizing learning situations

- Culturally competent communication among team members
- Increased opportunities for student mastery of emerging skills.

Each benefit is discussed in the sections that follow.

Inclusion of Children With Disabilities

Meaningful participation of students with special needs in classroom learning and social activities requires collaboration from all individuals in a student's education (Odom, Boyd, & Buysse, 2007). The IDEA mandates that children with disabilities must have access to the general education curriculum (see Resource Box 1.1). A team approach, focused on helping students with disabilities participate in school activities and lessons with their peers, leads to positive outcomes for students and satisfaction and support for the education team (Table 1.3; Fisher, Roach, & Frey, 2002; Idol, 2006; Thousand & Villa, 2000). Children are exposed to and learn from other children who have a wide range of strengths, talents, and learning needs. They also learn that membership in a group and participation in school is a right, regardless of one's mental or physical ability. Rather than setting one apart, individual differences are embraced as part and parcel of the various strengths and capacities inherent within a group. Educating children with their same-age peers unites an entire classroom as a learning community that respects and adapts to the individual differences of all children rather than viewing learning as a one-to-one relationship between a teacher and a student "with problems" (Lipsky & Gartner, 2001).

Student Voices: Inclusion vs. segregation

First of all, I wanted to go to a regular school about ten miles from my home because, for me, I guess that represented being valued. Secondly, I was offended by the stigma of being in a special class. . . . I prefer to think of my disability as a type of diversity rather than deviance or deficiency: my disability is just one characteristic or attribute among many that make me who I am. People do not need to prove their worthiness.

—Norman Kunc (as quoted in Giangreco, 1995, pp. 2–3)

Shared Accountability to Reach Desired Outcomes

Students with disabilities often have complex needs, and most are expected to achieve specific federal, state, and local standards for education (No Child Left Behind Act of 2001 [NCLB]). Collaborative teaming unifies historically separate special and general education services to address how all students learn and interact in school (Hunt, Soto, Maier, & Doering, 2003). Opportunities are presented for general and special education staff and families to "share knowledge and skills to generate new and novel methods for individualizing learning, without the need for dual systems of general and special education" (Thousand & Villa, 2000, p. 255). As members of collaborative teams, occupational therapists must also take responsibility for assisting team members to meet required standards of education for all students.

Therapist Voices: Benefits for the entire team

Weekly consultation with other team members keeps me abreast of the children's progress, the curriculum expectations, and the issues that may interfere with the children's ability to access their environment. . . . If I know what they are studying, my interventions incorporate, support, and enhance the curriculum. . . . If there is a constructional task associated with the curriculum, I may be able to tweak it to improve the fine motor and sequencing skills specified on a particular child's IEP. (Bowen-Irish, 2006, p. 23)

Enhanced Team Competency by Sharing Knowledge and Resources

Opportunities to acquire and refine one's knowledge and experience are much more likely when team members collaborate. Through interviews with 30 educational teams that regularly engaged in collaboration, Thousand and Villa (1990) concluded that opportunities were created for the regular exchange of needed resources, expertise, and technical assistance, as well as professional growth through team supports such as peer coaching. Within education, and in the contemporary work world in business, health care, and social services, there has been an explosion of information via video conferencing, e-mail, Internet search engines, electronic mailing lists, DVDs, CDs, and periodicals and books.

Teacher Voices: It takes a team

As society has become increasingly complex, so have students' needs, and providing adequate educational programs has become almost a Herculean endeavor. . . . Teachers in today's schools work with each other, with specialists, with related services personnel, with parents, with community agencies, and with the business community. (Fishbaugh, 2000, p. 3)

School-based therapists must keep up with diagnostic modifications (e.g., autism spectrum disorder), intervention methodology (e.g., using assistive technology for student accommodations in high-stakes testing), and the changes in legal requirements for educating students with disabilities (e.g., early intervening services, discussed in Chapter 4). Recently, the profession's focus on evidence-based occupational therapy practice (Dunn, 2000; Holm, 2000) as well as the call for scientific-based research in IDEA and NCLB (Nanof, 2007; Swinth et al., 2007; Whitehurst, 2002) have further increased the need for therapists and other school personnel to stay abreast of the influx of information and research within school-based occupational therapy. *Scientifically based research* (e.g., peer-reviewed studies) refers to using intervention strategies that have demonstrated results and is analogous to occupational therapy's focus on *evidence-based practice* (Nanof, 2007). IEP teams should base their decisions about a student's needs for special education, related services, and supplementary aids and services on peer-reviewed research "to the extent practicable" (see the requirements for an IEP in Exhibit 1.1A in the Appendix). Peer-reviewed research is one method for establishing the efficacy of occupational therapy services and supports in education settings; other approaches are suggested in the sources identified in Resource 1.4.

Support for Individualizing Learning

Collaboration builds on the experience and knowledge of a variety of education and related services personnel and family members and increases the options for individualizing teaching strategies and supports for all students.

Therapist Voices: Understanding a student's context

By assisting a child initially in their classroom routines, I become aware of the process and environment in which they are really trying to perform. That makes it easier for me to talk to the teachers about strategies that are reasonable and effective for carryover of the intervention. . . . This planning with teachers is important. I need to hear their comments, perspectives, comments, and questions; offer ideas and strategies; and collaborate about how to implement the strategies we decide to try. (Wakefield, 2001, p. 3)

Students with unique or complex learning, medical, and behavioral issues must have teams that collaboratively plan, implement, and evaluate their education program on a regular basis. Examples include students with multiple health conditions or who have significant disabilities across developmental domains; students who require extensive modifications to materials and environment to participate in school; and students with low-incident disabilities (e.g., significant hearing and visual impairment).

> **Resource 1.4. Resources for Evidence-Based Practice in Schools**
> - Using evidence to guide decision making in the educational setting (Collins, 2006)
> - Using AOTA evidence-based practice resources to enter pediatric practice in the context of public schools (Polichino & Scheer, 2006)
> - Using evidence to inform school-based practice (Saracino, 2002)
> - Occupational therapy: Effective school-based practice within a policy context (Swinth et al., 2007).

Remember this . . .
Collaboration increases the options for individualizing teaching strategies and supports for all students.

Increased Opportunities for Student Mastery

Teamwork increases the opportunities for students to practice emerging skills and behaviors in "real-life" activities and routines throughout the school setting and at home. Practice in familiar contexts is the key to generalization and mastery (Fishbaugh, 2000; Schmidt & Lee, 2005). Students with disabilities need frequent opportunities beyond individualized therapy to generalize their emerging skills with a specialist to natural contexts with familiar materials and routines (McWilliam & Scott, 2001).

Therapist Voices: Practice makes perfect

We are often running from school to school, classroom to classroom, without much time to spare. One or two 30-minute sessions per week can act as a stimulus for change in a child, but if the child has the opportunity to practice these skills on a daily basis, the results can be amazing! (Bowen-Irish, 2006, p. 24)

[B]y collaborating with classroom staff members, pediatric practitioners may enhance the child's progress by maximizing appropriate practice opportunities throughout the school day. Pediatric practitioners may discover that motor learning terminology provides a common language that is understood by many educators and allows for increased integration of occupational therapy goals and objectives into the child's daily routine. (Baker, 1999, p. 3)

Culturally Competent Communication

"Cultural diversity must be recognized as a characteristic that resides in interactions and comparisons between persons rather than as a characteristic possessed by individual persons themselves" (Barrera, Corso, & Macpherson, 2003, p. 8). In other words, diversity is a dynamic and relational quality. A student, parent, or colleague can be considered "diverse" only in comparison to another person.

Teacher Voices: Explore values with team members

Understanding one's own value orientations is a critical first step for thinking about cross-cultural communication. Next, it is important to consider how these orientations influence communication. Then it is helpful to examine how these match the orientations of others in the school and community. . . . Your efforts to achieve cultural self-awareness will help you begin to develop culturally competent communication skills that will enhance your collaborative interactions with colleagues and parents. (Friend & Cook, 2007, p. 211)

When teams collaborate and share perspectives and information, they increase the opportunities for respectful, nonjudgmental communication that takes a wide-angle view of students' abilities and challenges regarding their learning and socialization (see Chapter 2 for further discussion). Team members can inform one another and bridge cultural gaps in understanding due to unfamiliarity with language, customs, roles, educating and parenting children with disabilities, and providing services and supports in a school environment.

Challenges to Effective Collaboration

Three kinds of challenges—interpersonal, personal, and system—can create barriers to team collaboration in a school setting. Chapters 3, 5, and 6 provide additional strategies for addressing the challenges and barriers to effective collaboration that inevitably arise.

Interpersonal Challenges to Collaboration

Interpersonal challenges arise when one or more team members lack effective communication or social skills. Communication skills, particularly recognizing the potential for conflict and what to do about it, can also present significant challenges to team collaboration. Expect interpersonal challenges when team members begin to jointly plan and implement intervention outside their traditional comfort zone in separate classrooms and therapy spaces.

Some professionals mistakenly equate conversation with collaboration and caring with teaming (Friend, 2000). Successful collaboration among team members is measured by student outcomes, not how often teachers, families, and therapists talk to one another, share resources, or jointly plan and implement interventions. It is not

Remember this . . .
Successful collaboration among team members is measured by student outcomes, not how often people talk to one another or share resources.

unusual for the following interpersonal challenges to arise when people commit to working together:

- Loss of control of one's physical environment and preferred materials or equipment

- Changing the status quo, that is, known routines and procedures, even when the anticipated outcome is positive

- Fear of being viewed as incompetent (e.g., "What will people think about my teaching or therapy?"; Brownell, Adams, Sindelar, & Waldron, 2006; Harris & Cancelli, 1991)

Personal Challenges to Collaboration

Personal variables that can challenge how effectively occupational therapists and other team members collaborate are rooted in one's knowledge and experience about

- Collaboration in education settings (e.g., collaborative consultation, coaching, co-teaching, and other team supports);

- Implementing inclusion and following the IDEA requirements for providing special education and related services in the least restrictive environment;

- Developing IEPs as a team with integrated goals; and

- Using evidence-based practices to provide educationally relevant services and supports.

Personal attributes and beliefs can also either support or challenge collaboration. One study reviewed how general educators incorporated new collaborative practices and found that those teachers who readily adopted new ideas and materials differed in important ways from those who did not (Brownell et al., 2006):

> Teachers who had a strong knowledge base to build on, who were able to consider the needs of individual students while responding to the whole class, and whose beliefs closely aligned with the innovations we presented seemed to understand how to adapt novel strategies for their students and were most likely to adopt them. (pp. 182–183)

Reflection 1.3

Expectations and Missions

What are your expectations for working in education settings? How do you define your personal and professional mission for school-based occupational therapy?

One's attitude and expectations about the preferred role for occupational therapists in a school setting will significantly affect personal actions and interactions with team members. For example, expecting to work one-on-one with children in a therapy space is far more conducive to success in private practice than providing hands-on/team supports in the least restrictive environment in the schools. Believing that traditional pull-out therapy is the only way to provide occupational therapy intervention in the schools will certainly influence the satisfaction of either a parent or a teacher when a therapist hopes to provide team supports such as co-teaching, collaborative consultation, or both. Another expectation that creates both personal and interpersonal challenges to collaboration is how therapists view their mission regarding occupational therapy in school settings (see Reflection 1.3). Is the outcome of occupational therapy intervention for a student to acquire a specific skill, raise scores on a certain test, participate in the general education curriculum with peers, to the extent possible, or all of these?

Resource 1.5. Potential Challenges to Collaboration Identified by Educators (Dettmer, Thurston, & Sellberg, 2005; Fishbaugh, 2000; Friend & Cook, 2007)

Interpersonal (challenges arise during interaction with others)

- Uncertainty with what and how to communicate with team
- Unwillingness of school personnel to share expertise
- Coming across as a boss or supervisor
- Being treated as a teacher's aide, "go-fer," or quick-fix expert
- Difficulty managing time and resources.

Personal (challenges arise from emotional reactions)

- Unrealistic expectations about collaboration role
- Fear of losing touch with students
- Reluctance to change familiar teaching and therapy practices
- Concern about being viewed as less than competent.

System (challenges within school operations and policies)

- Lack of time for planning and team discussion
- Collaboration viewed as secondary to hands-on services
- Inflexible curriculum and assessment procedures
- Lack of training for the role of collaborator
- An excessive caseload that short-circuits team supports.

System Challenges to Collaboration

System variables become challenges to collaboration when there is insufficient time and resources to address and maintain positive team dynamics (Dettmer, Thurston, & Sellberg, 2005; Hanft & Place, 1996; Chapter 5 discusses strategies for managing time, workload, and providing flexible services and supports). All stakeholders in a school setting—families, administrators, therapists, and educators—must understand and embrace collaboration as an essential approach to facilitate student learning. Family acceptance of blending team and system supports and hands-on services is crucial to the success of collaborative team functioning (discussed further in Chapter 7). Obviously, therapists must also understand the art and science of collaboration and work to achieve its potential benefits.

Other challenges described by educators involved in collaboration are identified in Resource 1.5; knowing to watch for these potential challenges can help educators and therapists use the strategies for collaborative teaming identified throughout this book.

Conclusion: A Framework for Collaboration in Education Settings

Collaboration is an interactive team process dependent on the communication and interpersonal skills and knowledge of its individual members. Students and their families are the center of each school team. Each student has his or her own resources, interests, abilities, and challenges that determine current and desired educational performance. Gathering and integrating all team members' perspectives about a student's ability profile and future education needs is a critical first step for team collaboration. Collective decision making at this juncture ensures a more comprehensive profile of a student than could be collected by a single therapist, educator, or family member. It also provides the critical foundation for teams to work together to develop student goals, implement intervention, and review progress together.

Team members must learn to skillfully engage in the basics of team interaction, that is, share ideas to develop and implement a course of action to reach specified goals, and then assess outcomes. The traditional service model of providing only pull-out therapy to students with disabilities in therapy spaces and places is no longer considered effective practice.

To function effectively in a collaborative role, occupational therapists and their education partners must learn to

- Blend hands-on services for a student, when needed, with team supports, system supports, or both;

- Solicit student interests, preferences, and needs from team members, including students, as appropriate;
- Respect the diverse cultural, professional, and experiential backgrounds of team members as well as their perspectives and suggestions for interventions;
- Share knowledge and resources to assist team members in implementing suggested strategies, as appropriate to their role, education, and experience; and
- Use evidence-based practices and scientifically based research to evaluate the effectiveness of their services and supports in helping students reach their identified goals and participate in typical school lessons and activities.

Collaboration is the engine that drives flexible team decisions about when, and how, to provide occupational therapy services and supports to promote the academic achievement and functional performance of all students. As two partners described their collaboration:

Teacher Voices: Benefits for my students

We sit down and talk about things . . . tasks [students] would need to learn to do before they could go out and get a job; brainstormed about what activities we could come up with, swapped materials, worked together on a timeline to introduce different skills; [decided] what kind of adaptations could be used to produce the same results. (Dillon et al., 1996)

Therapist Voices: Joy of collaboration

It's a partnership—you get so much more done when you have two people focused and you're going the same way. It's just a pleasure to work with this teacher and things get done. You see progress! (Dillon et al., 1996)

Acknowledgments

This chapter was produced in collaboration with Jake Cashion, Melanie Cashion, Judy Davis, Ed Feinberg, Christine Knippenberg, Crystal Mallory, Dottie Marsh, Roland McDevitt, Christy Moser, Carol Olson, Jean Polichino, Jo Read, Judith Schoonover, and Maritza Villegas. Thanks to all for blending their team supports with our hands-on writing!

Selected Resources

Brownell, M., Adams, A., Sindelar, P., & Waldron, N. (2006). Learning from collaboration: The role of teacher qualities. *Exceptional Children, 72,* 169–185.

This study suggests that general educators may need different levels of assistance to adapt and adopt strategies learned in a collaborative professional development project to improve instruction for students with disabilities. Occupational therapists should consider the lessons learned about teachers who were most open to implement new learning, that is, they had a strong knowledge base to build on, they were able to consider the needs of individual students while responding to the whole class, and their professional beliefs aligned closely with the suggested strategies.

Polichino, J. (2004). "Moving Out of the 'Therapy Room.'" In Y. Swinth (Ed.), *Occupational therapy in school-based practice: Contemporary issues and trends* (AOTA Online Course, Lesson 7). Bethesda, MD: American Occupational Therapy Association.

> Written to complement an online continuing education course about school-based practice for occupational therapists, this lesson highlights the legal requirements for providing related services in education settings and describes strategies for selecting and implementing in-context services and supports to students in all school places and spaces.

Swinth, Y., Hanft, B., DiMatties, M., Handley-Moore, D., Hanson, P., Schoonover, J., et al. (2002, September 16). School-based practice: Moving beyond 1:1 service delivery. *OT Practice,* 12–20.

> This article presents five success stories from occupational therapists across the country who have found creative ways to blend hands-on services with team supports in the context of daily school environments. It is a good communication tool for opening the dialogue about collaborative practice with administrators, teachers, and families.

Thousand, J., & Villa, R. (2000). Collaborative teaming: A powerful tool in school restructuring. In R. Villa & J. Thousand (Eds.), *Restructuring for caring and effective education* (pp. 254–291). Baltimore: Paul H. Brookes.

> This chapter presents a rational for collaborative teams as well as a detailed description with suggestions for sustaining five core elements of the collaborative teaming process: face-to-face interaction, mutual goals, interpersonal skills, regular assessment of team functioning, and accountability for meeting responsibilities and commitments.

References

American Occupational Therapy Association. (1989). *Guidelines for occupational therapy services in school systems.* Bethesda, MD: Author.

American Occupational Therapy Association. (2002). Occupational therapy practice framework: Domain and process. *American Journal of Occupational Therapy, 56,* 609–639.

Baker, B. (1999). Principles of motor learning for school-based occupational therapy practitioners. *School System Special Interest Section Quarterly, 6*(2), 1–4.

Barnes, K., & Turner, K. (2000). Team collaborative practices between teachers and therapists. *American Journal of Occupational Therapy, 55,* 83–89.

Barrera, I., Corso, R., & Macpherson, D. (2003). *Skilled dialogue: Strategies for responding to cultural diversity in early childhood.* Baltimore: Paul H. Brookes.

Bayona, C., McDougall, J., Tucker, M., Nichols, M., & Mandich, A. (2006). School-based occupational therapy for children with fine motor difficulties: Evaluating functional outcomes and fidelity of services. *Physical and Occupational Therapy in Pediatrics, 26*(3), 89–110.

Bennis, W., & Biederman, P. (1997). *Organizing genius: The secrets of creative collaboration.* Reading, MA: Addison-Wesley.

Bowen-Irish, T. (2006, June 12). The orchestra of the classroom: Are you a member? *OT Practice,* 23–24.

Brownell, M., Adams, A., Sindelar, P., & Waldron, N. (2006). Learning from collaboration: The role of teacher qualities. *Exceptional Children, 72,* 169–185.

Campbell, P. (2000). Promoting participation in natural environments by accommodating motor disabilities. In M. Snell & F. Brown (Eds.), *Instruction of students with severe disabilities* (5th ed., pp. 291–329). Upper Saddle River, NJ: Prentice Hall.

Campbell, P., & Milbourne, S. (2006). Promoting children's participation through adaptive interventions. *Pennsylvania Early Intervention Newsletter, 17*(1), 1–3. Retrieved July 11, 2007, from www.pattan.k12.pa.us/files/Newsletters/EINewsWinter200.pdf

Case-Smith, J. (2002). Effectiveness of school-based intervention on handwriting. *American Journal of Occupational Therapy, 56,* 17–25.

Case-Smith, J., & Cable, J. (1996). Perceptions of occupational therapists regarding service delivery models in school-based practice. *Occupational Therapy Journal of Research, 16,* 23–43.

Cipollone, B., & Harris, J. (1999). Commentary: Teachers. *School System Special Interest Section Quarterly, 6*(3), 3.

Clark, G., Polichino, J., & Jackson, L. (2004). Occupational therapy services in early intervention and school-based programs. *American Journal of Occupational Therapy, 58,* 681–685.

Collins, A. (2006). Using evidence to guide decision making in the educational setting. *School System Special Interest Section Quarterly, 13*(3), 1–4.

Daniel R. R. v. State Board of Education, 874 F.2d 1036 5th Cir. (1989).

Davies, P., & Gavin, W. (1994). Comparison of individual and group consultation treatment methods for preschool children with developmental delays. *American Journal of Occupational Therapy, 48,* 155–161.

Deboer, A., & Fister, S. (1994). *Strategies and tools for collaborative teaching* (Participant's handbook). Longmont, CO: Sopris West.

Dettmer, P., Dyck, N., & Thurston, L. (1999). *Consultation, collaboration, and teamwork for students with special needs* (2nd ed.). Boston: Allyn & Bacon.

Dettmer, P., Thurston, L., & Sellberg, N. (2005). *Consultation, collaboration, and teamwork for students with special needs* (5th ed.). Boston: Allyn & Bacon.

Dillon, M., Flexman, C., & Probeck, L. (1996). *Examining the role of the occupational therapist and the educator in the transition planning process.* Unpublished master's research project, Virginia Commonwealth University, Richmond.

Donovan, S., Bransford, J., & Pellegrino, J. (Eds.). (1999). *How people learn: Bridging research and practice.* Washington, DC: National Academies Press, Committee on Learning Research and Educational Practice.

Dreiling, D., & Bundy, A. (2003). A comparison of consultative model and direct–indirect with preschoolers. *American Journal of Occupational Therapy, 57,* 566–569.

Dunn, W. (1985). Therapists as consultants to educators. *Sensory Integration Special Interest Section Newsletter, 8*(1), 1–4.

Dunn, W. (1988). Models of occupational therapy service provision in the school system. *American Journal of Occupational Therapy, 42,* 718–723.

Dunn, W. (1990). A comparison of service-provision models in school-based occupational therapy services: A pilot study. *Occupational Therapy Journal of Research, 10*(5), 300–320.

Dunn, W. (1991). Integrated related services. In L. Meyer, C. Peck, & L. Brown (Eds.), *Critical issues in the lives of people with severe disabilities* (pp. 353–377). Baltimore: Paul H. Brookes.

Dunn, W. (2000). *Best practice occupation therapy.* Thorofare, NJ: Slack.

Fertel-Daly, D., Bedell, G., & Hinojosa, J. (2001). Effects of a weighted vest on attention to task and self-stimulatory behaviors in preschoolers with pervasive developmental disorders. *American Journal of Occupational Therapy, 55,* 629–640.

Fishbaugh, M. (2000). *The collaboration guide for early career educators.* Baltimore: Paul H. Brookes.

Fisher, D., Roach, V., & Frey, N. (2002). Examining the general programmatic benefits of inclusive schools. *International Journal of Inclusive Education, 6,* 63–78.

Friend, M. (2000). Myths and misunderstanding of professional collaboration. *Remedial and Special Education, 21,* 130–132.

Friend, M., & Cook, L. (2007). *Interactions: Collaboration skills for school professionals* (5th ed). Boston: Allyn & Bacon.

Gersten, R., Morvant, M., & Brengelman, S. (1995). Close to the classroom is close to the bone: Coaching as a means to translate research into practice. *Exceptional Children, 62,* 52–67.

Giangreco, M. (1995). *The stairs don't go anywhere: A self-advocate's reflections on specialized services and their impact on people with disabilities.* Retrieved May 16, 2006, from www.normemma.com/arstairs.htm

Giangreco, M., Prelock, P., Reid, R., Dennis, R., & Edelman, S. (2000). Roles of related services personnel in inclusive schools. In R. Villa & J. Thousand (Eds.), *Restructuring for caring and effective education* (pp. 360–388). Baltimore: Paul H. Brookes.

Goodrich, B. (2004). Universal design for learning and occupational therapy. *School System Special Interest Section Quarterly, 11*(1), 1–4.

Gretz, S. (1999). Commentary: Parents. *School System Special Interest Section Quarterly, 6*(3), 2–3.

Hanft, B. E., & Place, P. A. (1996). *The consulting therapist.* Austin, TX: Pro-Ed.

Hanft, B., Shepherd, J., & Read, J. (in press). Competence in numbers: Working on pediatric teams. In S. Lane & A. Bundy (Eds.), *Kids can be kids: Supporting the occupations and activities of childhood.* Philadelphia: F. A. Davis.

Harris, A., & Cancelli, A. (1991). Teachers as volunteer consultees: Enthusiastic, willing, or resistant participants? *Journal of Educational and Psychological Consultation, 2,* 217–238.

Hasbrouck, J., & Christen, M. (1997). Providing peer coaching in inclusive classrooms: A tool for consulting teachers. *Intervention in School and Clinic, 32,* 72–77.

Holm, M. (2000). Our mandate for the new millennium: Evidence-based practice. *American Journal of Occupational Therapy, 54,* 575–585.

Hunt, P., Soto, G., Maier, J., & Doering, K. (2003). Collaborative teaming to support students at risk and students with severe disabilities in general education classrooms. *Exceptional Children, 69,* 315–340.

Idol, L. (1990). The scientific art of classroom consultation. *Journal of Educational and Psychological Consultation, 1,* 3–22.

Idol, L. (2006). Toward inclusion of special education students in general education: A program evaluation of eight schools. *Remedial and Special Education, 27*(2), 77–94.

Idol, L., Nevin, A., & Paolucci-Whitcomb, P. (1987). *Collaborative consultation* (2nd ed.). Austin, TX: Pro-Ed.

Idol, L., Nevin, A., & Paolucci-Whitcomb, P. (1996). *Collaborative consultation* (3rd ed.). Austin, TX: Pro-Ed.

Individuals With Disabilities Education Improvement Act of 2004, Pub. L. 108-446, 20 U.S.C. § 1400 *et seq.* (2004).

Jackson, L. L. (Ed.). (2007). *Occupational therapy services for children and youth under IDEA* (3rd ed.). Bethesda, MD: AOTA Press.

Jirikowic, T., Stika-Monson, R., Knight, A., Hutchinson, S., Washington, K., & Kartin, D. (2001). Contemporary trends and practice strategies in pediatric occupation and physical therapy. *Physical and Occupational Therapy in Pediatrics, 20*(4), 45–62.

Johnson, D., & Johnson, R. (1987). Research shows the benefit of adult cooperation. *Educational Leadership, 45*(3), 27–30.

Kemmis, B. L., & Dunn, W. (1996). Collaborative consultation: The efficacy of remedial and compensatory interventions in school contexts. *American Journal of Occupational Therapy, 50,* 709–717.

King, G., McDougall, J., Tucker, M. A., Gritzan, J., Malloy-Miller, T., Alambets, P., et al. (1999). An evaluation of functional, school-based therapy services for children with special needs. *Physical and Occupational Therapy in Pediatrics, 19*(2), 5–29.

Knippenberg, C., & Hanft, B. (2004). The key to educational relevance: Occupation throughout the school day. *School System Special Interest Section Quarterly, 11*(4),1–4.

Lipsky, D., & Gartner, A. (2001). Education reform and early childhood inclusion. In M. Guralnick (Ed.), *Early childhood inclusion: Focus on change* (pp. 39–48). Baltimore: Paul H. Brookes.

McWilliam, R. A., & Scott, S. (2001, November). *Integrating therapy into the classroom.* Retrieved December 21, 2006, from www.fpg.unc.edu/~inclusion/IT.pdf

Nanof, T. (2007). Education policy, practice, and the importance of OT in determining our role in education and early intervention. *School System Special Interest Section Quarterly, 14*(2), 1–4.

No Child Left Behind Act of 2001, Pub. L. 107-110, 115 Stat. 1425 (2002).

Odom, S. L., Boyd, B., & Buysse, V. (2007). Promising practices to support effective early childhood inclusion for Pre-K to Grade 3. In V. Buysse & L. Aytch (Eds.), *Early school success: Equity and access for diverse learners* (Executive Summary from the FirstSchool Diversity Symposium, pp. 14–17). Chapel Hill: University of North Carolina, FPG Child Development Institute. Retrieved November 2, 2007, from www.fpg.unc.edu/~firstschool/assets/FirstSchool_Symposium_ExecutiveSummary_2007.pdf

Oliver, C. E. (1990). A sensorimotor program for improving writing readiness skills in elementary-age children. *American Journal of Occupational Therapy, 44,* 111–117.

Palisano, R. (1989). Comparison of two methods of service delivery for students with learning disabilities. *Physical and Occupational Therapy in Pediatrics, 9,* 79–99.

Polcyn, P., & Bissell, J. (2005). Flexible models of service using the sensory integration framework in school settings. *Sensory Integration Special Interest Section Quarterly, 28*(1), 1–4.

Polichino, J. (2004). Moving out of the "therapy room." In Y. Swinth (Ed.), *Occupational therapy in school-based practice: Contemporary issues and trends* [AOTA Online Course, Lesson 7]. Bethesda, MD: American Occupational Therapy Association.

Polichino, J., Clark, G., & Chandler, B. (2005, February 21). Meeting sensory needs at school: Supporting students in the natural environment. *OT Practice,* pp. 11–15.

Polichino, J., & Scheer, J. (2006). Using AOTA EBP resources to enter pediatric practice in the context of public schools. *OT Practice, 10*(3), 11–15. Retrieved January 30, 2007, from www.aota.org/pubs/otp/features/2005/f-022105.aspx

Priest, N., & Waters, E. (2007). "Motor magic": Evaluation of a community capacity-building approach to supporting the development of preschool children (Part 2). *Australian Occupational Therapy Journal, 54,* 140–148.

Rainforth, B., & York-Barr, J. (1997). *Collaborative teams for students with severe disabilities: Integrating therapy and educational services* (2nd ed.). Baltimore: Paul H. Brookes.

Samaha, N., & DeLisi, R. (2000). Peer collaboration on a non verbal reasoning task by urban, minority students. *Journal of Experimental Education, 69,* 5–21.

Sandler, A. (1997). Physical and occupational therapy services: Use of a consultative therapy model in the schools. *Preventing School Failure, 41,* 164–167.

Saracino, T. (2002). Using evidence to inform school-based practice. *School System Special Interest Section Quarterly, 9*(2), 1–4.

Schmidt, R., & Lee, T. (2005). *Motor control and learning: A behavioral emphasis* (4th ed.). Champaign, IL: Human Kinetics.

Shasby, S., & Schneck, C. (2005). Use of sensorimotor theme groups to enhance developmental skills in preschool and kindergarten children. *School System Special Interest Section Quarterly, 12*(4), 1–3.

Shepherd, J. (1999). Commentary: Practitioners. *School System Special Interest Section Quarterly, 12*(4), 1–3.

Snell, M., & Janney, R. (2005). *Collaborative teaming* (2nd ed.). Baltimore: Paul H. Brookes.

Swinth, Y., Chandler, B., Hanft, B., Jackson, L., & Shepherd, J. (2003). *Personnel issues in school-based occupational therapy: Supply and demand, preparation, and certification and licensure.* Gainesville, FL: Center on Personnel Studies in Special Education. Retrieved August 12, 2006, from www.coe.ufl.edu/copsse/docs/IB-1/1/IB-1.pdf

Swinth, Y., Spencer, K. C., & Jackson, L. L. (2007). *Occupational therapy: Effective school-based practice within a policy context* (COPSSE Document No. OP-3). Gainesville: University of Florida, Center on Personnel Studies in Special Education.

Thousand, J., & Villa, R. (2000). Collaborative teaming: A powerful tool in school restructuring. In R. Villa & J. Thousand (Eds.), *Restructuring for caring and effective education* (pp. 254–291). Baltimore: Paul H. Brookes.

Turnbull, R., Stowe, M., & Huerta, N. (2007). *Free appropriate public education* (7th ed.). Denver: Love.

VandenBerg, N. (2001). The use of a weighted vest to increase on-task behavior in children with attention difficulties. *American Journal of Occupational Therapy, 55,* 621–628.

Van Meter, P., & Stevens, R. (2000) The role of theory in the study of peer collaboration. *Journal of Experimental Education, 69,* 113–127.

Villa, R., Thousand, J., Nevin, A., & Malgeri, C. (1996). Instilling collaboration for inclusive schooling as a way of doing business in public education. *Remedial and Special Education, 17,* 169–181.

Wakefield, L. (2001, November). *Integrating occupational therapy.* Retrieved December 21, 2006, from www.fpg.unc.edu/~inclusion/IT.pdf

Walther-Thomas, C., Korinek, L., McLaughlin, V., & Williams, B. (2002). *Collaboration for inclusive education: Developing successful programs.* Boston: Allyn & Bacon.

Westling, D., & Fox, L. (1995). *Teaching students with severe disabilities.* Upper Saddle River, NJ: Prentice-Hall.

Whitehurst, G. J. (2002, October). *Evidence-based education (EBE).* Presented at the Student Achievement and School Accountability Conference. Retrieved July 28, 2006, from www.ed.gov/nclb/methods/whatworks/eb/edlite-index.html

Wiggins, K., & Damore, S. (2006). "Survivors" or "friends"? A framework for assessing effective collaboration. *Teaching Exceptional Children, 38,* 49–50.

CHAPTER 2

Team Faces and Spaces

Jayne Shepherd, MS, OTR, FAOTA, and
Barbara Hanft, MA, OTR, FAOTA

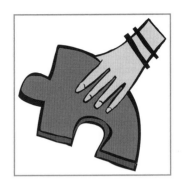

*M*y relationships with Matt's OTs were always special. They could see that
Matt was struggling, as was I, to make sense of some overwhelming problems.
Matt was not willful, just a great kid at heart, who had to deal with "overloads to
his system" in the best ways he could.

—Betty Thompson, parent of Matt, Virginia

Collaboration depends on three key elements of team process:

1. The *faces,* or people involved
2. The *places* and *spaces* where teamwork occurs
3. How the team and student *pace* their interactions to meet their expectations and goals.

Team members respect, affiliate with, and appreciate one another and embrace the student and the family as the heart of the team. Assessing and understanding the context in which the team works together is essential in providing educationally relevant services and supports. How students and other team members meet each other's expectations and pace their interactions and routines requires systematic analysis. This chapter discusses these concepts and provides worksheets to help therapists and their team members evaluate the impact of the school context on the collaborative process.

After reading this material, readers will be able to

- Identify key characteristics that influence collaborations with teachers, students and families, paraprofessionals, and other team members;

- Identify how different contexts influence how occupational therapists work on teams for students from preschool through graduation;

- Determine a variety of strategies to assess contextual influences on team collaboration;

- Recognize how to adapt and evaluate education contexts to facilitate students' participation in school lessons and activities; and

- Identify the key elements that affect the collaborative process: the *faces* on the team; the *places* and *spaces* in which team members interact and work

Key Topics

- *Faces:* Core and extended school teams

- *Places and spaces:* School environments

- *Paces:* Routines, schedules, classroom culture

- Contextual influences on collaboration

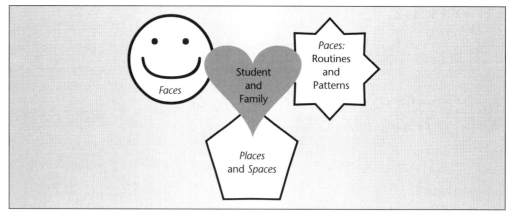

Figure 2.1. Essential elements of team collaboration.

with students; and the routines and habits (current and expected) of students and team members that affect how they *pace* their interactions.

Each element of collaborative teaming (i.e., the faces, places and spaces, and paces) is illustrated in Figure 2.1 and described in the sections below.

Part 1: Understanding the Faces on the Team

Team collaboration rests on the premise that a student and his or her family is the heart of the team. The other faces on the team include core and extended team members such as educators, administrators, related services personnel, school staff, classmates and friends, volunteers, and community partners (Giangreco, Cloninger, & Iverson, 1998). Both core and extended members contribute different perspectives to a team's vision for a child and can collectively brainstorm a variety of strategies, options, and ideas for developing and implementing meaningful intervention (Hanft, Shepherd, & Read, in press). When choosing team members, the areas of expertise and abilities of various members and how they contribute to promote the academic achievement and functional performance of a particular student are considered (Giangreco, 2001). Occupational therapists contribute their wisdom and experience to the discussion of who needs to be on each student's team.

Occupational therapists may function either as core or as extended team members of student-focused teams (Thousand & Villa, 2000). When occupational therapists are *core* members of a student's team, they work on a regular basis (from one to several times per week) with the student while also providing team supports. Sometimes the therapist is an *extended* team member, providing team supports on a monthly basis or on an as-needed basis (Hanft et al., in press; Thousand & Villa, 2000). Depending on the goal being addressed, core and extended teams may change composition so that team members are involved only when needed.

In the following example, Heidi, an occupational therapist, collaborates with both core and extended team members to help Jonell negotiate the lunch routine in the cafeteria.

Collaboration in Action: Core and extended team members

Core team members who collaborate to achieve this goal include

- Jonell, who decides if and how peer assistance can help her with the lunch routine (e.g., opening packages, pulling out the chair, picking up any items that fall);
- Jonell's parents, who make suggestions and practice lunchroom skills at home;
- Jonell's special education and kindergarten teachers, who decide on seating arrangements, communicate with team members about progress, and provide help to Jonell when asked;
- Anita, the speech–language pathologist, who helps Jonell communicate with the cafeteria staff and her peers; and
 - Heidi, the occupational therapist, who works with all the team members to modify the cafeteria tasks and environment to meet Jonell's needs.

Extended team members include

- The cafeteria manager who assigns Jonell's class to sit close to the lunch line;
- The custodian who helps find the right chair for Jonell (e.g., has arms at the appropriate height, slides easily on the floor, and fits at the end of the cafeteria table);
- The nutritionist or school cafeteria manager who chooses the food menu;
- The cafeteria worker who serves the food and decides where to place liquid foods on the tray for Jonell; and
- The administrator who approves the purchase of cafeteria tables, chairs, and lunch trays with dividers and deep cavities.

Therapists collaborate with key core and, possibly, extended members. (Chapter 3 focuses on how therapists pace their collaborations with team members in school routines.) Rarely are all the faces mentioned above on a student's team at one time. For example, once Jonell has learned the cafeteria routine, many extended team members may step back; if this is the only goal for Jonell that Heidi works on, she may no longer function as a core team member.

75% TS
25% HO

Faces: Students and Families

Family Voices: Part of the team

All the OTs through the years, with only one exception, felt like allies. They didn't think I had rocks in my head for looking at environmental factors in behavior. They validated me and came up with helpful suggestions about modifications. The OTs made me feel like a team member, because they would listen, affirm my observations, and offer things to try that fit my lifestyle.

—Betty Thompson, parent of Matt, Virginia

Reflection 2.1

Imagine Yourself as a Student or Family Member

Imagine yourself as a student or family member on one of your school teams:

• How would you like everyone to make decisions about you but never ask for your opinion or include you in the decision-making process?

• How would you talk with your team members if everyone spoke a different language and there was no interpreter? (Professional jargon can also sound like a foreign language.)

• What if you arrived at an IEP meeting and your spouse is not there, and you are asked to decide how your child would be educated?

• What if your team members greeted you with hugs and kisses or called you "Honey" or "Mom" or by your nickname without your permission? Or no one looked at you when they spoke?

• What if teachers and therapists focused on independence when suggesting goals, when in your culture interdependence is expected and valued?

Students and families are the heart of the collaborative team (Hanft et al., in press). They are recognized and valued for their knowledge about the child or themselves and provide a refreshing perspective about how the child functions in everyday life outside of school (Segal & Hinojosa, 2006; Thousand & Villa, 2000). All families have expectations for how their members will communicate and interact with others within and outside the family (Hanft & Place, 1996). In the multicultural environment of schools, team members need to make it their business to respect and support these communication styles so students and families are able to participate as full team members. Families and students are more invested in collaborating when they are respected for their values, knowledge, and interaction style; understanding between all team members is then possible (Turnbull, Turbiville, & Turnbull, 2000). Learning about student and family interests, desired goals, and typical routines helps teams select collaborative goals embedded in everyday routines (Cohn, Miller, & Tickle-Degnen, 2000; McNamara & Humphry, 2007). Reflection 2.1 asks team members to imagine their personal answers to practices that may occur to their students and families.

By gaining insight about family culture, team members can meaningfully structure the blended role of hands-on services with team and system supports for occupational therapists in school settings. Many parents may have never experienced collaborative services and supports for their children and will need assistance to appreciate how an occupational therapist can provide team supports and still achieve student outcomes. Figure 2.2 can assist parents and other team members with visualizing the outcomes of hands-on services with team and system supports for students,

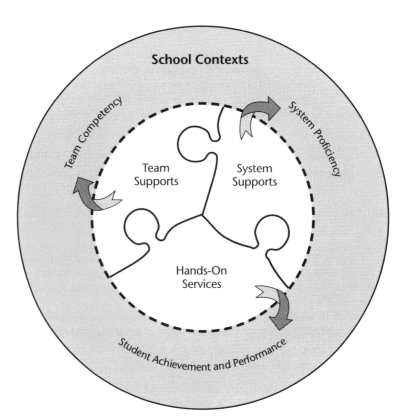

Figure 2.2. Collaboration in school-based practice.

teams, and the school system. Occupational therapists help students improve their academic achievement and functional performance, team members enhance their competency, and school systems offer proficient education programs. (Chapter 7 assists therapists in understanding the different perspectives team members may have about collaborative occupational therapy supports and services.)

Strategies for helping occupational therapists learn about and respect students and families as the heart of a team are highlighted in the following sections, which discuss student and family interviews, student self-assessment, student-centered team assessment, and inclusion of families and students in team decisions. These strategies emphasize collaboration by including families and students in collective team decisions.

Student and Family Interviews

Team members learn about individual students, and their families, in a variety of ways and share this information during meetings and informal discussions. Interviews, checklists, observations, conferences, or previous interactions with a student and family, together with formal student assessments, help answer an essential question, "What does this student want and need to learn to participate in school?"

Interviews may be conducted with a student, a parent, an educator, or other team members to understand a student's educational needs. First, it is important to decide whom to interview and what information to gather. Keep the purpose of the interview in mind—for example, find out what strategies a teacher has already tried or what a student would like to do better, faster, or like everyone else. If possible, speak with a student first, using the informal interview questions identified in Figure 2.3. Students as young as 6 or 7 years old understand when they are having difficulty in school and can often say what they wish they could do without any prompting from others:

- "I want to write like Joshua."
- "Why can't I play with my friends on the playground?"
- "I don't want to be treated differently. . . . I will not leave early for art class."
- "I want to be in the chorus like my brothers were."
- "I want to go to Jump Rope Club in the mornings with my friend."

In Chapter 4, Figure 4.2 provides additional questions that guide therapists in developing an occupational profile for a student to share with team members.

Remember this . . .
Related services personnel collaborate effectively when they provide services that

- **Are contextually relevant for each school place and space;**
- **Are related to current instructional lessons;**
- **Are integrated in natural routines and schedules and are flexible;**
- **Facilitate active student participation using adaptations and equipment as appropriate; and**
- **Are acceptable to the student and other team members (Giangreco, Prelock, Reid, Dennis, & Edelman, 2000; Snell & Janney, 2005).**

---

1. What do you like best about school?
2. What do you like least about school?
3. What is important to you about school?
4. What is hard for you in school?
5. What is easy for you in school (what are you good at)?
6. What is your favorite part of the day?
7. If you could change one thing about school, it would be. . . ?

Figure 2.3. Student Interview Questionnaire.

Note. Adapted with permission from Judie Sage, occupational therapist, Wisconsin.

Sometimes parents or guardians do not speak English and rely on their older children or other family member to interpret what is being said in an IEP meeting or school conference. Obviously, this communication barrier can influence collaboration, as the team may be unsure of a family's concerns or expectations related to their child. In the vignette below, consider how a translator provided a team with insight about working with parents whose only language was Farsi.

Therapist Voices: Learning preferences

It was very beneficial to have a Farsi translator at the IEP meeting. It became evident that if there was to be follow-through at home, then we needed to make sure that the father was informed and willing to participate. This was not the impression I had prior to the meeting because the mother always dropped off and picked up her child, and therefore she was primarily the parent I interacted with. Furthermore, it became clear that the parents did not entirely agree on what was best for the child. However, in this family's culture, the father was entitled to make all the final decisions. Following the IEP meeting, the team made a point to include and contact both parents about their child's intervention.

—Inbal Fraiman, occupational therapy student,
University of Southern California

Remember this . . .
An essential question that guides team decisions is, "What does this student want and need to learn to participate in school?"

Student Self-Assessment

How students perceive their performance of the student role, in a variety of environments, is the focus of the School Setting Interview (SSI; Hemmingson, Egilson, Hoffman, & Kielhofner, 2005). The SSI is a semistructured interview for elementary through high school students (Hemmingson, Kottorp, & Bernspang, 2004). Through a series of questions, a student describes how he or she is doing in academic, class, and schoolwide environments as well as in interpersonal relationships. Following each descriptive statement, the student decides whether the item is a need, not a need, or a need that is already being addressed. This interview helps the team consider the student–environment fit to help plan necessary accommodations to address student-identified needs.

The Child Occupation Self Assessment (COSA; Keller, Kafkes, Basu, Federico, & Kielhofner, 2005) is another instrument that assesses a child's or adolescent's feelings of self-competency related to home, school, and community. By using a card sort or simple checklist version of the COSA, a student identifies meaningful occupations and his or her perceived occupational competency in each task (e.g., "how important this is to me" and "do I have a problem with this"). At least half the questions on the COSA relate to school, and responses to all the questions provide therapists with a more holistic view of the child's activities and environments than just the student role. For example, the COSA asks a student whether he or she has a problem with dressing or bathing and then asks the student to rate the importance of the task.

Student-Centered Team Assessment

Another collaborative assessment that may be used by an entire team is the Vermont Interdependent Services Team Approach (VISTA; Giangreco, 1996). A team uses the

VISTA to identify valued life outcomes and then considers a checklist of student skills to guide their discussion of what supports are needed to achieve the student's goals. This assists teams in choosing student- and family-centered goals and helps determine which team members to involve in assessment and intervention, based on their skills and availability (Resource 2.1 identifies Internet sites for further information about the SSI, COSA, and VISTA; additional collaborative assessments for school practice are described in Exhibit 2.1A in the Appendix.)

Past experiences with therapy services often influence the expectations of students, parents, or both regarding school-based occupational therapy. Hanft and Place (1996) suggested that therapists can gain many insights from students and their parents by asking the following questions:

Resource 2.1. Where to Find St[...] Assessments

- Child Occupation Self Assessment (C[...] & Kielhofner, 2005): www.moho.uic.edu/as[...]
  Sample: www.moho.uic.edu/images/assessments/ COSA%20summary%20form.pdf
- *Making Action Plans* (*MAPS;* Falvey, Forest, Pearpoint, & Rosenbury, 2004): www.inclusion.com/artcommonsensetools .html
- *Planning Alternative Tomorrows With Hope* (*PATH;* Pearpoint, O'Brien, & Forest, 1995): www.inclusion.com/ pkpathinactionpack.html
- School Setting Interview (Hemmingson et al., 2005): www.moho.uic.edu/assess/ssi.html
  Sample: www.moho.uic.edu/images/assessments/ SSI%20Summary%20Form.pdf
- Vermont Interdependent Services Team Approach (Giangreco, 1996): www.uvm.edu/%7Emgiangre/vista.html

- *For families:* What experiences have you had with an occupational therapist or other related services personnel? What did you like doing with that occupational therapist? What did you dislike? What could have made this experience more helpful for you?

- *For students:* "How would you like an occupational therapist to work with you at school?" or "What help do you need from me?"

The answers to these questions help occupational therapists and their team members understand what intervention to suggest. For example, middle schooler Raj explained that with his previous occupational therapist, "I liked playing games but I hated missing class. I don't want all that equipment stuff! It makes me look different from my friends." This information helps his therapist understand that Raj only knows therapy in a pull-out model and wants to fit in with his peers. Perhaps he needs more guidance to explain his needs so that his occupational therapist can select adaptive aids or make environmental modifications that are acceptable to him. If, on the other hand, Raj had said, "I loved therapy because I got out of class," his therapist would have a different task helping Raj buy into hands-on therapy with team supports in school places and spaces. Respond to Reflection 2.2 and give examples of adaptations that are appropriate for Raj.

Including Student and Family Members in Team Decisions

After identifying the faces on the team and becoming more familiar with their roles, ask core team members about a student's strengths, school challenges, and educational goals. Rather than select discipline-specific goals, team members should identify individualized goals to address each student's educational needs while respecting his or her culture. This information is also essential for determining what assessments or interventions may work for a particular student or family. Open discussion and clear communication (e.g., "What exactly do you mean by Roberto *will be more social?*") helps the team clarify behaviors, maintain curriculum standards,

Reflection 2.2

Adaptations for Raj

Raj has difficulty producing legible writing within the time frame allowed for in-class assignments. The occupational therapist has identified that his grip, strength, vision, and visual–perceptual skills limit his handwriting output, yet Raj wants to "look like his friends." Using Figure 1.3 in Chapter 1, as a guide, what adaptations would you suggest to meet Raj's needs and desires?

and focus on key education outcomes. The following questions can help teams generate collaborative goals for a student:

- What are this student's strengths?

- What are our concerns about this student?

- What education outcomes are desired by and for this student?

- What is the parents' vision for their child's participation in school?

- How can we help this student participate in the general curriculum and meet the required academic standards?

Reflection 2.3

Helping a Student and Family Feel Part of Their Team

Choose one student and family you work with in your school district, and consider how they might answer the questions in Worksheet 2.1A (in the Appendix). Would they consider your team to be student centered or family centered?

Teams can use Worksheet 2.1A (located in the Appendix) to consider how family friendly their services and supports are. Reflection 2.3 asks teams to consider whether their practices and policies include students and families as full team members.

Teams use numerous strategies to ensure that the student and family feel valued as key collaborators. Communication with the family may be accomplished through home and school notebooks, e-mail, phone calls, online IEPs, IEP meetings, videos, actual visits to the classroom, or soliciting and sharing family vision statements for their child. After reading the following portion of a vision statement from Brooke's parents, consider whether the Yarbroughs will value out-of-context hands-on services:

Family Voices: Our vision

We envision a future for Brooke that is full of richness and diversity, one in which she determines her own destiny. We offer the support of loving parents and promise her that through life's many challenges, we will stand by her; be there when she needs us. May Brooke be rich in what truly is of value: relationships, friendships, and a deep sense of belonging. We believe in a world that will accept Brooke for who she is.

- Brooke is healthy; she is not in need of remedy, therapy, or cure.

- Brooke is not broken; she does not need to be fixed.

- Brooke loves chicken nuggets; swimming; sweet iced tea; and playing with her dog, family, and friends. She also likes the computer and listening to music.

- Brooke has blue eyes; light brown hair; an infectious smile and giggle; and physical, intellectual, and sensory disabilities.

Having disabilities is only a small part of who Brooke is, and it is our vision not to change Brooke . . . but to change the world around her.

—Dana and John Yarbrough, parents of Brooke, Virginia

Some teams appoint one person as the main contact between the family and school. Before a child study or an IEP meeting, a list of questions to prompt thinking about a student's performance may be shared with parents or a student may be prepped to participate in, or lead, the IEP meeting to promote self-determination (National Dissemination Center for Children with Disabilities, 2002a, 2002b). Chapter 6's Resource 6.3 provides additional information to involve students in the IEP process and plan for transitions. Vignettes about helping students learn how to lead their IEP meetings are presented in Chapter 5 (the vignette of Susannah) and in Chapter 6 (the vignette of Pedro).

Faces: Education Team Members

Therapist Voices: Understanding schools

You have to understand how a school system works, what the politics are like, and how the personalities work in order to find a way to fit yourself into the system and be effective. (Mendoza-Smith, 2005, p. 118)

In addition to student and family partners, therapists work with a variety of team members: educators, paraprofessionals, physical therapists, speech–language pathologists, nurses, psychologists, social workers, administrators, and community agency staff. Prior to hiring an occupational therapist, schools want to know whether the therapist will "fit" with their school's philosophy and team. Administrators may ask interview questions to understand the applicant's prior experiences with school-based practice and his or her examples of working with a variety of faces on the educational team. Reflection 2.4 provides sample questions a special education administrator may ask a therapist to determine how he or she will work with the team members in various places and spaces.

Learning from team members about their previous experiences with occupational therapists' professional training, interests, and areas of expertise helps therapists collaborate more effectively. Likewise, seeking similar information from colleagues and actively listening to their responses helps team members feel respected and more willing to discuss issues, ideas, and concerns. Once the members of a student's core team are identified, two key questions may facilitate a conversation with *selected* team members to find common ground (Hanft & Place, 1996).

Reflection
2.4

Questions of a Director of Special Education

A director of special education asks therapists the following questions during interviews to understand their experience with school-based practice and their willingness to work on educational teams. How would you answer them?

• What is your experience working with children and youth?

• What age group do you like best, and why?

• What kind of settings have you worked in?

• What interests you about working in a school setting? What experiences have you had?

• How do you see your role as a registered occupational therapist or certified occupational therapy assistant in a school setting?

• Describe how you have collaborated with teachers and principals.

• Tell me about a family collaboration or interaction you have initiated.

• How have you provided occupational therapy to promote a child's participation in the general curriculum?

• What specializations (e.g., assistive technology, transition post–high school, pediatrics, sensory integration) do you have, and how would you use these skills in a school setting?

• For registered occupational therapists: Describe how you have (or might) work with a certified occupational therapy assistant.

• Are you willing to supervise an occupational therapy student interested in completing a school affiliation?

Interview with Jo Read, director of student services, Colonial Heights Public Schools, Virginia, September 13, 2006.

Question 1: What Are the Experiences of Education Partners Collaborating With an Occupational Therapist in School Places and Spaces?

Try to understand teachers' and paraprofessionals' history of collaboration, particularly in typical school places and spaces, with therapists or other team members to find out about the "ghosts of the past." Ask about the therapists' hands-on services and team supports, their effectiveness, and how communication occurred. Perhaps a teacher does not like messy activities or really enjoyed the co-teaching she and the occupational therapist carried out. Or the teacher may tell you she or he always reads e-mail or only wants face-to-face meetings on a regular basis. Using questions similar to those suggested for understanding student and family expectations about occupational therapy, ask education personnel the following:

- What worked well?
- What would you have changed to make this experience better?
- What were the benefits of working together in the classroom?
- How would you like an occupational therapist to work with you this year?

If a team member has never had any experience with occupational therapy, this presents an opportunity to explain school-based occupational therapy. Therapists may use "*Wh . . .*" questions to explain occupational therapy in the schools: *What* is it; *who* is seen and *why; when* and *where* does therapy occur; and *who* does what to provide educationally relevant therapy? For example, if a preschool team includes a physical therapist, an occupational therapist may focus less on mobility issues and more on the student's social, self-care, and tool usage issues.

Sometimes, the occupational therapist or occupational therapy assistant is the only team member who has previously worked with a student.

Teacher Voices: Long-term perspective

With a lot of the kids, she [the occupational therapist] worked with them in preschool, and now they're 14. She's able to re-establish rapport quickly with the parents. This is really advantageous both with the parents and the teacher. She can say to the teacher, "He's been doing this since he was 5." Having a long-term perspective has been really helpful.

—Teacher working in transition (Dillon, Flexman, & Probeck, 1996)

Question 2: What Knowledge or Experiences Do Education Partners Contribute to Team Collaboration?

Diverse educational backgrounds, lifestyles, professional and family experiences, values, and beliefs about working on teams and educating children with and without disabilities all influence team members during their interactions. General and special education teachers and paraprofessionals work with a student far more often than does the occupational therapist. Therefore, looking for information about a teacher's philosophy of classroom or behavior management, past experiences, learning style, and tolerance for new ideas or materials is helpful when planning intervention strategies (Hanft & Place, 1996). Knowing that a teacher is an expert on positive behavior supports or has had numerous students with autism in his or her class provides an entirely different context for team supports than working with a first-year special education teacher or guidance counselor who has had limited training or experience with children with autism. On the other hand, a first-year special education teacher may not have worked with children with autism but may have extensive experience developing visual schedules for students with intellectual disabilities, a valuable organization strategy for students who do not read. By looking for teammates' education and expertise, common ground is often found for sharing information and ideas.

Besides their disciplinary knowledge and expertise, team members may bring to the team process valuable *personal* experiences and interests (Hanft & Place, 1996). Personal stories and experiences may help all team members understand one another's perspectives and open communication lines, as illustrated in the following examples:

- A teacher who has adopted children can inform team members about positive adoption terminology and help them understand how classroom assignments (e.g., family trees or writing a birth announcement) may upset students who are adopted. This team member may also have knowledge or access to a variety of adoption resources.

- A physical therapist who plays the clarinet could help adapt a clarinet stand for a student who is too weak to hold the instrument without support during band performances. This physical therapist may then consult with the adaptive physical education teacher to incorporate arm-strengthening activities to improve the student's strength and ability to hold the clarinet for longer periods of times.

- An occupational therapist who has studied origami or travels extensively can contribute to classroom lessons about countries visited.

Knowing how to tap or expand the knowledge, expertise, experience, or interests of team members increases the opportunities to influence student participation and learning throughout the school environment. It also multiplies the opportunities for personal growth for all team members and encourages acceptance of the complementary roles that educators, occupational therapists, and other related services personnel play on collaborative teams. It is essential that occupational therapists clearly explain their roles and contributions to all team members. (See Chapters 3 and 7 for additional ideas about explaining occupational therapy services and supports.)

Soliciting Team Members' Perspectives and Assumptions

At times, team members make assumptions about one another's perspectives and expertise. Teachers may assume that feeding techniques, assistive technology, and positioning or equipment adaptations are part of every occupational therapist's expertise. In actuality, another team member may be equally or more knowledgeable about these areas (Giangreco et al., 2000; Giangreco, Cloninger, Dennis, & Edelman, 2002). Likewise, therapists may also make assumptions about teachers' areas of expertise that need clarifying.

Remember this . . . **Learning about a teacher's philosophy of classroom or behavior management, past experiences, learning style, and acceptance for new ideas or materials is critical when planning intervention strategies (Hanft & Place, 1996).**

In the following scenario, consider the efforts an occupational therapist made to understand the perspectives of a specific teacher on one of her teams and how she provided team and system supports to meet the teacher's and students' needs.

Therapist Voices: Asking what's needed

I was asked to add a school that had a lot of OT turnover to my workload. The school lacked a good leader, and many OTs didn't want to work there as they felt the teachers didn't value them. When I entered the setting, one team was obviously skeptical of working with OT.

I decided to go to one of the lead teachers and find out why she was ambivalent. We agreed to meet for 20–30 minutes after school, and I asked, "Can you help me understand why the team members seem to disregard OT services for their students? There seems to be a reluctance to collaborate with me." The teacher immediately replied with a question of her own. "Are you going to be here next year?" I then understood that the turnover in this school did not encourage trust and collaboration as the teachers always felt the OTs were there for the short term. So we talked; I explained how I saw my role and solicited comments from her about what would work for her and her students.

As our relationship developed, about mid-semester, I again asked this teacher how I could help her with the class. She needed more support for using the technology in her classroom. I had assumed that this teacher had a good handle on technology since she was using so much of it in her class. So I hadn't spent much time on it. Well, it just shows assumptions can lead down the wrong path. I learned she wanted to call a vendor to ask a question but was having a terrible time finding time to do it. I offered to make the call, and then together we figured out how to use the information to solve the problem the student was having with technology.

Later that year, we worked together to start a swimming program for the students. We asked the administration for support and secured funding from the physical education and special education departments. This assured us that the swimming program would remain part of the regular school activities no matter who the OT was at the school.

> — Darcie Votipka, occupational therapist,
> director of student services, Colorado

Faces: Cultural Considerations

Each year, as the population of the United States becomes more and more diverse, school teams are expected to educate students and interact with families and colleagues from many cultural groups (Federal Interagency Forum on Child & Family Statistics, 2006). Barrera, Corso, and Macpherson (2003) described *cultural diversity* as a "dynamic and relational reality that exists between persons rather than any single person" (p. 3). Becoming *culturally competent* is a process of learning to understand the meanings of diverse behaviors and to support interactions among team members that are respectful, reciprocal, and responsive.

Key Principles of Culturally Competent Practice

Culturally competent practice encompasses five key principles (Barrera et al., 2003) for consideration by all team members:

1. Anticipate and appreciate variances in individual interaction styles, values, and parenting or teaching practices.
2. Identify potential personal biases or barriers that may interfere with collaboration when interacting with students, families, and education staff.
3. Be aware of language and behaviors that have specific meanings for a parent or teacher, and find ways to support these behaviors and communications.
4. Build relationships that are responsive, respectful, and shared.
5. Use specific strategies (i.e., anchored understanding of diversity and third-space dialogue) to develop a concrete and empathetic understanding of a team member's cultural context.

Anchored understanding of diversity occurs when two or more people from diverse cultural groups interact and consciously accept another's behavior as meaningful *to that person,* even though it may be very different from one's own behavior. For example, consider the following vignette:

> Dina, a preschool teacher, wants Adoria to put her coat and shoes on herself and recognizes that Adoria's parents do not share this goal for her. In fact, the mother, Maya, helps Adoria take her coat off when she drops Adoria off in the morning, and Adoria waits for her mother to put it back on at the end of school. Dina understands that Adoria is an only child and that in her parents' culture, children are not expected to dress themselves until much older. The parents' expectation about helping Adoria makes as much sense to them as Dina's expectation (of Adoria putting on her own coat) makes to her.

Both the parents and teachers must recognize that they are each anchored in their own cultural beliefs before they can begin to communicate effectively about helping Adoria.

Third-space dialogue is a second tool for viewing another person's culturally based behaviors and perceptions as complementary to one's own behavior so that new options or actions may be generated to facilitate collaboration (Barrera et al., 2003). Rather than negotiate whether "my view" or "your view" is the correct one, both parties agree to look for the *third space*—that is, a third perspective that builds on the common ground between each person's perspective, or an entirely different one that both people can accept. Continuing the previous vignette:

> Adoria refuses to help with shoe tying and putting on her coat and usually throws herself on the ground crying. Her mother, Maya, picks her up and hugs her, saying softly, "You are so young, you don't have to do this yet; I'll help you." Dina thinks that Maya's actions reinforce Adoria's immature behavior.

What can Dina say to Maya to open a third-space dialogue? One option is to look for a way to compliment Maya, rather than admonish her, and recognize her nurturing

Resource 2.2. Learning About Different Cultures

- IRIS Center (Special Education Resources for Inclusion, Research-to-Practice Instructional Strategies): http://iris.peabody.vanderbilt.edu/onlinemodules.html
- National Center for Culturally Responsive Educational Systems (NCCRESt): www.nccrest.org/
- Culturally and Linguistically Appropriate Services: Early Childhood Research Institute: www.clas.uiuc.edu/search.html

attitude and support of Adoria. This approach conveys an attitude of "Let's work together" instead of "Don't you see how wrong your behavior is?" Another option is to acknowledge their different expectations and ask Maya whether there is anything she would like Adoria to learn to do for herself, and then offer to help. If Maya were to say no, then Dina might look for common ground by describing some other parts of the preschool curriculum related to independence and see if these areas are more acceptable to Maya. Anchored understanding of diversity and third-space options are based on conversations that demonstrate respect for others' perspectives, reciprocity or sharing of perspectives, and responsiveness to reflect understanding of unfamiliar perspectives.

Self-Reflection About Cultural Competency

Culturally competent school-based providers analyze and reflect on their interactions with a variety of team members. Barrera et al. (2003) and Hanft (2004) suggested that therapists consider the following questions with team members:

- Does my perspective of a student or teacher match or supplement that of the team?
- Do I describe a student or teacher positively in words that team members can accept?
- Do I understand a student's, family's, or other team member's expectations, hopes, and dreams?
- Can I describe what participation in school or family life means to each student or team member I work with?
- Do I recognize possible communication barriers when a teacher's or family's story is not congruent with my story about the student?

Cultural competency takes time and is always evolving as students and team members change. Resource 2.2 provides online sources for learning more about the cultural beliefs of various groups.

Faces: Collaborating With Paraprofessionals in Schools

Paraprofessional Voices: Holding it together

The range and flexibility of paraeducator positions make it difficult for most folks to understand exactly where our role begins and ends. We are the mortar that fits where it needs to fit to keep the whole structure together.

—Sandie Blankenship, special education paraeducator, Rhode Island (as quoted in National Education Association, 2004, p. 2)

Definition of *Paraprofessionals*

Paraprofessionals "are the individuals who provide instructional and other services to students and who are supervised by licensed professionals who are responsible for student outcomes" (Friend & Cook, 2007, p. 141). They may be called *para-*

professionals, paraeducators, supplementary aides, teacher aides, personal aides, or *instructional* or *teaching assistants*. They may have had on-the-job training and, as mandated by No Child Left Behind (NCLB), they must have a secondary degree and at least 2 years of college coursework, an associate's degree in education or another field, or a way to document their knowledge (U.S. Department of Education [ED], Office of Elementary and Secondary Education, 2002). In this volume, we have chosen the term *paraprofessional* to describe this team member.

Over the past decade, more school districts have hired paraprofessionals to support students with disabilities in inclusive classrooms, and paraprofessional research and resources have mushroomed (Chopra et al., 2004; French, 2003; Giangreco & Doyle, 2007; Pickett, Likins, & Wallace, 2003). In one study, paraprofessionals described themselves as the connectors between team members (Chopra et al., 2004). They facilitated parent–teacher communication and family–community connections and linked students to teachers, peers, and the curriculum. One paraprofessional described her connections with parents:

Paraprofessional Voices: Contact person

Typically, . . . you can go to the schools and see that we're the ones in the lunchrooms, on the playground, meeting them at the bus, walking [students] down the hallway, wiping their noses, as truly the support thing. . . . I've always been the contact person, and parents just come to expect that as the role.

—Paraprofessional (as quoted in Chopra et al., 2004, p. 225).

Paraprofessionals' Roles and Responsibilities in School

Many researchers have voiced concerns about the overuse of paraprofessionals within inclusive classrooms. This overuse may affect all team members. Students with disabilities who work with paraprofessionals demonstrate less socialization and interaction with teachers and peers as well as stigma, isolation, and dependence on the paraprofessional (Broer, Doyle, & Giangreco, 2005; Giangreco, Edelman, & Broer, 2001; Hemmingson, Borell, & Gustavsson, 1999). Teachers often ask the paraprofessional to spend most of his or her time instructing students, but they offer little guidance or supervision (Broer et al., 2005; French, 2003; Giangreco & Doyle, 2002, 2007).

Paraprofessionals may feel like they do all the work with the students but are not respected or asked to collaborate or give an opinion when teams are making decisions (Giangreco et al., 2001; Patterson, 2006). Often, paraprofessionals do not have designated time to attend team meetings or even talk with occupational therapists and other consulting team members except while assisting students in school lessons and activities. It is thus not surprising that paraprofessionals are often not on board with the team's vision or goals for the student with whom they work (Chopra & French, 2004). Resource 2.3 provides Internet resources on soliciting knowledge from paraprofessionals and including them in team interactions and activities.

Resource 2.3. Paraprofessional Internet Resources

- National Education Association's Summary of Needed Qualifications for Paraprofessionals: www.nea.org/esea/eseateach.html
- National Clearinghouse for Paraeducator Resources: www.usc.edu/dept/education/CMMR/Clearinghouse.html
- Paraeducator Resource and Learning Center: www.uvm.edu/~cdci/prlc/
- Supporting paraprofessionals working in the schools: http://ici.umn.edu/products/curricula.html
- Railsback, J., Reed, B., & Schmidt, K. (2002). *Working together for successful paraeducator services: A guide for paraeducators, teachers, and principals.* Northwest Regional Education Laboratory. Retrieved January 3, 2007, from www.nwrel.org/request/may2002/paraeds.pdf

Remember this . . .
Team members need to respect and show their appreciation for the daily work of paraprofessionals and collaboratively supervise, guide, and coach them to help meet the student goals.

Occupational therapists often depend on paraprofessionals to implement their suggestions for students in school places, spaces, and paces and should consider a teacher's classroom etiquette and preferences for engaging in hands-on services and team supports. Some teachers prefer to be informed about any suggestions or interventions by occupational therapists before they collaborate with the paraprofessional working in their classroom with a specific student; others prefer therapists to interact directly with the paraprofessional. Positioning, equipment set up, assistive technology, self-care, mobility, written or augmentative communication, job coaching, or behavior management are important areas in which collaboration is always necessary. When working with paraprofessionals, occupational therapists need to follow AOTA's (2004) *Guidelines for Supervision, Roles, and Responsibilities During the Delivery of Occupational Therapy Services.*

As required by NCLB, school districts need to reexamine how they hire and supervise paraprofessionals to meet the requirements of "highly qualified" personnel (ED, Office of Elementary and Secondary Education, 2002). Occupational therapists can collaborate with team members to find effective ways to learn from paraprofessionals and build on their strengths. Occupational therapists should consider how to

- Solicit the input of paraprofessionals in team discussions and informal contacts or meetings, especially about the impact of occupational therapy services and supports;
- Assist paraprofessionals to interact effectively with students (e.g., provide objective feedback and coaching to enhance their skills and promote self-determination); and
- Celebrate the positive student outcomes paraprofessionals have helped to achieve (Giangreco et al., 2001).

Therapists and all team members need to respect and show their appreciation for the daily work of paraprofessionals and collaboratively supervise, guide, and coach them to help meet the student goals. Table 2.1 provides specific examples of how occupational therapists can provide team and system supports to enhance the competency of paraprofessionals in their student-related tasks.

Part 2: Spaces and Places in School

Therapist Voices: Ecosystems change

Every school is its own ecosystem . . . as an OT, you have to understand what you are walking into each day and realize how it changes from place to place.

—Jan Emerick-Brothers, occupational therapist, Virginia

Students participate in a variety of environments, or *spaces* and *places,* during the school day, providing the best context for occupational therapists to observe students' actual school performance (Polichino, 2004; Polichino, Clark, & Chandler, 2005). Spaces and places include the classroom, bathroom, cafeteria, library, playground, bus, gymnasium, auditorium, hallways, or a community setting for a field trip or a job.

Table 2.1. Team Supports for Paraprofessionals

Support Category	Examples of Occupational Therapy Team and System Supports
1. Job description listing paraprofessional responsibilities, expectations, and supervision	• Contributes input to school committee that develops job descriptions (system supports). • Develops a checklist for setting up Intellikeys keyboard or other adaptive equipment (team supports). • Schedules a biweekly consult with a paraprofessional to review data collection forms, student progress, answer questions, and review the communication log between school and the family (team supports).
2. In-service education or coaching for the paraprofessional	• Collaborates with physical therapist on in-service training (e.g., transfers), body mechanics, using videos, and practice (system supports). • Observes paraprofessional, demonstrates and solicits self-reflection (e.g., using a slant board), organizing work space, slowing down to make letters a specific way (team supports). • Provides on-site coaching through demonstration and reflection to facilitate student self-determination or peer-to-peer friendships (hands-on and team supports).
3. Communication with the teachers, parents, students, or related service providers	• Asks paraprofessional to review data collection forms, student progress, and communication logs between school and the family and provide team with an update (team supports). • Uses e-mail for pressing questions or concerns (team supports).

Note. These examples for occupational therapists are based on some of the support recommendations of Giangreco, Edelman, and Broer (2001).

The arrangement of school environments affects student performance and social participation (Schenker, Coster, & Parush, 2005) and careful analysis of the interaction of the environment, the tasks required, and the student's ability to meet the demands of school occupations is essential (Muhlenhaupt, 2003; Rempfer, Hidenbrand, Parker, & Brown, 2003). Consider Margot, who is sitting on the classroom floor; is she meeting the demands of the environment? Yes, if she is 4 years old and in a preschool classroom during morning circle time and is able to sit, socially participate, and manipulate the materials being used. No, if Margot is 12 and in a physical education class and is sitting on the floor away from her peers when she is expected to run a relay with her teammates.

School environments contain explicit and implicit social and cultural expectations; team members need keen awareness of those expectations while working together. Expectations and the actual physical environment change from one teacher, class, grade level, or school to another, and therapists adjust the type of hands-on services and team supports accordingly. For example, a third-grade teacher who has a structured teaching style may prefer the occupational therapist to provide services at a specific time and place (e.g., provide hands-on services and team supports for tool usage on Tuesdays during art class or computer class but not during math class). A special education resource teacher who is less structured may willingly incorporate hands-on services and team supports to practice tool usage at any time or place (e.g., in the resource room, in the classroom, or during math class; Griswold, 1993). A student in middle school may request no hands-on/team supports from his or her therapist during class time but is willing to use team supports to participate in after-school activities.

In addition to analyzing student performance in school spaces and places within cultural, virtual, and temporal contexts, it is important to realize that political (e.g., laws, policies, regulations, initiatives, and agendas), attitudinal, and financial factors (e.g., funding sources, budgets, who controls the monies) can influence how places and spaces are used (Hemmingson & Borell, 2002; Pivik, McComas, & Laflamme, 2002). For example, if the school district's focus is on early literacy to improve standardized scores for school accreditation, monies may not be available for adaptive playground equipment or revamping computer stations according to ergonomic standards. In working with a Head Start program to craft an inclusive playground, Ideishi, Ideishi, Gandhi, and Yuen (2006) described the importance of matching person, task, and environment characteristics to design a meaningful space and learning about the political environment. Essential to collaboration was learning about the history of the program and its the mission and objectives; budget; typical activities, routines, and schedules; and perceived needs. A related services provider emphasized the importance of understanding the political environment as follows: "You have to know the politics because you won't survive here without knowing what to say, to whom and when and how to say it" (Mendoza-Smith, 2005, p. 175).

Observations in Natural Contexts

A student's daily routines and contexts provide the primary setting for all occupational therapy services and supports. (See Chapter 1's section "In-Context Services and Supports," which reviews the research and laws related to observing and providing services in natural contexts.)

Before observing a student in context, occupational therapists should request permission from a teacher and a student (as appropriate) to visit the classroom. Explaining the purpose of an observation to each student, in words matched to their age and communication level, is important. For example,

> *For a high school student with a neuromuscular disorder:* "Hillary, I'm going to visit chemistry today, so I can see what procedures the students use for the lab. While in the class, I will look for ideas to help you manipulate the test tubes and other materials but will wait till later, outside of class, to talk about any options that may be helpful for you and the class."

> *For an elementary school student with a developmental disability:* "Jon, I'll be in PE today to play some games with you and your class."

When occupational therapists routinely spend their time providing in-context services and supports, their classroom observations become much less obtrusive and may not require a special student explanation.

Setting up a time and place to visit should also be coordinated with key team members. Perhaps Franz, a kindergartner, has difficulty manipulating small fasteners, so his teacher suggests that the occupational therapist come before art class when Franz has to put on his smock or at the beginning or end of the day when he puts on or takes off his coat. Keep in mind that occupational therapists are invited guests in the classroom, even when they routinely provide collaborative supports and services, and must respect the teacher's places and spaces. The following professional behaviors convey the desire to make "helpful" school observations (Hanft & Place, 1996):

- Give nonjudgmental feedback even when there are some areas that are obviously in need of change (e.g., be careful not to show negative body language or facial expressions or make critical comments about the classroom environment or teacher's instructional methods during the observation period).

- Understand that each observation is just a snapshot of the student's day; what you see may be an atypical lesson or interaction.

- Use a structured or systematic observation (see examples in Chapter 4) to determine a student's ability to carry out roles, performance patterns, and routines; if possible, try to observe at different times or on different days to understand the student's typical performance and possible needs.

- Jot down initial impressions of a student's behavior, organization, routine, and patterns, and then ask other team members for corroboration of your observations ("Was Suzy's behavior and performance today what you typically see?").

- Try a variety of different observation formats to see what works for the team, and adapt structured observation formats accordingly.

- Consider using a time geographic diary to record where (place) the activity occurs, the time of day (pace), and any social interactions that occur (Kellegrew & Kroksmark, 1999).

Remember this . . .
Occupational therapists are invited guests in the classroom, even when they routinely provide collaborative supports and services, and must respect the teacher's places and spaces.

The following sections describe the physical and social environments within the cultural, virtual, and temporal contexts of school places and spaces. Although described separately, the characteristics of the environment are intertwined with each other and influence a student's participation in school. Asking a student, "How does the environment make it easier or harder for you to . . . ?" provides the student perspective to the team (Mihaylov, Jarvis, Colver, & Beresford, 2004). Structured observations also help occupational therapists assess the influence of the environment. Worksheet 2.2A in the Appendix provides key questions to guide an assessment of the characteristics of school places, spaces, and paces. Therapists may adapt this structured observation form according to their team's needs.

Physical Environment

Therapist Voices: Optimizing engagement

Inclusive participation requires adapting and matching the needs, interests, and abilities of the children and teachers with the environmental and activity qualities that optimize engagement. (Ideishi et al., 2006, p. 3)

The *Occupational Therapy Practice Framework: Domain and Process* (AOTA, 2002) describes the physical environment as including accessibility and availability of the building, objects, tools, and devices; space dimensions and traffic pathways; and sensory characteristics of the materials or environment. Classrooms are often set up with standard furniture, blackboards, computer workstations, and cubby or locker areas for personal belongings. Teachers will arrange these items in a variety of ways, typically following their own preferences for promoting social interaction, movement patterns, and learning. Where objects are placed determines whether the child has access to (i.e., can reach or get to) school tools and materials. How the space is arranged may affect a child's ability to perform school tasks in the environment and participate in social activities (Evertson, Emmer, & Worsham, 2003; Schenker et al., 2005). For instance, for a child in a wheelchair, a lack of defined and wide traffic pathways may limit access to other students, materials, different spaces in a classroom (e.g., reading corner, cubby), or places in the school (e.g., boy's bathroom). If the intent of a space is clearly marked with designated furniture or dividers, preschoolers may quickly learn where the reading, construction, or art centers are in the room. Teams can reconfigure space by moving or adding furniture, removing unneeded items, establishing "niches" for different classroom activities, or considering the temporal sequence of activities. The IRIS Center (see "Selected Resources" at the end of this chapter) provides teams with free, evidence-based, online, and interactive training modules, case studies, and handouts and activities to learn about other environmental considerations for students with disabilities.

The following scenario illustrates how an occupational therapist provided team supports to assist a teacher in adapting the physical environment for her students while considering the temporal context.

Therapist Voices: Finding flow in the environment

A teacher for a class of students with autism asked me to help her figure out how to improve the behavior of her students. Her main complaint was that they had difficulty with self-regulation and transitions and before half the day was over, they were emotionally and behaviorally unable to do anything else.

I observed the morning routine to get a feel for the classroom organization and structure. As I watched the class come in, I, too, became disorganized. The teacher had wonderful stations set up all over the room for hanging up coats, collecting lunch money, putting papers away, reading stories, completing centers, etc. As I watched, the students wandered from one end of the room to the other, then back again, to where they began, then to another corner of the room. The "flow" of the physical boundaries and set up of activities was nonexistent. No wonder the kids were losing it.

As I discussed my observations with the teacher, she was willing to try a different arrangement of the same centers and stations. Together, we organized the physical space according to the temporal context of when activities happened during the day. The children learned that their activities went clockwise around the room, and this gave them the structure they needed to ease transitions. The calm, predictable flow also seemed to help keep arousal levels on a more even keel.

—Judith Schoonover, occupational therapist and
assistive technology specialist, Virginia

Universal Design for Environments and for Learning

Therapists should also consider the framework of *universal design (UD)* for promoting accessibility of environments, products, or classroom materials (Schoonover, Levan, & Argabrite Grove, 2006). *Accessibility* refers to the widest range of students, regardless of their abilities, using school tools, materials, and environments in school activities without adaptations or specialized designs (Goodrich, 2004; Rose & Meyer, 2002,

2006). If teams use UD principles (Connell et al., 1997) when considering materials, equipment, or structural designs (e.g., a new playground, an addition to school, the remodeling of the locker room or life skills room), more students will be included to participate in a variety of school places and spaces. Examples of applying UD to school environments are provided in Table 2.2.

Universal design for learning (UDL) is a teaching–learning theory suggesting that people have many ways of engaging in learning. UDL provides learners with multiple and flexible means of representation (e.g., presentation media), expression of knowledge, and engagement in learning (Goodrich, 2004; Rose & Meyer, 2006). The principles of UDL are illustrated in Table 2.3. While observing or bringing materials and equipment to classroom teachers, therapists should consider how UD or UDL is supported (Schoonover et al., 2006). This is a critical area in which occupational therapists can provide team and system supports, particularly when schools are considering purchasing playground equipment, computer furniture, computers, or curriculum materials; building new environments; or modifying current space. Reflection 2.5

Reflection 2.5

Using Universal Design for Least Restrictive Environment

In the scenario on p. 54, how did Judith use the principles of universal design and select in-context strategies to assist the teacher in creating the least restrictive environment for a specific student with disabilities that benefited all children in the classroom? (see Figure 1.2 in Chapter 1).

Table 2.2. Principles of Universal Design Related to Schools

Principle of Universal Design	Example of School Setting
1. Equitable in use	• Accessibility of the building, classrooms within the building, buildings within the campus, and the playground • Adaptable seating in auditorium or cafeteria so students with wheelchair can participate • Elevated plant beds for children in wheelchairs or who cannot squat down
2. Flexibility in use	• Materials or equipment used by people with a large range of abilities and preferences, such as scissors or paper punch usable by either right- or left-handed users • Elevator has visual, tactile, and auditory feedback when buttons are pushed
3. Simple and intuitive design	• Bathrooms identified with words and universal symbols for girls' and boys' bathrooms (understandable by all) • Arrows and lanes marked on playground for a running or bike lane to delineate traffic patterns • Equipment controls (e.g., TV, computer, lab) clearly marked with words and symbols
4. Perceptible information	• Materials available in alternative formats (e.g., closed-caption TVs, computer accessibility options, videos with closed captions) • Morning announcements are announced (auditory) and projected on television screen (visual) simultaneously
5. Tolerance for error	• Learning games or computer programs that allow "undo" without penalty or with hints for success • Unbreakable lab equipment
6. Low physical effort	• Power-assist doors; easy-to-open doors; or faucets in bathroom with lever or loop handles • Touch switches or lamps for task lighting • Microscope is connected to computer display screens
7. Size and space for approach and use	• Hallways, playgrounds, and classrooms have enough space for multiple users with equipment • Students have a clear line of sight to the teacher and material being displayed

From Bremer, C. D., Clapper, A. T., Hitchcock, C., Hall, T., & Kachgal, M. (2002). Universal design for learning: A strategy to support students' access to the general education curriculum. *Information Brief, 1*(3). Retrieved February 15, 2007, from www.ncset.org/publications/viewdesc.asp?id=707. Copyright © 2002 by National Center on Secondary Education and Transition Institute on Community Integration. Adapted with permission.

Table 2.3. Universal Design for Learning (Rose & Meyer, 2002)

Universal Design for Learning: All students can benefit from a flexible curriculum so it can be digitally changed to meet learner needs (from audio to visual, from visual to audio, to be accessed through voice, or specialized hardware such as keyboards or switches or other technology).

Principle	Example
1. Multiple and flexible represen-tation of knowledge and infor-mation (presentation)	A math lesson about fractions may use manipulatives, a chart, or other graphic representation, such as a computer assignment with digital capabilities to be manipulated, enlarged, or presented orally.
2. Multiple and flexible means of expression to demonstrate knowledge	A math lesson about fractions may have students express their knowledge by completing worksheets (e.g., write a number, circle the correct answer, put a mark above the right answer, work with a peer buddy), color in a chart or diagram, use manipulatives, express answers using a computer exercise or activity, or give oral answers.
3. Multiple means of engage-ment for affective learning (using interests and motiva-tion and providing challenges)	Fractions may be taught using the student's favorite food and dividing the pieces among classmates; relate fractions according to interests (e.g., student genetic characteristics, class likes and dislikes, money); discuss throughout the curriculum, not just during math.

challenges therapists to think how to incorporate universal design into classroom in-terventions. The IRIS Center (see "Selected Resources" at the end of this chapter) pro-vides free online and interactive training modules, case studies, and handouts and activities that teams can use to arrange the physical and social environments for stu-dents with disabilities.

Sensory Features of Physical Spaces

The tactile, kinesthetic, auditory, visual, proprioceptive, or temperature characteristics of the spaces and places may affect learning. Overly stimulating visuals on the bulletin board, fluorescent lights, noise from a nearby peer typing on a computer, or a cold room may distract the attention of a student with sensory over-responsiveness or attention-deficit/hyperactivity disorder. The texture of a rug sat on for circle time may irritate a student and may need to be removed or covered with a towel. Occupational therapists can assist team members in reviewing all classroom materials and school environments for their sensory features as well as for UD or UDL. For example,

> *Collaboration in Action: Considering sensory characteristics*
>
> Tyrone, an occupational therapist, chose puzzles for a preschool classroom that incorporated UDL. The puzzles had large knobs, a bumpy surface, and lit up and made sounds when put into the correct hole. All students, including Joshua, who has cerebral palsy, and Yuri, who is deaf–blind, could use the puz-zles with their peers. However, Tyrone observed that this puzzle was too stim-ulating for Ashley, who cried at new noises in the class, so he turned off the sound feature on the puzzle when she participated in the activity. While in the classroom, the teacher and Tyrone shared their observations about the student's responses to the sensory aspects of the environment.

Careful analysis and selection of the sensory features of environments, materials, and information help therapists provide team supports by sharing their insight and suggestions with team members. Some suggestions are as follows:

- Modifying the sensory characteristics of the environment or objects being used (e.g., using a weighted pen, using a sticker to amplify the enter key on the keyboard, placing elastic bands on the bottom of a chair, or organizing a desk)

- Changing the demands of the school activity (e.g., presenting less information on a worksheet, using plastic gloves to finger paint, using a stamp for writing the date on a paper)

- Implementing a self-regulation program (e.g., Alert Program; Williams & Shellenberger, 1996)

- Writing a Sensory Story (e.g., giving students a visual and auditory aid to prepare for different sensations in their daily school routine; Marr, Mika, Miraglia, Roerig, & Sinnott, 2007; Marr & Nackley, 2007).

> **Resource 2.4. Universal Design for Learning and Virtual Environment Resources**
> - Alliance for Technology Access: www.ataccess.org/
> - The Access Center: Improving Outcomes for All Students K–8: accesscenter@air.org
> - Center for Implementing Technology in Education: www.cited.org/
> - Loudoun County Public Schools Assistive Technology—Review one school system's comprehensive resources for academics, ergonomics, and communication as well as "Tips 'N Tricks" videos: http://cmsweb1.loudoun.k12.va.us/50910068152053/site/default.asp
> - National Education Technology Plan: www.ed.gov/about/offices/list/os/technology/plan/2004/site/edlite-default.html
> - National Instructional Materials Accessibility Standard (NIMAS) Resources: http://nimas.cast.org/about/resources/index.html
> - Universal Design for Learning: www.cast.org/research/udl/index.html

Resources for learning more about UD and UDL, as well as information on other technology, are provided in Resource 2.4.

Cultural Context

Administrator Voices: All for student success

I like to promote the culture that all the children, in or out of special education, belong to all of us at school . . . together as a team, we can become better educators for student success.

—Ilene Banker, assistant principal, Virginia

When entering a school, the climate and culture of a school is immediately evident. *School climate* refers to the effect of the learning atmosphere or expectations on students, and *school culture* relates more to the attitude or acceptance of diversity and relationships among students, families, and staff (McBrien & Brandt, 1997). The school climate may be welcoming or nurturing, or it may feel authoritarian or somewhere in between. Culture includes customs, beliefs, values, ethnicity, teaching practices, and behavior standards of personnel within a particular school, as described in "Faces: Cultural Considerations" in this chapter.

Classroom Culture

Within a school, every teacher has his or her own culture regarding teaching practices and behavior standards. Because occupational therapists typically provide services and supports within many classrooms and schools, understanding the cultural expectations of each school or classroom and respecting diversity are extremely important. Mendoza-Smith (2005) conducted a 10-month qualitative case study of Sara, a school-based occupational therapist and identified school culture as a theme heard from multiple team members: "I must learn the rules that govern behavior" (p. 175). Additional results from Mendoza-Smith's dissertation are identified in Exhibit 2.1.

Exhibit 2.1. Becoming Part of the School Community

In *The Socialization of a Professional Stranger: The Work of an Occupational Therapist in a Public School,* Mendoza-Smith (2005) described the experiences of one occupational therapist in an elementary school over the course of 10 months as she sustained and managed relationships with parents, administrators, and peers. Key ingredients for becoming an integral part of a school community include

- Communication and interpersonal skills that develop and nurture effective relationships within a school community, especially with classroom teachers and school administrators, and
- Patience, diplomacy, and perseverance.

Building interdependent professional relationships in the school is one of the most complex and challenging aspects of practice in educational settings and is in need of greater attention from occupational therapy practitioners, researchers, and educators.

—Maria Mendoza-Smith, occupational therapist,
personal communication, June 27, 2007

Hanft and Place (1996) suggested that therapists find out what classroom etiquette is expected of students and visitors when observing and working in a specific place in a school. It may be fine to sit down and talk to children during lunch, but such behavior would be considered blatantly disruptive in some classrooms, even during free time. Are there posted rules or schedules or certain procedures that the teacher expects of all the children (e.g., how to address adults or interact with each other or visitors)? Brief questions concerning the timing of an observation and interaction and that convey a desire to fit into a teacher's environment while observing students and working with them include

- "When is the best time to see Carly during a group activity (or at home)?"
- "Are there certain days or times that are better than others to see how Carly...?"
- "What's the best way for us to communicate?"
- "Are there certain days or times that are better for us to meet or talk on the phone?"
- "When do other therapists work with Carly?"
- "How do students in your class address visiting adults?" (e.g., Mrs. Shepherd, Jayne, Miss Barbara, Mrs. H); and
- "If other students ask for help while I'm here, how would you like me to respond?"

Besides teacher timing and communication preferences, therapists need to ask what types of activities are acceptable to the teacher during an observation. Questions concerning a choice of activities or communication methods and that convey interest in following a teacher's classroom culture during the observation include

- "Is it all right with you if I take notes while I'm observing? Will it bother the children?"
- "Where would you like me to sit during an observation? Where would you like me to set up our joint activity?"
- "When I'm in your class to work with Joan, what can I do to help you carry out your planned activities and lessons?"

- "Is there a particular piece of equipment or classroom materials you would rather I not use while working with you?"

- "I'm thinking about using shaving cream or pudding for the activity today; is that okay with you?"

- "How would you like me to handle misbehavior while I'm in the classroom?"

- "I'm unfamiliar with Onan's language; can you tell me a little about what you've learned about his culture?" and

- "When would you like me to give suggestions to Myra (the paraprofessional)?"

Social Environment

Social environments are influenced by the cultural expectations evident in the classroom as students interact with peers and adults and attempt to follow routines while fulfilling their student roles. The number of students and teaching personnel in the classroom and their personal characteristics (e.g., whether they are verbal, aggressive, friendly, competitive, or anxious) may influence the type of social interactions within the classroom (Ellison, Boykin, Towns, & Stokes, 2000). Teachers often talk about the personality of a class that affects the activities and interactions students engage in. For example, a class of students with four or five leaders vying for attention or power can dramatically affect how students interact. Social participation may be influenced by

- The organization of space and time;

- The amount of supervision or assistance the student receives from others;

- Attitudes or behaviors of others toward the student (stigma);

- Bullying from peers; and

- The supports (e.g., peer to peer, assistive technology for communication) available to the student (Hemmingson & Borell, 2002; Mihaylov et al., 2004; Pivik et al., 2002; Simeonsson, Carlson, Huntington, McMillen, & Brent, 2001).

Considerations for selecting hands-on services and team supports to promote social interactions and to educate students in the least restrictive environment (IDEA 2004) are as follows:

- Does the teacher encourage social interaction between students, and are opportunities and time built into the day to encourage reciprocal interactions between children (Richardson, 2002)?

- What are the expected social norms or routines within a class?

- What are the proportions of students with and without disabilities, and how does this influence the social norms and routines?

- What are the attitudes of peers, teachers, and administrators toward the student with a disability?

- What is the person–environment–occupation fit for particular students (Muhlenhaupt, 2003)? Are these students reinforced and given positive feedback for their effort to participate? How do they respond to adults and peers in the environment?

By examining the expected social norms and the students' relationships with peers and adults, therapists assist classroom teachers to assess what in the social environment is supporting, limiting, or neutral in promoting student participation and interaction (Muhlenhaupt, 2003; Richardson, 2002). Specific suggestions for improving social interaction in the least restrictive environment by adapting materials, equipment, and the environment include

- Moving a table, seat, or desk;
- Assigning a peer buddy;
- Giving choices;
- Suggesting changes in a schedule;
- Modeling ways to decrease assistance;
- Educating peers and the team about the student's disability;
- Promoting sharing of interests, ideas, and materials; and
- Providing positive reinforcement and changing the demands of the environment (e.g., all students greet each other in the morning; Muhlenhaupt, 2003).

Worksheet 2.3A in the Appendix and Figure 1.3 in Chapter 1 also illustrate ways to consider whether students are included in the least restrictive environment.

Virtual Context

With the benefits of technology, highly trained teachers, a motivated student body and the requirements of *No Child Left Behind,* the next 10 years could see a spectacular rise in achievement—and may usher in a new golden age for American education. (ED, 2004, p. 46)

Virtual environments—that is, using information technology and communication networks—are becoming more prominent in today's schools. Team members must keep abreast of what is available and learn how to use and apply technology principles to help students succeed as well as to communicate with each other (ED, 2004). Federal and state initiatives provide funds to place computers with Internet access in every classroom and encourage schools to investigate virtual learning environments and administrative paperwork alternatives (ED, 2005). Students frequently own (or may use loaned) laptops, hand-held devices, cell phones, and other electronic memory or communication devices that connect to the airways. Many school tasks are now accomplished in the virtual environment:

- Take notes on a portable word processor and send the notes to the computer through an infrared signal
- Read books in an electronic format
- Research and complete written assignments over time
- Submit, revise, and share assignments with peers and teachers

- Participate in online discussion boards

- Communicate with teachers and peers via e-mail

- Complete assessments, assignments, or entire courses online.

In addition, students may use one access device (e.g., infrared switch, joystick) to control their assistive technology. For example, the integrated joystick may control a student's computer, power wheelchair, augmentative communication device, and electronic aids for daily living (EADL; e.g., controls the lights; turns on a classroom TV, computer, or kitchen appliance during life skills; answers phones at work). Understanding how students interface with the virtual environments at school and home helps occupational therapists provide team supports. Refer again to the excerpt of an assistive technology evaluation in Exhibit 1.2A in the Appendix and Figure 1.3 in Chapter 1.

Many classrooms are also equipped with whiteboards connected to computers (instead of blackboards) and computer projection systems to support virtual assignments and lessons. How often are these devices used in various classrooms? Consider how a student or teacher is positioned while using them; how the devices facilitate students' homework, writing production, and socialization; and help students to organize and follow the routines of the day. A parent of a 16-year-old adolescent describes how using a personal digital assistant (PDA) has improved her son's performance at school and work:

Family Voices: Incorporating outside resources

OT has been of great benefit to Noah's life during high school. Through a grant program at a state University, Noah's natural ability in using a Palm device was revealed by a community-based OT. Although Noah has Asperger's, he has grown by leaps and bounds with the Palm to remember tasks, download a good book, and keep himself on schedule.

When the school system was skeptical about using the Palm, the community OT wrote a compelling letter to the school administration, describing the benefits of this assistive technology for Noah and the current research with PDAs and students with autism. Luckily, the school team was willing to hear the opinion and advice from an "outsider," and Noah now uses his Palm at school every day. In fact, Noah is using his Palm at his summer job with a videographer. He is the go-fer and is being trained to do computer editing with software unique to the business. He is taking notes on the Palm about the dos and don'ts on his new job.

—Donna Cannon, parent of Noah, Virginia

Part 3: Paces: Temporal Context in School

Teacher Voices: Fit within the routine

Educational settings are very different from a lot of other places; recommendations need to fit into the routine, there needs to be order, because teachers are dealing with lots of children at one time.

—Linda, teacher (as quoted in Mendoza-Smith, 2005, p. 91)

School personnel, students, and families *pace* their interactions with each other to meet their common goals and expectations. This temporal context for collaboration includes the timing, duration, organization, and sequencing of student instruction and routines to ensure that they are age appropriate and acceptable within a school's cultural and social environments. Personal preferences for different environments also may influence student participation in educational and social activities (Eriksson, 2005). Interviews with students, family members, and school personnel and observation of students within school places and spaces often shed light on expected and preferred paces and routines and how a student meets these expectations. Temporal expectations are often externally controlled within the home and school environment, but students also have personal, internal expectations for how fast they should learn a subject or how long an activity should last. In home and school environments, timelines for homework, projects, and school activities are often set by parents or teachers. As students learn how to meet school demands, study habits are practiced and routines become established that affect student learning (Segal & Hinojosa, 2006). Students may incorporate those habits into their own routine and impose their own deadlines on homework or how much time they will spend on school lessons and activities.

The temporal context (e.g., personal biorhythms; time of day, month, or year; pace, duration, or sequence of an activity) should always be considered to embed instruction within the places and spaces where students or teams work together (Odom, Boyd, & Buysse, 2007). When entering a classroom, therapists need to be aware of the time of day and whether it is a convenient time to observe or work with the teacher and student. In the following scenario, the time of day the therapist observed the student was essential to addressing the teacher's concerns and suggesting effective interaction.

Collaboration in Action: Timing is key

In April of one school year, Renata, a teacher, asked me to help her figure out why Jacob, a student with sensory defensiveness, was suddenly so irritable and inattentive after having settled down so well through the winter. We had selected a spot at the back of the room for Jacob's desk because he liked to see all the comings and going of his classmates. However, we did not factor in warm weather in the spring, lunch recess, and his desk's proximity to the water fountain. After lunch, the kids made a beeline for the fountain, and I watched girls with long hair bending over to drink, flipping their hair right across the back of his neck. The timing of my observation was the key to figuring out what was going on. This situation only occurred in the afternoon, so if I had observed him in the morning, I still would have been clueless about what was triggering Jacob's discomfort and off-target behavior.

—Barbara Hanft, occupational therapy consultant, Maryland

Similar or overlapping schedules of team members and the physical location of classrooms and staff and therapy work spaces can also facilitate or impede collaboration. It often takes time and creativity to learn a teacher's schedule, his or her time preferences for collaboration, and how classroom instruction is paced. Chapter 4 gives examples of how to work within classroom routines.

Therapist Voices: Ask when to come

Recently I have really been trying to understand the rules (paces) of each class-room and the teacher's preferences for my interaction within her class. Being in and out of so many classrooms, sometimes it is difficult to remember which teacher prefers what. I developed a therapist–teacher communication weekly log to understand how each classroom works [see Figure 2.4].

—Sara Cassone, occupational therapy student,
University of Southern California

How Routines and Habits Support Temporal Demands of School Activities and Lessons

Successful interventions are ones that can be woven back into the daily rou-tine; they are the threads that provide professionals with the means to rein-force, rather than fray, the fabric of everyday life. (Bernheimer & Keogh, 1995, p. 430)

During observations and intervention, the primary question related to student progress and achievement is, Are expected performance patterns completed in a timely manner using appropriate routines and habits? When beginning school, tem-poral organization is mostly structured by the teacher, who determines the schedules and routines; later, the student makes the routine his or her own and expects certain

Occupational Therapy–Teacher Communication Weekly Log
Teacher: ___Mrs. Cassiopia___
Student Name: ___Shaniiqua and Jermiah___
Week of _____

School-based occupational therapy at its best is working in the classroom, which is often the least restrictive environment for students. By coordinating with teachers, I am trying to collaborate as much as possible to keep up with the curriculum standards. ☺

It would be great if you would please fill in the topic/theme/activity that is planned during the highlighted time when I will be in your class-room. Please return this form to the OT mailbox in the teacher's lounge at least one day prior to the scheduled OT time.

Please be as specific or as general as you'd like; I really appreciate your help! Thank you.

Sara Cassone, OTS

Mondays (date)		Thursdays (date)	
8–8:30		8–8:30	
8:30–9		8:30–9	
9–9:30	Social Studies: Jamestown	9–9:30	
9:30–10	Recess on playground	9:30–10	
10–10:30		10–10:30	
10:30–11		10:30–11	
11–11:30		11–11:30	
11:30–12		11:30–12	Resource: Music
12–12:30		12–12:30	Lunch

Figure 2.4. Sample occupational therapy–teacher communication weekly log.

Note. Adapted with permission from Sara Cassone, occupational therapy student, University of Southern California.

events to occur (e.g., snack, circle time, art class; McNamara & Humphry, 2007). The following sections suggest observations to make with team members to understand the temporal influences on student performance.

Age-Appropriate Expectations for Routines

Routines and expectations for students change as they mature and progress to higher grade levels in school. As children negotiate more complex physical and social environments, they develop occupational patterns (Pierce, 2003). As observers, occupational therapists ask the following questions:

- *What are the routines and expectations in this class?* Is this an age-appropriate routine or expectation? For example, in a fifth-grade class, students are expected to clean up after themselves in a timely manner, manage their own lunch money, or go to the office for their medications without teacher reminders. If observing a class for students with significant disabilities in high school, are student routines embedded in the daily schedule while using age-appropriate materials and habits (e.g., using a fidget toy instead of a stuffed animal to self-calm during an assembly)?

- *How are class, student, and teacher routines initiated and stopped?* Review how the class typically begins and ends a specific lesson or period. Are there implicit or explicit markers for students? Do they understand and follow the routines? For example, preschool teachers use a special song or music chord to signal start and stop signs; bells ring in middle and high school; and physical education teachers use whistles to signal "stop." For individual students, therapists may suggest using auditory or visual timers such as a kitchen timer, an hour glass, digital watches, a timer on a handheld organizer, or a timer that shows elapsed time as well as time remaining (e.g., a Time Timer [Time Timer, LLC, Cincinnati, OH]) or a visual schedule board with removable pieces.

- *Do routines change, and if so, how often?* Some children thrive on consistent routines and do not transition well if there are numerous changes to a schedule or limited time to adapt to new expectations. Others may become bored with the same routine every day or challenged by higher expectations for performance patterns. For example, is there enough time to accommodate to the change in expected performance patterns? Are team members given an explanation for this change?

In the following vignette, Jessica engages in an age-appropriate and meaningful activity within typical spaces and places in her high school.

Family Voices: Open minds

Jessica struggled with learning to tie her shoes through elementary and junior high school. It always was an annual OT goal for her to learn to tie her shoes. When she was in high school, a classmate attending her IEP meeting suggested she join SADD [Students Against Drunk Driving], where the other kids could help her tie ribbons around car door handles and antennas. Jessica's OT not only was open to trying something new but was enthusiastic.

With her support and direction, the plan was put into operation for Jessica and her friends. Jessica was tying her own shoes by the end of the football season. The open minds on Jessica's team solved a vexing problem. Jessica's OT was at the center of that resolution.

—Tricia and Calvin Luker, parents of Jessica, Michigan

Sequencing and Timing of Classroom Instruction and School Activities

Individuals have preferences for timing and organizing activities and following routines. When team member preferences oppose one another, conflict may occur. Consider a parent who wants his son to complete his paper 3 days in advance to reduce stress at home or a child who dawdles in the bathroom before the school bus arrives. In school, a student who needs time to process directions will experience problems if the teacher's time is on fast mode (e.g., he or she talks fast, moves fast, and expects students to pick up the pace so they can get more things done). Recognizing the difference in pacing routines and interactions is essential for all parties involved and may take some team problem solving to work out the differences (see Chapter 6).

Keeping up with the pace often relates to student characteristics (body functions, body structures, or personal preferences) and the type of school demands. Further analysis of the social and physical environment and the cultural expectations of family, peers, and teachers may reveal that a student moves too quickly or slowly to either avoid or prolong an activity (Griswold, 1993; Kellegrew & Allen, 1996; Richardson, 2002). The following questions help determine whether the student can meet the pace and demands of school faces, places, and spaces:

- *Is there a class schedule, and is it structured or unstructured?* Is it posted on the walls, and do students know what to expect from day to day? How does this schedule influence a student's participation and performance?

- *Is the schedule followed?* How flexible is the teacher with changes in the schedule? Some teachers are always on time and expect their classroom routine to be followed to the letter, and others change the schedule frequently. A teacher's interaction style and temporal values and expectations must match a student's need for organizational structure.

- *Are there a variety of activities and lessons with quiet and active times available?* Do students have opportunities to move throughout the day and change positions, or are classroom routines fairly sedentary?

- *What is the duration of each activity and lesson?* How long are the students expected to attend without a break? Some students never want certain activities to end (e.g., playground time or lunch). For others, meeting any temporal demand to maintain engagement, even in an enjoyable activity, is difficult. In the following vignette, the therapist provided team supports by helping a classroom assistant reframe her interpretation of a student's behavior.

Remember this . . .
The main question to answer is, Does the student meet expected performance patterns in a timely manner using appropriate routines and habits?

Therapist Voices: Time choices

One of the most influential suggestions I made for Johanna, a first grader with hemiplegia, was to time (with a stop watch held in my pocket) how long she sat in a chair and attended to the activity at hand before jumping up. The classroom assistant interpreted this behavior as disruptive, whereas I observed fatigue and a desire for sensation from assuming a new position. In all situations, Johanna could tolerate about 10 minutes sitting before needing to change her position. I shared this information with the teacher and assistant and suggested they keep track of time and after 9 minutes, give her a choice to stand up or finish her reading in a bean bag chair. Now her same behavior was viewed as appropriate, and she was no longer considered a distractible child.

—Barbara Hanft, occupational therapy consultant, Maryland

How Routines and Habits Influence Student Performance

Teacher routines and habits and the school culture may support or hinder a student's success with participating in daily school activities. By understanding the preferences of the team, occupational therapists provide suggestions to embed instructional or environmental adaptations within the day-to-day routines. Therapists might ask the following questions:

- *How are academic subjects scheduled and reviewed?* Consider what time of day they occur, how they are introduced, and how materials are managed during these times. For example, is there a place and a specific time when students turn in homework, have homework checked, bring materials to group, or have a weekly spelling test? Are students aware of these time factors, and have they developed the habits or been provided with supports to follow these expectations? Occupational therapists may recommend a peer buddy, a memory aid, visual supports, or a change in the physical environment to make expectations explicit and to cue students. Carrying a divided pocket folder or having pocket dividers in notebooks may also assist the student's temporal organization for homework assignments.

- *Do the external temporal expectations match a student's biorhythms* (Pierce, 2003)? Although this is difficult to do for all students, it is an area to consider if a student is having a difficult time in a subject. For example, if Nathan has difficulty in Spanish, is he more alert in first period at 7:25 a.m. or at a later period of the day? If his school uses a block schedule, is Spanish a class that meets every day or every other day? Will daily repetition help Nathan retain his learning? If schedules are inflexible, an occupational therapist might help Nathan enhance his state of alertness by suggesting a routine for the early morning class. Suggestions could include sitting in front of the class near the window, so that the bright light will be alerting; using a nondistracting fidget toy, such as a pencil or a malleable art eraser; using a special gel pen; or modifying the morning routine so he lifts weights or gets other physical exercise prior to school.

- *What is the timing for self-care tasks?* Are routines established (with enough time) for a student to go to the bathroom, pick up food in the cafeteria line, find his or her coat and put it on in time to make the bus, or go to the office for medication? If time is problematic, do adult expectations or a student's abilities (e.g., client factors), such as motor skills (strength, endurance, paces) or process skills (temporal organization, paces) limit performance? Does a student use automatic routines and habits to become more efficient using those skills in school contexts? Suggestions for a student who is not keeping up with the pace might include giving additional time, changing the time or sequence of routines (e.g., going to the bathroom first, then having a snack; completing two assignments before center time), developing a visual sequence and checklist to be used at school and home, using mnemonics to remember the sequence, or grading the activity difficulty and amount of time allowed.

- *What is the pacing and routine for going to and from classes or different areas of the school?* Can Libby manage the hallways in a timely fashion with her walker, or does she need to be released early to give her enough time to get to her next class? Are visual or verbal cues given for transitions? Suggestions might include using a Time Timer or another visual cue to signal transitions, planning an alternative route to the next class, working with the guidance counselor to schedule classes near each other, considering alternative means of transportation or adaptive equipment, or enlisting a peer buddy to leave with her.

Therapist Voices: Routines

By assisting the child initially in their classroom routines, I become aware of the process and environment in which they are really trying to *perform.*

—Linn Wakeford, occupational therapist,
North Carolina (Wakeford, 2003, p. 3)

When observing student routines within the natural environment, occupational therapists must consider the implicit meaning of behavior as well as the observable aspects of the school environment.

Systematic Analysis for Teams and Students

Team Meeting Environments

Consider all aspects of the environments discussed above and think about where team members interact to conduct team business. They may meet formally or informally in a set place each week; on the fly in the hallway, the bathroom, the teacher's lounge, the office, or the copy room; or during school events (Snell & Janney, 2005). Recognizing the physical, social, cultural, virtual, and temporal aspects of meeting environments is essential for effective communication. Knowing how and when to interact in school environments promotes collaboration among therapists and other team members. For example, a staff lounge where teachers and staff move in and out may be a great place to share a student's success story but is probably not conducive to resolving a conflict. A teacher's break or teaching session is not an acceptable time to begin a negotiation. Chapter 3 provides additional information about team structure, and Chapter 4 gives examples of how to consider the school context to plan collaborative intervention.

Tying Faces, Spaces, and Paces Together for Student Success

Think about a student on your team, and complete the Faces, Spaces, and Paces Worksheet (Worksheet 2.4A in the Appendix). Consider the educational needs of this student, based on the information collected, and consider what hands-on services and team and system supports you could bring up for discussion with other team members to help this student succeed in school.

Analyzing the Faces, Spaces, and Paces in School Environments

Collecting information on the faces, spaces, and the paces of the team interaction in school requires a systematic analysis. Worksheet 2.4A in the Appendix provides a format for occupational therapists to record their observations and make suggestions for team and system supports. Specific examples of how to use the worksheet are presented in Leo's vignette in Chapter 4 and Susannah's vignette in Chapter 5. Refer to Reflection 2.6 and use Worksheet 2.4A to assess the faces, spaces, and paces of a team.

Summary

Collaboration embraces a student and family as the heart of a team, which functions within the context of typical routines in school places and spaces. As team members work together, they learn to appreciate all the faces on the team by sharing information about previous experiences, knowledge, cultural expectations and concerns, and student goals. Assessing and understanding the context, or the places and spaces where the faces on the team work together, are essential to providing educationally relevant services and supports. By observing physical, cultural, social, and virtual environments within the natural context of instructional lessons and school activities, therapists assess how the environments affect the pacing of team interactions and student performance. Appropriate services and supports can then be selected by the team to facilitate a student's learning and participation in typical school lessons and activities.

> *Paraprofessional Voices: Everyone is equal*
>
> In our school, everyone is valued, from the custodian to the principal. Everyone is considered the same. If there is something going on, everyone is informed. I don't think anyone feels inferior at all. That's just the way our principal runs our school.
>
> —Paraprofessional (as quoted in Chopra et al., 2004, p. 227).

Acknowledgments

This chapter was produced in collaboration with Betty Thompson, Dana and John Yarbrough, Tricia Luker, Calvin Luker, Jan Emerick-Brothers, Ilene Banker, Sara Cassone, Darcie Votipka, Inbal Fraiman, Judie Sage, Jean Polichino, Jo Read, and Judith Schoonover. Thanks for providing the faces to help others understand the places and spaces where we work.

Selected Resources

Barrera, I., Corso, R., & Macpherson, D. (2003). *Skilled dialogue: Strategies for responding to cultural diversity in early childhood.* Baltimore: Paul H. Brookes.
   The authors discuss culture and cultural diversity and present specific strategies for learning how to understand another's culture. This book is based on a field-tested research model and discusses the concept and process of developing a "skilled dialogue" to help team members understand their students and families. A reproducible critical incident analysis worksheet is provided.

Dettmer, P., Thurston, L. P., & Sellberg, N. J. (2005). *Consultation, collaboration, and teamwork for students with special needs* (5th ed.). Needham Heights, MA: Allyn & Bacon.

Written for educators, this book addresses collaboration and teamwork issues that are critical to all team members. Successful techniques for collaboration, such as team communication, problem solving, and the day-to-day routine of collaboration, are discussed in detail. Related services are discussed in Chapter 11, which provides helpful examples of how to be partners in inclusion.

Hanft, B., & Place, P. (1996). *The consulting therapist: A guide for occupational and physical therapists in schools*. Austin, TX: Pro-Ed.

This book was written by a therapist–educator team to help physical and occupational therapists learn the art of consultation in a school setting. Nine chapters, with reproducible forms, focus on assessing the consultation situation (student performance, human resources, and the context), developing a consultation plan with team members, a six-step decision model for choosing consultation, stages of the consultation process with typical conflict situations encountered and strategies for resolving them, and the interpersonal skills needed for effective consultation.

Swinth, Y. (Ed.). (2004). *Occupational therapy in school-based practice: Contemporary issues and trends* [AOTA Online Course]. Bethesda, MD: American Occupational Therapy Association.

This online self-study course provides a variety of ideas and resources to help therapists collaborate with the team members in the many contexts of the school setting. Lesson topics related to school-based practice include policies and educational philosophies, overview of the framework, clinical reasoning, evaluation of occupational performance, differences between education and occupational intervention plans, effectiveness and efficiency in intervention, reviewing intervention, evidence-based practice, developing and maintaining competencies, and applying knowledge in school-based case studies. Ten additional supplementary lessons are available.

Vanderbilt University, IRIS Center, http://iris.peabody.vanderbilt.edu

This national center provides free online and interactive training modules, case studies, and handouts and activities about students with disabilities. Modules related to this chapter include accommodations, classroom design, collaboration, and diversity. The resources are evidence-based practice and are developed for trainers in professional development or college and university faculty. Each of the STAR legacy modules has five components: challenge, initial thoughts, perspectives and resources, assessment, and wrap up.

References

American Occupational Therapy Association. (2002). Occupational therapy practice framework: Domain and process. *American Journal of Occupational Therapy, 56,* 609–639.

American Occupational Therapy Association. (2004). *Guidelines for supervision, roles, and responsibilities during the delivery of occupational therapy services*. Bethesda, MD: American Occupational Therapy Association. Retrieved September 4, 2006, from www.aota.org/Practitioners/Resources/Docs/Popular/36202.aspx

Barrera, I., Corso, R., & Macpherson, D. (2003). *Skilled dialogue: Strategies for responding to cultural diversity in early childhood*. Baltimore: Paul H. Brookes.

Bernheimer, L. P., & Keogh, B. K. (1995). Weaving intervention into the fabric of everyday life: An approach to family assessment. *Topics in Early Childhood Special Education, 15,* 415–433.

Bremer, C. D., Clapper, A. T., Hitchcock, C., Hall, T., & Kachgal, M. (2002). Universal design for learning: A strategy to support students' access to the general education curriculum. *Information Brief, 1*(3). Retrieved February 15, 2007, from www.ncset.org/publications/viewdesc.asp?id=707

Broer, S. M., Doyle, M. B., & Giangreco, M. F. (2005). Perspectives of students with intellectual disabilities about their experiences with paraprofessional support. *Exceptional Children, 71,* 415–430.

Chopra, R. V., & French, N. K. (2004). Paraeducator relationships with parents of students with significant disabilities. *Remedial and Special Education, 25*(4), 240–257.

Chopra, R. V., Sandoval-Lucero, E., Aragon, L., Bernal, C., Berg de Balderas, H., & Carroll, D. (2004). The paraprofessional role of connector. *Remedial and Special Education, 25*(4), 219–231.

Cohn, E., Miller, L. J., & Tickle-Degnen, L. (2000). Parental hopes for therapy outcomes: Children with sensory modulation disorders. *American Journal of Occupational Therapy, 54,* 36–43.

Connell, B. R., Jones, M., Mace, R., Mueller, J., Mullick, A., Ostroff, E., et al. (1997). *The principles of universal design.* Retrieved June 6, 2006, from http://design.ncsu.edu/cud/about_ud/udprinciples.htm

Dillon, M., Flexman, C., & Probeck, L. (1996). *Examining the role of the occupational therapist and the educator in the transition planning process.* Unpublished master's project, Virginia Commonwealth University, Richmond.

Ellison, C. M., Boykin, A. W., Towns, D. P., & Stokes, A. (2000). *Classroom cultural ecology: The dynamics of classroom life in schools serving low-income African American children* (Report No. CRESPAR–R–44). East Lansing, MI: National Center for Research on Teacher Learning. (ERIC Document Reproduction Service No. ED442886)

Eriksson, L. (2005). The relationship between school environment and participation for students with disabilities. *Pediatric Rehabilitation, 8,* 130–139.

Evertson, C. M., Emmer, E. T., & Worsham, M. E. (2003). *Classroom management for elementary teachers* (6th ed.). Boston: Allyn & Bacon.

Falvey, M., Forest, J., Pearpoint & Rosenbury, R. (2004). *All my life's a circle: Using the tools: circles, MAPS & PATHS.* Toronto: Inclusion Press.

Federal Interagency Forum on Child & Family Statistics. (2006). *America's children in brief: Key national indicators of well-being.* Washington, DC: U.S. Government Printing Office. Retrieved February 2, 2007, from www.childstats.gov/pubs.asp

French, N. K. (2003). *Managing paraeducators in your school: How to hire, train, and supervise non-certified staff.* Thousand Oaks, CA: Corwin Press.

Friend, M., & Cook, L. (2007). Paraeducators. In M. Friend & L. Cook (Eds.), *Interactions: Collaboration skills for school professionals* (5th ed., pp. 139–163). Boston: Allyn & Bacon.

Giangreco, M. F. (1996). *Vermont Interdependent Services Team Approach (VISTA).* Baltimore: Paul H. Brookes.

Giangreco, M. F. (2001). Interactions among program, placement, and services in educational planning for students with disabilities. *Mental Retardation, 39*(5), 341–350.

Giangreco, M. F., Cloninger, C. J., Dennis, R., & Edelman, S. W. (2002). Problem-solving methods to facilitate inclusive education. In J. S. Thousand, R. A. Villa, & A. I. Nevin (Eds.), *Creativity and collaborative learning: The practical guide to empowering students, teachers, and families* (2nd ed., pp. 111–134). Baltimore. Paul H. Brookes.

Giangreco, M., Cloninger, C., & Iverson, M. (1998). *Choosing outcomes and accommodations for children (COACH,* 2nd ed.). Baltimore: Paul H. Brookes.

Giangreco, M. F., & Doyle, M. B. (2002). Students with disabilities and paraprofessional supports: Benefits, balance, and band-aids. *Focus on Exceptional Children, 34*(7), 1–12.

Giangreco, M. F., & Doyle, M. B. (2007). Teacher assistants in inclusive schools. In L. Florian (Ed.), *SAGE handbook of special education* (pp. 429–439). London: Sage.

Giangreco, M. F., Edelman, S. W., & Broer, S. M. (2001). Respect, appreciation, and acknowledgement of paraprofessionals who support students with disabilities. *Exceptional Children, 67,* 485–498.

Giangreco, M. F., Prelock, P. A., Reid, R. R., Dennis, R. E., & Edelman, S. W. (2000). Roles of related services personnel in inclusive schools. In R. Villa & J. Thousand (Eds.), *Restructuring for caring and effective education: Piecing the puzzle together* (2nd ed., pp. 360–388). Baltimore: Paul H. Brookes.

Goodrich, B. (2004). Universal design for learning and occupational therapy. *School System Special Interest Section Quarterly, 11*(1), 1–4.

Griswold, L. A. (1993). Ethnographic analysis: A study of classroom environments. *American Journal of Occupational Therapy, 48,* 397–402

Hanft, B. (2004). *Early childhood tutorial: Module on developing and implementing IFSPs with families.* Baltimore: Maryland Infants & Toddlers Program. Retrieved June 1, 2007, from www.cte.jhu.edu/ecgateway/

Hanft, B., & Place, P. (1996). *The consulting therapist: A guide for occupational and physical therapists in schools.* Austin, TX: Pro-Ed.

Hanft, B., Shepherd, J., & Read, J. (in press). Competence in numbers: Working on pediatric teams. In S. Lane & A. Bundy (Eds.), *Kids can be kids: Supporting the occupations and activities of childhood.* Philadelphia: F. A. Davis.

Hemmingson, H., & Borell, L. (2002). Environmental barriers in mainstream schools. *Child: Care, Health, and Development, 28,* 57–63.

Hemmingson, H., Borell, L., & Gustavsson, A. (1999). Temporal aspects of teaching and learning: Implications for pupils with physical disabilities. *Scandinavian Journal of Disability Research, 1,* 26–43.

Hemmingson, H., Egilson, S., Hoffman, O., & Kielhofner, G. (2005). *School Setting Interview (SSI,* Version 3.0). Chicago: MOHO Clearinghouse.

Hemmingson, H., Kottorp, A., & Bernspang, B. (2004). Validity of the school setting interview: An assessment of the student–environment fit. *Scandinavian Journal of Occupational Therapy, 11,* 171–178.

Ideishi, S. K., Ideishi, R. I., Gandhi, T., & Yuen, L. (2006, June). Inclusive preschool outdoor play environments. *School System Special Interest Section Quarterly, 13*(2), 1–4.

Individuals With Disabilities Education Improvement Act of 2004, Pub. L. 108-446, 20 U.S.C. § 1400 *et seq.* (2004).

Kellegrew, D. H., & Allen, D. (1996). Occupational therapy in full-inclusion classrooms: A case study from the Moorpark model. *American Journal of Occupational Therapy, 50,* 718–724.

Kellegrew, D. H., & Kroksmark, U. (1999). Examine school routines using time-geography methods. *Physical and Occupational Therapy in Pediatrics, 19,* 79–91.

Keller, J., Kafkes, A., Basu, S., Federico, J., & Kielhofner, G. (2005). *Child Occupational Self Assessment (COSA,* Version 2.1). Chicago: MOHO Clearinghouse.

Marr, D., Mika, H., Miraglia, J., Roerig, M., & Sinnott, R. (2007). The effect of sensory stories on targeted behaviors in preschool children with autism. *Physical and Occupational Therapy in Pediatrics, 27,* 63–78.

Marr, D., & Nackley, V. (2007). *Sensory stories.* Framingham, MA: Therapro.

McBrien, J. L., & Brandt, R. S. (1997). *The language of learning: A guide to education terms.* Alexandria, VA: Association for Supervision & Curriculum Development.

McNamara, P., & Humphry, R. (2007). Now this is what you do: Developing structured routines. *OTJR: Occupation, Participation, and Health, 27*(Suppl.), 88S–89S.

Mendoza-Smith, M. (2005). *The socialization of a professional stranger: The work of an occupational therapist in a public school.* Unpublished doctoral dissertation, New York University.

Mihaylov, S. I., Jarvis, S. N., Colver, A. F., & Beresford, B. (2004). Identification and description of environmental factors that influence participation of children with cerebral palsy. *Developmental Medicine and Child Neurology, 46,* 299–304.

Muhlenhaupt, M. (2003). Enabling student participation through occupational therapy services in the schools. In L. Letts, P. Rigby, & D. Stewart (Eds.), *Using environments to enable occupational performance* (pp. 177–196). Thorofare, NJ: Slack.

National Dissemination Center for Children With Disabilities. (2002a). *Helping students develop their IEPs (2nd ed.) Technical assistance guide (TA2B).* Retrieved June 3, 2007, from www.nichcy.org/pubs/stuguide/ta2book.htm

National Dissemination Center for Children With Disabilities. (2002b). *A student's guide to the IEP.* Retrieved June 3, 2007, from www.nichcy.org/pubs/stuguide/st1book.htm

National Education Association. (2004). *Results-oriented job descriptions: How paraeducators help students achieve.* Washington, DC: Author. Retrieved June 1, 2007, from www.nea.org/esphome/nearesources/rojd-paras.html

No Child Left Behind Act of 2001, Pub. L. No. 107–110, 115 Stat. 1425 (2002).

Odom, S. L., Boyd, B., & Buysse, V. (2007). Promising practices to support effective early childhood inclusion for Pre-K to Grade 3. In V. Buysse & L. Aytch (Eds.), *Early school success: Equity and access for diverse learners* (Executive Summary from the FirstSchool Diversity Symposium, pp. 14–17). Chapel Hill: University of North Carolina, FPG Child Development Institute. Retrieved November 2, 2007, from www.fpg.unc.edu/~firstschool/assets/FirstSchool_Symposium_ExectuiveSummary_2007.pdf

Patterson, K. B. (2006). Roles and responsibilities of paraprofessionals: In their own words. *TEACHING Exceptional Children Plus, 2*(5), Article 1. Retrieved July 9, 2007, from http://escholarship.bc.edu/education/tecplus/vol2/iss5/art1

Pearpoint, J., O'Brien, J., and Forest, M. (1995). *PATH: A workbook for planning positive possible futures: Planning alternative tomorrows with hope for schools, organizations, businesses, families.* Toronto: Inclusion Press.

Pickett, A., Likins, M., & Wallace, T. (2003). *The employment and preparation of paraeducators, the state of the art.* Logan: Utah State University, National Resource Center for Paraprofessionals. Retrieved July 1, 2007, from http://eric.ed.gov/ERICDocs/data/ericdocs2sql/content_storage_01/0000019b/80/1a/e0/c8.pdf

Pierce, D. (2003). *Occupation by design: Building therapeutic power.* Philadelphia: F. A. Davis.

Pivik, J., McComas, J., & Laflamme, M. (2002). Barriers and facilitators to inclusive education as reported by students with physical disabilities and their parents. *Exceptional Children, 61,* 97–107.

Polichino, J. (2004). Moving out of the "therapy room." In Y. Swinth (Ed.), *Occupational therapy in school-based practice: Contemporary issues and trends* (AOTA Online Course, Lesson 7). Bethesda, MD: American Occupational Therapy Association.

Polichino, J., Clark, G., & Chandler, B. (2005, February 21). Supporting students in the natural environment. *OT Practice,* pp. 11–15.

Railsback, J., Reed, B., & Schmidt, K. (2002). *Working together for successful paraeducator services: A guide for paraeducators, teachers, and principals.* Northwest Regional Education Laboratory. Retrieved January 3, 2007, from www.nwrel.org/request/may2002/paraeds.pdf.

Rempfer, M., Hidenbrand, W., Parker, K., & Brown, C. (2003). An interdisciplinary approach to environmental intervention: Ecology of human performance. In L. Letts, P. Rigby, & D. Stewart (Eds.), *Using environments to enable occupational performance* (pp. 119–136). Thorofare, NJ: Slack.

Richardson, P. K. (2002). The school as social context: Social interaction patterns of children with physical disabilities. *American Journal of Occupational Therapy, 56,* 296–304.

Rose, D., & Meyer, A. (2002). *Teaching every student in the digital age: Universal design for learning.* Association for Supervision & Curriculum Development. Retrieved January 2, 2007, from www.cast.org/teachingeverystudent/ideas/tes/

Rose, D., & Meyer, A. (Eds.). (2006). *A practical reader in universal design for learning.* Cambridge, MA: Harvard University Press.

Schenker, R., Coster, W., & Parush, S. (2005). Participation and activity performance of students with cerebral palsy within the school environment. *Disability Rehabilitation, 27,* 539–552.

Schoonover, J., Levan, P., & Argabrite Grove, R. (2006). Occupational therapy and assistive technology in school-based practice: Supporting participation. *OT Practice, 11*(1), CE1–CE8.

Segal, R., & Hinojosa, J. (2006). The activity setting of homework: An analysis of three cases and implications for occupational therapy. *American Journal of Occupational Therapy, 60,* 50–59.

Simeonsson, R., Carlson, D., Huntington, G., McMillen, J. S., & Brent, J. L. (2001). Students with disabilities: A national survey of participation in school activities. *Disabilities Rehabilitation, 23,* 49–63.

Snell, M. E., & Janney, R. (2005). *Collaborative teaming* (2nd ed.). Baltimore: Paul H. Brookes.

Thousand, J., & Villa, R. (2000). Collaborative teaming: A powerful tool in school restructuring. In R. Villa & J. Thousand (Eds.), *Restructuring for caring and effective education* (pp. 254–291). Baltimore: Paul H. Brookes.

Turnbull, A., Turbiville, V., & Turnbull, R. (2000). Evolution of family–professional partnerships: Collective empowerment as the model for the early 21st century. In J. P. Meisels & S. J. Shonkoff (Eds.), *Handbook of early childhood intervention* (2nd ed., pp. 630–650). New York: Cambridge University Press.

U.S. Department of Education. (2004). *Toward a new golden age in American education: How the Internet, the law, and today's students are revolutionizing expectation.* Retrieved January 31, 2007, from www.ed.gov/about/offices/list/os/technology/plan/2004/index.html

U.S. Department of Education. (2005). *10 facts about K–12 education funding.* Washington, DC: Author.

U.S. Department of Education, Office of Elementary and Secondary Education. (2002). *No Child Left Behind: A desktop reference.* Washington, DC: Author.

Wakeford, L. (August, 2003). *Integrating occupational therapy (p. 3) National individualizing preschool inclusion project.* Retrieved September 1, 2007, from www.collaboratingpartners.com/docs/R_Mcwilliam/Integrated%20Services%20-%20April.pdf

Williams, M. S., & Shellenberger, S. (1996). *How does your engine run? A leader's guide to the Alert Program for Self-Regulation.* Albuquerque, NM: TherapyWorks.

CHAPTER 3

Teamwork vs. the Lone Ranger

*Jayne Shepherd, MS, OTR, FAOTA, and
Barbara Hanft, MS, OTR, FAOTA*

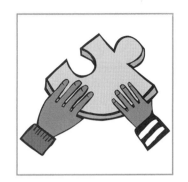

I remember dialoguing with a teacher and thinking, "This is really working!" Collaboration is the most exciting thing I do as an OT—you get two or more professionals problem solving together, and you come up with a solution for a student that is so much better than what one person alone could do.

—Judie Sage, occupational therapist, Wisconsin

It is essential that occupational therapists and related services personnel collaborate with teachers to meet students' educational needs (American Occupational Therapy Association [AOTA], 2004; Villa, Thousand, Nevin, & Malgeri, 1996) and not be "Lone Rangers" trying to do it all by themselves. Chapter 3 focuses on the interactive process of team collaboration and what makes it work for various team members. Six major collaborative characteristics of teams (DeBoer & Fister, 1995) are discussed in relation to team structure and interaction. Written and unwritten rules about getting along, a structure for meetings and communication, a decision-making model, a team evaluation strategy, and a mentoring–coaching program to promote team collaboration are described.

After reading this material, readers will be able to

- Identify team characteristics that promote collaboration between members;

- Recognize and select team structures and strategies to create collaborative partnerships for effective student and team outcomes;

- Identify, select, and apply different team-building strategies and decision models to work with children and school teams;

- Analyze and apply a variety of strategies for assessing interpersonal communication; and

- Identify components of mentoring and coaching programs to promote team collaboration

Key Topics

- Characteristics of collaborative teams

- Collective decision making

- Team operations and communication

- Mentoring and coaching

1-2-3-4-5: Keeping Team Collaboration Alive

What keeps team collaboration alive and working in inclusive environments? According to Odom, Boyd, and Buysse (2007), early childhood research suggests the following:

Collaboration among professionals that is built on communication, mutual respect, common vision, adequate time for planning and resources, training, and administrative support will provide the necessary and sometimes invisible (if one were to only look in the classroom) infrastructure necessary for inclusion. (p. 15)

Occupational therapists often have the daunting role of collaborating on a variety of teams in the school system, and those teams may not possess the characteristics described above (Hanft, Shepherd, & Read, in press). School-based occupational therapists can contribute and provide leadership to assistive technology, prereferral, and response to intervention (RtI) teams as well as departmental, system, and school–community teams. This multiteam involvement requires a therapist to analyze each team's structure and goals and the communication skills and perspectives of a team's faces. Figure 3.1 identifies possible teams and committees that therapists may join in school settings.

Team structure sustains team interaction by defining its organization and purpose, its membership, how it will operate, and how its work is evaluated. School policies, administrator leadership style, and individual team members help define the team's organization and how it will operate (Friend & Cook, 2007; Johnston, Knight, & Miller, 2007; Snell & Janney, 2005). Administrator support from principals, special education coordinators, therapy coordinators, and other supervisors is essential. These team members may implement policies and procedures that affect team structure (e.g., time and place to meet during the school day, team membership, school or team climate, responsibilities, financial resources; Hargreaves, 1994; Johnson et al., 2007; Khorsheed, 2007; Rafoth & Foriska, 2006; Salisbury & McGregor, 2002).

The six core characteristics of collaborative teams help build the structure that sustains team interaction: voluntary participation, equality among members, common purpose, joint responsibility for outcomes, shared resources, and collective decision making (DeBoer & Fister, 1995). Although distinct, these characteristics overlap to build the structure for collaborative teamwork. The following sections discuss how teams develop each characteristic.

Voluntary Participation

Occupational therapists often join ongoing or preexisting student or school teams (e.g., eligibility, individualized education program [IEP], grade level, professional development teams), with a variety of faces on the team. At other times, in addition to the student-focused teams, they volunteer to be part of a new team at the building level (e.g., school beautification, fundraising, parent–teacher association, playground committees) or the district (e.g., assistive technology committee, accessibility task force, continuing education). Either way, an agreement to join a team and collaborate means that an occupational therapist identifies and accepts particular responsibilities and considers how to support other team members.

Members of collaborative teams voluntarily choose to engage in an interactive relationship (DeBoer & Fister, 1995). When an occupational therapist is a member of a student's team, participation is expected by virtue of the services identified on the student's IEP. How the therapist chooses to engage with the team—that is, as a collaborator or as a lone ranger—is voluntary.

Remember this . . .
Team structure sustains team interaction by defining

• **Organization and purpose,**

• **Membership,**

• **Operation rules, and**

• **How the team's work is evaluated.**

Student Focused	System Focused
• Individualized education program (IEP) teams	• Curriculum
• Early childhood special education or special education department teams	• Department (e.g., high school English, science, math, foreign language)
• Assessment accommodations	• Eligibility
• Assistive technology	• Occupational therapy department
• Prereferral	• Professional development committee
• Response to intervention (RtI)	• School committees (e.g., library, extracurricular activities, public relations)
• Transition	• School improvement
	• School–community committees
	• Task forces or ad hoc committees on school policies and procedures
	• Transportation

Figure 3.1. School teams and committees in which occupational therapists may participate.

When joining a team, members must actively commit to participate in collaborative relationships and together decide how the team will function and work together for the benefit of all students. Collaboration does not just happen without a concerted effort by all team members to define and nourish an interactive process. Frequent face-to-face and impromptu interactions occur during teaming, and team membership may change over time, depending on a team's or a student's needs. Therefore, careful considerations must be given to

- Who should be on the team and why (4–6 is an optimal size for a core team);

- Who should attend team meetings (ask preferences, who is needed?);

- Where, when, and how often will the team meet and for how long (a place, agenda, and schedule of meetings); and

- How will the team communicate during the meeting and inform a team member who cannot attend (rules of engagement, recording, and reporting procedures). (Rainforth & York-Barr, 1997; Snell & Janney, 2005; Thousand & Villa, 2000)

Remember this . . .
Collaboration does not just happen without a concerted effort by all team members to define and nourish an interactive process.

Equality Among Members

On collaborative teams, parents and students are the experts about their own needs (Thousand & Villa, 2000). No one team member is more important than the child and parent, who are the heart of the team. Even though teams may define their structure differently (e.g., purpose, membership, operations), team members' specific responsibilities, opinions, ideas, and needs are respected and given equal consideration (Snell & Janney, 2005; Thousand & Villa, 2000). Equality among team members is often supported by accepting team ground rules, sharing leadership responsibilities, and arranging the physical environment to facilitate collaboration (e.g., arrange seating so all members can see one another, use circular seating to emphasize equality; Thousand & Villa, 2000). All team members have various professional (and personal) backgrounds and experiences that influence which team member(s) may be best to work with a student (Giangreco, 1995, 1996, 2001). Giangreco, Prelock, Reid, Dennis, and Edelman (2000) cautioned therapists to avoid "the expert trap" (p. 364). As part of a collaborative team, an occupational therapist must relinquish an expert approach ("Only I know how to help this student") and contribute to shared decision making ("Together, we can help this student learn"). This can be a challenge when a team member expects a therapist to assume an expert role or a therapist chooses to act as an expert. At the same time, team members value each other's experience and advice, as described by administrator Ilene Banker:

Administrator Voices: Start at the beginning

It is my responsibility to help all children succeed. Why wouldn't I bring together my specialists who have the experience to suggest if this child needs simple adaptations to the curriculum or may need an additional evaluation or services? I value what they bring to the team and see that we are more effective by having their input from the beginning.

—Ilene Banker, assistant principal, Virginia

Common Purpose

To guide their work, collaborative teams develop a shared vision or purpose that reflects their professional and personal values and beliefs. These values and beliefs help unify team members when planning and selecting common goals for a student or team (DeBoer & Fister, 1995; Rainforth & York-Barr, 1997). For example, if a team values student self-determination, then when developing student goals, members will naturally consider what choices or types of decisions are offered to students. Did a team include students in planning and leading their IEP meetings, as appropriate? Did the students have opportunities to choose activities or reinforcers for learning new skills?

Another value supporting collaborative teaming is to jointly assess and develop one IEP with integrated goals for each student (Giangreco, Prelock, et al., 2000). Using only discipline-specific assessments to evaluate student performance and determine baseline behavior, such as the Peabody Developmental Motor Scales II (PDMS–2; Folio & Fewell, 2000), precludes the development of integrated educational outcomes and intervention for students. These assessments may provide a therapist with information about underlying learning challenges for a student, but when used alone they promote domain-specific thinking rather than academic and functional goals for students. In the following comment, Judith Schoonover reiterates the need to work on integrated goals.

Therapist Voices: Wasted time on isolated goals

How many students have performed in the 10th percentile of the [PDMS–2], yet can write their name or manipulate their school materials with adaptive equipment or techniques? Valuable time is wasted on isolated goals and treatment when a therapist removes a child from the classroom and works on "her" goals. It sends the message that the OT is the expert and the only one that can work on specific areas with the child as opposed to one of the team members addressing a need all team members are supporting.

—Judith Schoonover, occupational therapist and
assistive technology specialist, Virginia

School-based therapists should never have separate therapy goals stapled to the end of the student's IEP document (Chandler, 2007; Polichino, Clark, & Chandler, 2005). Such separate, isolated goals and intervention often have a negative impact on student progress because these goals are often unrelated to the educational program, and only the expert helps a student work on identified skills once or twice a week instead of every day (Giangreco, Prelock, et al., 2000). It also reinforces autocratic instead of collaborative decision making. When therapists do not work collaboratively in the classroom on contextually purposeful tasks, students miss other educational opportunities for learning and participation (Dunn, 2000; Jackson, 2007; Polichino, 2004). In addition, the teachers and paraprofessionals do not learn from the occupational therapist how to give specific student supports (e.g., equipment set-up, verbal or gestural cues, sequencing of steps; Giangreco, Edelman, & Dennis, 1991; Jackson, 2007; Knippenberg & Hanft, 2004; Swinth et al., 2002).

Joint Responsibility for Outcomes

On collaborative teams, each team member is responsible for specific student outcomes and is held accountable for commitments made to the team, for example, talking to the parents, arranging the schedule, or setting up the meeting room (Demchak, Alden, Bergin, Ting, & Lacey, 1995; Johnson & Johnson, 1999; Snell & Janney, 2005). School teams work together to select goals that answer the question "What does this student need to learn to participate in school and in meaningful educationally relevant occupations?" (Hanft & Place, 1996; Polichino et al., 2005). When evaluating how well a team collaborates, the critical measure is not that the team "feels" they worked well together but that they can affirm that student outcomes were achieved. The team is held accountable for the success or failure to meet outcomes, and no one person is blamed if outcomes are not met (DeBoer & Fister, 1995). Data are collected and jointly reviewed to assist all team members in working together. Both student progress and the team process may be evaluated, celebrated, and rewarded when teams succeed in reaching their mutual goals (Thousand & Villa, 2000).

Mutual purpose and joint responsibility for student outcomes create positive attitudes, interdependence among team members, and decreased disciplinary boundaries and turf conflicts (Giangreco, St. Denis, Cloninger, Edelman, & Schattman, 1993; Thousand & Villa, 2000). By sharing a purpose or vision for helping students achieve their outcome, team members learn to work together and forestall potential conflicts by asking at regular intervals, "Are we effectively meeting our goals?"

Sharing Resources to Learn From One Another

In collaborative teams, all team members learn from one another and participate in lifelong learning. Team members are expected to reflect on their practice and share their skills, talents, knowledge, and materials with each other (DeBoer & Fister, 1995).

Remember this . . .
Another value supporting collaborative teaming is to jointly assess and develop one IEP with integrated goals for each student. There are no isolated occupational therapy goals.

This "positive resource interdependence" (Thousand & Villa, 2000, p. 267) is characteristic of collaborative teams and is an example of how leadership is shared, created, and perpetuated as team members make the effort to work together.

Educate Others About Possible Occupational Therapy Contributions to the Team

In collaborative teams, occupational therapists often educate parents, teachers, and administrators about what occupational therapy has to offer to the team to help a student succeed in school, and they listen to the input and contributions of other team members. When this does not occur, student teams miss opportunities for team and system supports from occupational therapists and other related services providers. Each team member brings a different point of view to educational teams. How many times do occupational therapists assist teams with addressing behavior that is influenced by sensory processing issues, poor positioning, or understanding of organizational cues? In many school divisions, related services personnel may have worked with a student for multiple years and know his or her strengths, needs, and preferences better at the start of the school year than a new teacher.

In the next vignettes, two therapists discuss how they teach others about their role in the public schools. In the first scenario, consider how a veteran therapist in a rural school district helps a new teacher feel comfortable with her class using a "hands-on/team supports" approach

Therapist Voices: How can I help?

I promise to see new teachers right away. This year when I learned Nancy was a brand new teacher in the class for children with multiple disabilities, I purposely went to meet her prior to school opening. I started a conversation by saying, "Hi, I'm Judie Sage, I'm the occupational therapist. How can I help you? Have you ever worked with an OT before? I have worked with most of the children in your classroom for many years, and I'd be happy to help you on the first day of school if you'd like."

During the teacher workdays prior to school opening, I talked with the other teachers who had children on my workload. I explained that I would be working with Nancy for the first few days of school, but I would get them set up with the equipment they needed for their students. I also let them know how to get in touch with me if they had any questions or concerns.

—Judie Sage, occupational therapist, Wisconsin

In the next vignette, a group of occupational therapists pooled their knowledge and provided system supports to educate others about occupational therapy.

Therapist Voices: Crafting the message

I called the OT staff together to produce a simple PowerPoint to share with related services personnel, teachers, or to use in other settings for hospital administrators, rotary clubs, and other community organizations to understand what OT does in our school district. The group determined the take home message they wanted others to know about OT. Together, we developed 16 slides to describe how OT works in the schools. Topics included early learning supports, understanding and interpreting sensory systems, life skills, environmental adaptations, school health and safety, classroom tool use, assistive technology, preparing for the future, and how to access therapists and their support. After the PowerPoint was developed, we all could bring a consistent message about OT to many of the schools in our district and the community.

—Jan Emerick-Brothers, occupational therapist, Virginia

Learn From Each Other

Collaboration is an interactive team process, and all the team members are interrelated. The key question to ask is, How can we help each other for the benefit of the student?

—Rebecca Argabrite Grove, administrator, occupational therapist, and assistive technology specialist, Virginia

As described above, learning is a joint responsibility between team members. Therapists must be willing to seek new information and learn new skills to understand how teachers and other educational personnel operate to help students learn. Occupational therapists must also understand how current trends or buzz words (e.g., *annual yearly progress, co-teaching, RtI*) affect the work demands and daily routines of the education team (see Resource 3.1 for suggested resources). Reading literature from other professions (e.g., education, special education, psychology) helps occupational therapists understand different education perspectives and buzz words.

Understanding basic curriculum content, state standards and testing, different teaching techniques, general and special education laws and regulations, and new research or methods in education are just a few things therapists must learn. In a study of related services personnel by Giangreco et al. (1991), families of children with disabilities appreciated coordinated services and personnel who admitted what they did or did not know, worked together to solve a problem, and took action to solve the problem. By taking joint responsibility for learning new skills, team members have more resources to support student progress (Snell & Janney, 2005).

Like any professional, educators approach the teaching process guided by theories and frameworks specific to their discipline. Block and Chandler (2005) discussed the importance of understanding the relationship of occupational therapy and three learning theories—behaviorism, cognitivism, and constructivism—as a basis for communicating effectively with teachers and making recommendations that complement their professional frameworks. These education theories and perspectives influence "how the teacher will view recommendations, suggestions, routines, media, materials, and methods that the occupational therapist may use or provide to assist a student in meeting school-based experiences" (Block & Chandler, 2005, p. CE4). As a related services

Resource 3.1. Understanding the Influence of Education Buzz Words for Occupational Therapy Services

- *Response to Intervention (RtI):* http://interventioncentral.org
- *Annual yearly progress:* www.ed.gov/nclb/overview/intro
- *Standards for learning:* Web site for your state's department of education
- *Co-teaching:* www.dldcec.org/pdf/teaching_how-tos/murawski_36-5.pdf
- *Assessment accommodations:* www.teachervision.fen.com/teaching-methods/educational-testing/4170.html
- *Scientific research; peer-reviewed research:* www.canchild.ca/
- *Progress monitoring:* www.progressmonitoring.net

Remember this . . .
"Collaboration is a two-way street. . . . If you want teachers to carry over occupational therapy ideas, you must reinforce their strategies as well."
—Michelle Cullen, occupational therapist, New York

What Does Your Team Do?

• How do your team members share knowledge with each other?

• How do you relate your intervention suggestions to the curriculum?

provider, the occupational therapist's task is to "work with teams to ensure that a student is receptive to what the teacher has to offer and can benefit from the teacher's skills in manipulating learning theory to stimulate the acquisition of knowledge" (p. CE6). For example, many teachers believe that children learn through self-discovery in a structured yet open classroom in which materials are selected by the teacher for students to use to prompt their learning. This theory of learning (known as *cognitivism*) complements an occupational therapy perspective that meaningful actions and activities motivate students to participate in school lessons and activities and improve their performance. Thus, a therapist could easily find common objectives with a teacher who embraces a cognitivistic approach. Together, they could identify multiple strategies to help a student learn a specific curriculum and demonstrate mastery of the knowledge. Consider how knowledge is shared in your team (see Reflection 3.1).

After observing a school-based occupational therapist for a year for her doctoral dissertation, Maria Mendoza-Smith emphasizes the need to consider teacher views and responsibilities:

Therapist Voices: Blending expectations

Teachers have a very different worldview in their values, beliefs, and understanding of a child. As OTs, we cannot assume that they look at a child or classroom in the same way we do. They think about their class of 25 or 30 students as a whole, what they need to cover in the curriculum so that their students perform well on the local and state standardized tests, and how they will meet the goals of the grade-level team. Often, they cannot focus on the one student that an OT has identified as needing to make friends or build up hand strength to succeed in writing assignments.

OTs must learn the language, rules, and expectations of their school, community, and educational teams. Know how to present activities and suggest interventions [team supports, hands-on services] that tie into the curriculum, grade expectations, and team goals. For example, the increased emphasis on literacy in the recent federal legislation can be viewed as another obstacle or as an opportunity to explore the role of occupational therapists in supporting literacy.

—Maria Mendoza-Smith, occupational therapist, Connecticut

Use Principles of Adult Learning and Give Feedback to One Another

In collaborative teams, experiential learning with demonstrations and actual practice and coaching and mentoring are often used to help all team members learn new concepts and strategies (Hanft, Rush, & Shelden, 2004; Rainforth & York-Barr, 1997). Basic principles of adult learning are embraced, that is, adults are self-directed and goal oriented; they bring a variety of experiences to the learning environment; they appreciate relevant and practical suggestions; and they want to be treated respectfully (Comings, Garner, & Smith, 2007; Knowles, Holton, & Swanson, 2005). Adult learning depends on team members giving and receiving feedback about what they have learned or want to learn. Table 3.1 provides questions to prompt teams to consider how they use the principles of adult learning.

Table 3.1. Principles of Adult Learning and Application to Collaboration (Knowles, Holton, & Swanson, 2005)

Principles of Adult Learning	Application to Collaboration
1. Adults are self-directed and autonomous learners. By focusing on their interests and personal goals, they will be responsible for their own learning.	• What do you want to learn as we work together? • How can we work together effectively? • What would you like me to do? • Here's the information you requested. Let me know if you need anything else. (For those learners who really want self-discovery.)
2. Adults bring knowledge and a variety of life experiences to the learning environment. Previous work, education, family, cultural, or leisure experiences may influence how adults understand or respond to a learning experience.	• Tell me about yourself and your family (e.g., where you have lived, family, interests). Let me tell you a little about mine. • How long have you worked as a teacher or therapist? How long have you been at this school? • Tell me about your other work experiences. • Where did you go to school? Did your educational program have a certain emphasis (e.g., behavior analysis, assistive technology, inclusion)? • Have you ever worked with students similar to Johnny?
3. Adult learners are goal oriented. Adults usually have a clear idea of what they want to learn and why.	• What are your goals for us working together? • Do you have any personal goals for this year in teaching? • Do you feel my suggestions are relevant to your goals? • Have I given you some choices that will meet your goals?
4. Adult learners want practical and relevant information. New information is adopted more frequently if it makes sense, is doable, and appears helpful.	• I'd like to explain why I think this technique will work and how it will help Johnny meet his goals. • When would be the best time to try this idea in relation to your daily schedule? • This isn't something Johnny's aide can do every day, but if there is time two or three times a week, it would be helpful.
5. Adult learners want to be treated with respect. Adults want to be valued for their knowledge, opinions, and life experiences.	• I want to hear your opinion about this. • You played drums in high school; how can we help Natalie join the school band? • I only have a cursory knowledge of the curriculum; can you explain how you teach this reading concept? • I think you are great at managing behavior.

In the following vignette, an occupational therapy student recognized the importance of using principles of adult learning and making time to listen to the teacher's concerns. She also offered strategies and activities that could be incorporated into the typical classroom routine.

Therapist Voices: Working together

I do find team members are more receptive and willing to work with you if you incorporate and acknowledge their concerns and feedback. I have taught the teacher sensory strategies for a fifth-grade student, and we are also using these strategies with the whole class for the first 5 minutes before math. The teacher is very excited and willing to implement it after we worked out a plan that is both manageable for her and meets the needs of the student. She is even going to use these strategies with a few of her other students she feels could benefit from sensory breaks throughout the school day.

—Maritza Villegas, occupational therapy student,
University of Southern California

Sharing professional knowledge is a process of selecting information and informing another team member how to use it, as appropriate to his or her role and experience. If

Remember this . . .
"Building interdependent professional relationships in the school is one of the most complex and challenging aspects of practice in educational settings" (Maria Mendoza-Smith, personal communication, June 27, 2007).

a therapist's recommendations to other team members could potentially harm a student if implemented inappropriately, then specific plans must be made for initial training and follow-up team supports, preferably within the context of a student's daily activities and routines. Hanft et al. (2004) suggested asking the following questions when considering if, and how, professional knowledge and experience can be shared among team members (p. 178):

- What does a team member want to learn?

- If experience or foundational knowledge is desired, what does a team member already know?

- How will the team member use this knowledge and skills, and will it improve student outcomes?

- How can the desired information be shared with the appropriate team member?

- In what context will a team member apply the new knowledge and skills with students?

- Who has the expertise in and knowledge of evidence-based practice to guide a team member in acquiring and using the desired knowledge?

- What strategies will help a team member acquire or refine his or her knowledge and skills?

- On the basis of adult learning principles, what strategies will assist a learner (e.g., observation, demonstration, print materials)?

Collective Decision Making

Collective decision making (i.e., all members agree on a course of action rather than the majority ruling) is a process used to determine the what, who, when, and where regarding student outcomes and team operations. Team members' perspectives and concerns are openly discussed, and any conflict is resolved through compromise for the best possible decision (see Chapter 6 for discussion of conflict resolution). Team members may still hold varied expectations about a student's potential achievement or possible needs for services and supports, but if they have no strong objections, they agree to accept the overall decision.

The contribution an occupational therapist makes to the team decision-making process will vary according to the knowledge and experiences of team members, the nature of a student's educational abilities and challenges, the contextual variables, and the collective team perspective regarding supports and services. Occupational therapists often reframe the team's perspective or share a perspective or strategy that other team members may have not considered (Case-Smith, 1997), as eloquently said below:

Therapist Voices: Shedding light

My role involves shedding light on what the possibilities can be . . . looking at quality of life, what gives meaning to a person, not focusing on deficits.

—Occupational therapist working in transition (field notes; as quoted in Dillon, Flexman, & Probeck, 1996)

Deciding Who Will Be Involved

Student outcomes should drive all team decisions. Education team meetings provide the context for developing educationally relevant and "doable" IEPs to meet outcomes for students. On collaborative teams, a process for joint decision making is usually part of the agreed-on structure. Using a structured approach is a good way to solicit information from all team members. When all team members share their input, occupational therapists find it easier to blend hands-on services with team and system supports, collaborating with one another to take responsibility for reaching identified student outcomes. Team members can use assessment tools and strategies that support collaborative decision making (described in Chapter 2 and in Exhibit 2.1A in the Appendix). Vignettes at the end of Chapters 5 and 6 highlight how two teams used Making Action Plans (MAPS; Falvey, Forest, Pearpoint, & Rosenbury, 2004) and Planning Alternative Tomorrows With Hope (PATH; Pearpoint, O'Brien, & Forest, 1995) to promote collaborative decision making. Resource 3.2 highlights a family perspective about team decision making.

Collective decision making also determines who will have ongoing involvement with the student to meet the integrated goals. Giangreco (1996) developed a formal process for school teams to make these collective decisions, the Vermont Interdependent Services Team Approach (VISTA). Decisions are based on student and family preferences, data, team discussion of pros and cons, and the expertise and availability of team members, not which discipline "should" be involved. If team members have similar knowledge and skills, a team may select one member who may already be working with a student to implement the identified intervention and supports. VISTA guides an IEP team to consider

- Whether related services (hands-on services and team supports) are necessary and educationally relevant for a student and
- Who can carry out the identified intervention with support from another team member or members (Giangreco, Cloninger, Dennis, & Edelman, 2000, 2002).

Team Collaboration Vignettes

Review the characteristics that describe the interactive process in collaborative teams: voluntary participation, equality among members, common purpose, joint responsibility for outcomes, shared resources, and collective decision making (DeBoer & Fister, 1995). In the following two vignettes, consider how each team could or did demonstrate the six characteristics of collaborative teams.

Collaboration in Action: Entering a team as a new therapist

Matt is an experienced occupational therapist who recently moved to a large school district after serving as the assistive technology coordinator for a small school in another state. Half his time is dedicated to the county's assistive technology team; the other half will be devoted to working on the autism

Resource 3.2. Family Perspectives on Decision Making
One family's perspective about using the MAPS to develop a collaborative individualized education program for their daughter Lindsey: www.inclusion.com/artfamilyperspective.html

65% TS
35% HO

team for self-contained preschool classrooms. Although Matt has worked on numerous teams serving children with neuromuscular disorders, he has not worked with preschoolers for at least 9 years and is unsure of all the new technology for preschoolers recently purchased by the school district.

Reflection 3.2 suggests possible answers to questions about the collaborative interactions between Matt and his team. In the above scenario, if Matt followed the suggestions in Reflection 3.2, he would demonstrate a genuine interest in becoming part of the interactive team process. In the following vignette, Judy Davis describes how her established collaborative team works together on the common vision to include Gretchen, a student with Down syndrome, in high school academics and activities.

Reflection 3.2

What Suggestions Do You Have for Matt?

When answering the following questions, remember that Matt is trying to blend his roles as an assistive technology team member and as a therapist working in the autism preschool program.

- *On what teams might Matt participate? Think individualized education program (IEP), school, and system.* Matt will be assigned to the early childhood special education assistive technology (AT) team. He may be a core member on many IEP teams for the preschool autism class if it is determined his services are needed (using the Vermont Interdependent Services Team Approach collective decision-making process). He has also volunteered to be on the preschool transition team so he can learn more about the programs in his large school district and be sure these students have the AT they need before starting kindergarten. After working for a semester in this school system, Matt works with a committee to help update the school Web page so teachers can easily access software programs.

- *How can Matt introduce himself to show equality between team members? (Does he share his previous experiences or lack of experiences?)* "Hi, I'm happy to be

here, but I'm in a little bit of culture shock in this large school system and with preschoolers. It's been a long time since I had to get down so low to the floor or relate to young kids! I hope you can show me some of the ropes and help me learn about your preschool curriculum and this school system. I've had a lot of experience with AT in the past, but I haven't heard of some of the new pieces of equipment you've ordered. Have you worked with them before? Maybe we can learn about them together?"

- *What common purpose or vision could guide the preschool team?* The team's common purpose could be to provide a safe and nurturing environment that supports the students learning preacademic, self-care, socialization, and communication skills or to use AT when necessary to promote communication between students and adults.

- *Who will Matt ask to teach him about the AT and decide how to use it?* Matt could ask the parents, the special education teacher in the autism class, the paraprofessional, the speech–language pathologist, and other members of the school system's AT team. Of course, he

will also observe students' preferences and skills to provide input to the preschool team during the collective decision-making process.

- *How might Matt provide hands-on services with team and systems supports to meet student outcomes and program challenges?* Matt will learn how to operate the AT devices with the teacher, and then they will use them with students to co-teach a lesson, singing "Wheels on the Bus" using an IntelliKeys programmable keyboard (Cambium Learning, Natick, MA) and actual objects. He will make a template for an overlay with pictures that can be used for other songs the students will be learning.

- *What professional resources will the team share?* The team will share curriculum guides, developmentally appropriate practice, previously used low-tech communication systems, pictures, laminating paper, behavior plans, data collection sheets, equipment (e.g., AT devices, positioning equipment, materials for different units, checklists for observations, videos), sensory activities, and so forth.

Collaboration in Action: Team collaboration
for high school inclusion

These are some of the ways that inclusion works for Gretchen, a high school student who is fully included:

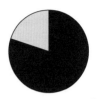

80% TS
20% HO

- Dressing skills are worked on when Gretchen dresses out for physical education [PE] daily, with a program set up by the OT. The physical therapist consults with the PE teacher to integrate strengthening, endurance, etc., into whatever the PE unit is. A paraprofessional assists for the dressing, then a peer/friend assists during the actual PE class.

- Gretchen follows a visual schedule (pictures of teachers and peers for each class period) to work on social skills, time management, and routines. With help from the speech–language pathologist, scripted interactions are used to help Gretchen greet a person, answer a simple prompt question, ask for materials, or make a choice. All team members use these with Gretchen throughout the day.

- Gretchen walks with a peer/friend to art and music, where she participates independently. The art teacher prepares separate projects (e.g., during still-life painting, this student does a simple paint-by-number still life) . . . similar to her peers. This is facilitated by the OT, emphasizing lifelong leisure opportunities.

- Gretchen attends a keyboarding/business class, where she is learning modified keyboarding and how to access the Internet for leisure, learning and, perhaps, some job skills for the future. She is assisted in the keyboarding during class by the teacher, paraprofessional, and OT, and then has Internet time with the other students and a peer buddy.

- Gretchen attends social studies with a paraprofessional, where she eagerly listens to stories about other cultures, countries, etc. (They eat a lot of ethnic food!) Then, during independent work on maps, people, etc., using adapted materials, she concentrates on her community and school, answering questions such as, Where is everything in town located? What is available?

- During work–study time, Gretchen job-shadows an employee (transition).

- Gretchen attends a life skills class in the resource room.

As you can see, she has a very full schedule that has friends, meaning, independence, and enhancement, and she is happy! It definitely isn't perfect, but it is a great team working toward meaningful inclusion.

—Judy Davis, occupational therapist, Colorado

Each of the above vignettes demonstrates the interactive process of team collaboration. In Reflection 3.3, review the six characteristics of collaborative teams and evaluate your team interaction or structures to support student success.

Reflection 3.3

Are We a Collaborative Team?

Choose one team of which you are a member. Review the characteristics of collaborative teams and consider how your team's interactions or structure support collaborative teaming:

- Voluntary participation
- Equality among members
- Shared purpose
- Joint responsibility for outcomes
- Shared resources
- Collective decision making (DeBoer & Fister, 1995).

Down, Set, Hut: Keep Teamwork Running

Teamwork drives the engine for the interactive team process, and team operations help keep it running. How teams are structured and carry out their responsibilities and functions also affects how well they collaborate and may vary dramatically even in the same school building. Team operations include the nitty-gritty details: schedules, meeting agendas, and rules of engagement during meetings, such as note taking, sharing of leadership, and communication methods and expectations (Wiggins & Damore, 2006). Collaboration depends on effective interpersonal and communication skills that enable all team members to express ideas and concerns and listen to each other respectfully (Friend & Cook, 2007). Preservice education for occupational therapists includes coursework in communication skills, group dynamics, and managing multiple team projects (Accreditation Council for Occupational Therapy Education, 2006). However, trust building, communication, leadership, problem solving, and conflict management are skills that collaborative teams must learn, use, and evaluate together (Thousand & Villa, 2000; Wiggins & Damore, 2006). Creative problem solving and conflict resolution are discussed further in Chapter 6. Resource 3.3 illustrates team interactions that promote effective collaboration.

Initiating Collaboration

Collaboration is built and sustained by trusting relationships that often begin with a student evaluation or screening. When first meeting a team member, it is helpful to bring something to the table to welcome a new person as well as to introduce oneself. This may be a piece of equipment, a book, a resource, or perhaps food. Darcie Votipka, a Colorado therapist, often brings her Kahlua cake to the first team meeting to break the ice and share her love of cooking. Below, three school therapists describe how they begin the collaborative team process with the team. First, Rebecca discusses how she might enter a new school.

Resource 3.3. Actions of Effective Team Members

- Listen and respect each other.
- Interact well with each other.
- Share values and beliefs for purpose of the team and team member roles.
- Have a flexible process to facilitate communication.
- Use rules of engagement for the team.
- Define roles and responsibilities for team members.
- Understand team members' roles and talents.
- Embrace role release.
- Trust each other.
- Use collective decision making.
- Identify and resolve concerns and conflicts.
- Expect all team members to learn from each other and participate in lifelong learning (Hanft, Rush, & Shelden, 2004).

Dettmer, Thurston, & Sellberg, 2005; Dinnebeil, Hale, & Rule, 1996; Friend & Cook, 2007; Snell & Janney, 2005; Thousand & Villa, 2000.

Therapist Voices: Getting in

To get involved with the team, I try to move out of discipline-specific knowledge and learn about the recent issues or ideas are in other professions so I can be more transdisciplinary. If I am entering a new school, I may target the school administrator first and offer handouts or training for the school's teachers, offer to attend child study, or write a blurb for the school newsletter related to their interests.

I become very proactive as I reach out to people and I tell them who I am and what OT can offer, and give examples of common referrals. I also ask the administrator to invite me to a schoolwide faculty meeting.

—Rebecca Argabrite Grove, administrator, occupational therapist, and assistive technology specialist, Virginia

Another approach to beginning the collaborative process is to find common ground with the teacher, as discussed by Judith Schoonover:

Collaboration in Action: Finding common ground

I begin my interactions by acknowledging the teacher or paraprofessional as a person first, and then I find common ground. As a former teacher, I understand how hard it is to teach, and I may comment on the materials he or she has developed, how the classroom is arranged, or something more personal such as talking about an item she is wearing. Soon I ask, "What would you like me to address with Jacob?" Then, "What have you tried?" If the teacher doesn't know what to do next, I describe my role as an occupational therapist or assistive technology trainer in the school.

Before I make a suggestion, I ask the teacher, "Have you heard about this approach?" If the teacher has, it affirms my recommendations and promotes buy-in for a strategy we may try together. If a teacher hasn't seen it, I will loan some information or provide a reference to look at when I leave.

—Judith Schoonover, occupational therapist and
assistive technology specialist, Virginia

Watching others collaborate helps team members understand and visualize the process of blending hands-on services, team supports, and system supports. In the scenario below, Judy Davis, an occupational therapist for five rural districts in Colorado, explains how she models collaboration for other related services providers:

Therapist Voices: Model collaboration

If at all possible, I try to get teachers and other related services personnel involved in a collaborative effort. Some teachers and therapists need to see collaboration in operation, so I volunteer to do in-services such as handwriting programs for preschool or I model how to provide services in the classroom for self-regulation or behavior management. While encouraging a speech–language pathologist (SLP) to buy into a collaborative process, I suggested we look at the teacher's thematic unit and go over each other's objectives and craft the lesson together. For example, the SLP reviews the objective with the teacher and together they figure out visual phonics, while I develop finger plays to emphasize the sounds while working on hand movements. Fairly soon, the SLP is saying, "Isn't this cool what I can do in class!"

If there is a reluctant teacher who doesn't want me in the classroom, I bring them lots of things, such as an Alphasmart [portable word processor] or a slant board or various types of writing implements that many of her students can use, not just the student in special education. After introducing these items to the teacher and students, I tell the principal, "Go see

Mrs. Crocker using the Alphasmart with her students." Soon the teacher starts asking me questions, and then we begin to share information with each other and true collaboration begins.

—Judy Davis, occupational therapist, Colorado

There are many ways to approach collaboration with different team members, and therapists need to find their signature for beginning the collaborative process. Initiating collaboration will vary according to the faces, places, and paces of the team.

Basic Communication Skills Essential for Team Membership

Hanft and Place (1996) suggested, at a minimum, using "active listening, a common language, and reading verbal and nonverbal messages appropriately" (p. 98). *Active listening* conveys an interest in another team member's ideas by restating, paraphrasing, or summarizing what was said in a nonjudgmental way. For example, a teacher may say, "Even though I give my children lots of practice, I am frustrated with how poorly they use paper and crayons. There must be something else I can do." The occupational therapist, using active listening, can reply, "If I understand you correctly, you would like some information and additional materials to help your students learn to draw more skillfully." Paraphrasing and restating work best when offered as a communication bridge to assure the speaker that the listener has not just heard, but also understood, the listener's message. Words, body language, and genuine interest in the other person facilitate effective communication. Stone, Patton, and Heen (2004) suggested that authenticity is essential for good communication because people often detect when someone is not genuine or has false intentions, no matter what they say or do.

As team members learn to read one another's verbal and nonverbal cues, they assess how well they project a positive attitude and whether others understand what they are saying. Table 3.2 provides examples of what a team member may say to support collaborative team interactions; Worksheet 3.1A (included in the Appendix) reviews interpersonal and communication skills related to problem solving and professional development.

Communicate Through a Common Language

Speaking the same language helps therapists and educators focus their expertise to promote a student's progress in acquiring the knowledge and skills specified in a school's curriculum. Using jargon-free language, occupational therapists must be able to explain how they can help students participate in school activities and learn classroom lessons. Information and recommendations can be exchanged through informal (e.g., e-mail, newsletters, fact sheets) and formal (e.g., scheduled classroom consultations, in-services, meetings) communication networks. Brief descriptions and success stories can help families who are more familiar with medical services and teachers who expect pull-out therapy to understand school-based therapy. It is usually more helpful to explain the educational relevance of occupational therapy to team members than to offer formal definitions from state practice acts or professional documents. Table 3.3 translates professional terms into language readily understood by other team members (see Table 5.1 in Chapter 5 for suggestions for describing occupational therapy services and supports).

Table 3.2. Individual Communication Skills That Promote Collaborative Teaming

Essential Skill	Example of Collaboration
Initiating: Suggesting new ideas or another way of looking at the group problem or goal; proposing new activities	"It's time to take a look at how we're meeting IEP objectives. Let's set up a time to talk about what we all are seeing."
Information seeking: Asking for relevant facts or authoritative information	"Has anyone read any studies about the effectiveness of using this intervention with students in middle school?"
Information giving: Providing relevant facts or authoritative information or relating personal experience pertinent to the group task	"I just read an article in *AJOT* about providing preschool services in the least restrictive environment. The author emphasized that we use our expertise to support children in their everyday activities, not just do a therapy session ourselves."
Opinion giving: Stating a pertinent belief or opinion about something the group is considering	"I don't know if that assessment tool will give us the information we need to review progress. How have you used it to measure progress?"
Clarifying: Probing for meaning and understanding, restating something the group is considering	"What did you mean when you said. . . ?"
Elaborating: Building on previous comments, enlarging on them, giving examples or providing additional information	"I suggested we try positioning the student in the corner chair during circle time because then she would be at the same eye level as the other kids, and they would be more likely to see her and talk to her."
Coordinating: Showing or clarifying the relationship among various ideas, trying to pull ideas, action, and suggestions together	"How about we spend 10 more minutes on this issue, and then move on to the next child up for review?"
Orienting: Defining the progress of the discussion in terms of the group's goals and raising questions about where to go	"Let's get back to the issue on the table: How can we help classroom teachers recognize the basic fine motor skills needed for learning to print?"
Testing: Checking with the group to see whether it is ready to make a decision or to take some action	"Are we sure these strategies will help the student complete the written work more legibly?"
Summarizing: Reviewing the key points or essential action steps before moving on to a new topic during team discussion	"So everyone is saying they have the 10th open at 10:00 a.m. for a joint evaluation?"

From Hanft, B., Shepherd, J., & Read, J. (in press). Competence in numbers: Working on pediatric teams. In S. Lane & A. Bundy (Eds.), *Kids can be kids: Supporting the occupations and activities of childhood.* Philadelphia: F. A. Davis. Copyright © F. A. Davis. Used with permission.

Note. IEP = individualized education program; *AJOT = American Journal of Occupational Therapy.*

For example, therapists, educators, disability advocates, and parents in Wisconsin developed a brochure describing school- and community-based occupational and physical therapy for educational personnel, health practitioners, third-party payers, and families (Judie Sage, personal communication, January 7, 2007). Their brief and concise descriptors of school-based therapy emphasize therapists' collaborative roles and summarize how occupational therapy supports and services are provided within a school setting:

- "School-based therapy is provided to assist a child with a disability to benefit from special education."

- "Therapy takes place where the child receives education. Appropriate intervention may be provided in classrooms, hallways, gyms, playgrounds, lunchrooms, bathrooms, or in a separate therapy room."

- "Collaborating with educational staff to modify the child's environment and daily school activities is always a part of school therapy."

Refer to Resource 3.4 for where to obtain this brochure.

Resource 3.4. Wisconsin Therapy Brochure

The complete text of a brochure explaining how a 10-year-old student in special education benefits from both school and community occupational and physical therapy in Wisconsin is available at www.wcdd.org/dawn/maprioauthorization/MAAR4_School_Community_Therapy.cfm. The brochure was developed by state agencies, professional organizations, and advocacy groups.

Table 3.3. A Sample Translation of Occupational Therapy Terms Into Everyday Language

Occupational Therapy Term	Everyday Language Translation
Areas of occupational performance	*School tasks:* self-care; school roles or chores (e.g., clean up, taking attendance); socialization and play skills; and volunteer, prevocational, or vocational skills
Activities of daily living, or ADLs	*Self-care skills:* dressing; feeding; grooming; toileting; and anything related to personal care devices such as glasses, hearing aids, splints, wheelchairs, crutches, and so forth
Instrumental activities of daily living, or IADLs	Chores or tasks related to homemaking or personal health care such as cooking; cleaning; shopping; using money; taking care of others; getting around the community; following safety precautions; and using the phone, computers, and any special technology
Calibrates	How hard or soft the child presses down when using a pencil or pen or when using an object (e.g., does the child tear the paper or bang the musical instrument too hard or not enough?)
Tripod grasp	Holding the pencil, pen, or marker between the index finger and the middle finger and thumb while writing
In-hand manipulation	Moving a pencil or object in the palm of one hand and between the fingers to position the object to use it (e.g., pick up a pencil to write or put coins into a drink machine)
Temporal organization	How the child sequences and follows through on completing a task. Is there order or logic in how he or she begins, organizes, and finishes the task?
Communication physicality	How the child uses his or her body when talking: eye contact, touching, using posture or gestures, or distance of body between the child and the listener
Sensory processing	How a child responds to and interprets touch, pressure, movement, smells, sounds, and visual stimuli. The child may overreact or underreact to these sensations (e.g., "that bell hurts my ears" or "push higher on that swing")

Give and Receive Feedback Willingly

A basic prerequisite for effective collaboration is a willingness to give and receive feedback from colleagues (Fishbaugh, 2000). Collaborative relationships are not directive like those of supervisor–supervisee, and team members are not responsible for evaluating or judging the work performance of others. Rather, occupational therapists and their teammates, as peer collaborators, must respect one another and learn to invite constructive feedback in a manner that signals openness (Hanft et al., 2004). Shared information and strategies should be clear, concise, and individualized to enhance a specific team member's role and promote a specific student's (or group's) learning and socialization.

The following statements underscore the give-and-take that is a vital component of peer–peer relationships:

- I enjoy being part of a school team.
- My team members are knowledgeable people I can learn from.
- I am comfortable sharing my knowledge and experience with others.
- I offer objective feedback to team members.
- I am open to suggestions from team members.
- It's helpful when a team member observes what I do and gives me feedback.

These statements about giving and receiving feedback can prompt discussion among families, therapists, and educators regarding their expectations about collaborative services for their students.

Review Team Interaction

When teams are comfortable with receiving and giving feedback, they need to routinely evaluate their interpersonal and team process skills. Through experience, team members learn about each other's communication style and how to work together as a team. It is essential to review these concepts often and reflect on what's going right and consider any changes, as needed. Thousand and Villa (2000) suggested a variety of ways to sample team process procedures and give feedback to each other (pp. 281–282):

- *Checklists:* Each member reviews, completes, and shares how the team discussion illustrates the 5- to 10-item checklist of team characteristics (see Worksheet 3.1A).

- *Turn to your neighbor:* Each person turns to an immediate neighbor and compliments him or her on a task completed or a relationship skill. For example, "You explained how to help Shanika in jargon-free language so she understood what to do!" Consider Table 3.3 when thinking about interaction skills.

- *State the group's accomplishments:* At a designated time, the team leader or member states the group's main accomplishments for the meeting.

- *Fill in incomplete sentences to describe performance:* Each team member completes a list of open-ended statements about how the team functions, for example, "Our team addresses conflict by. . . ."

- *Role evaluation:* Each team member evaluates his or her role on the team using Worksheet 3.1A.

- *Strength bombardment:* Team members give oral and written feedback to each other using positive statements, for example, "You really know how to get Jasmine working on her assignments!"

With technology capabilities changing every day, videotaping, audiotaping, and e-mailing may be used. Thousand and Villa (2000) suggested that reflection time about team processing should be built into the team agenda and recording process. Teams may use Table 3.2 to reflect individually and as a team. Prompts for reflecting on team collaboration are identified in Worksheet 3.2A (included in the Appendix). Discussing this worksheet together or completing it individually and sharing comments assists team members in systematically evaluating their collaboration with one another.

Another way to prompt a team's reflection about its collaborative process is for a team member (or a trusted outside observer) to serve as an observer of the team interaction (Johnson & Johnson, 1999). This individual observer (team members can rotate this activity) may be considered a peer coach (discussed in more detail in the next section). He or she observes and records observations of interpersonal skills and interactions that move the team forward in their discussions and actions. Often two or three interpersonal or team skills are preselected as the focus of the observation (Thousand & Villa, 2000). Use a simple recording form to note how often each skill is demonstrated and how it may be improved (e.g., "When Sheila reviewed the new IEP policy, Omar asked for clarification about recording functional performance and academic achievement"). Before sharing observations, team members are first invited to reflect on their own interactions. Encouraging individual members' reflections is an important part of a team's self-assessment process and helps all members refine their communication skills. Some school districts use a team evaluation or 360-degree feedback as part of individual performance reviews:

Therapist Voices: Evaluating performance

By obtaining information from a variety of sources (e.g., team members, students, parents, educators, other related services personnel, paraprofessionals, supervisors, principals), the occupational therapist receives valuable input about his or her ability to provide hands-on, team, and system supports. This gives the therapist or any team member a more comprehensive and valid evaluation. It is not just one person evaluating the OT but a multisource evaluation from people who interact with the therapist on a daily or weekly basis.

> —Darcie Votipka, occupational therapist and
> director of student services, Colorado

Feedback must be constructive, descriptive, and nonjudgmental. Team members practice active listening by making eye contact, using one another's names, paraphrasing messages, and sharing genuine feelings (Hanft et al., 2004).

Facilitate Team Operations

Ground rules to facilitate team operations such as collective decision making give equal footing to all team members. For example, a team leader, or principal, is expected to be on time and present for a meeting, just like other members. Occupational therapists and other related service providers may be members of numerous teams, and each team may have its own individual guidelines (team operations) and expected roles and responsibilities for members. Typical ground rules for interaction address schedules for meetings, leadership roles for team members, expected interpersonal skills, flexible communication strategies, decision making, and ways to manage conflict (DeBoer & Fister, 1995; Johnson & Johnson, 2000; Snell & Janney, 2005). Table 3.4 provides a checklist to help teams evaluate team operations.

Two essential team operations are to decide on task roles and when and how to meet. Worksheet 3.3A in the Appendix can help teams organize their meetings by recording decisions and action steps individual team members need to take. Task roles for teams are determined and defined by consensus, the skills of individual members, and the team's purpose (Thousand & Villa, 2000). Five task roles typically used by collaborative teams are facilitator, recorder, timekeeper, jargon buster, and reflector:

1. The *facilitator* begins the meeting; reviews, leads, and focuses the discussion on agenda items; and at the end of the meeting, summarizes action plans.
2. The *recorder* takes notes about who was at the meeting, who assumes what roles, what decisions or action items were decided, and what the plans are for the next meeting.
3. The *timekeeper* tells the team when the meeting should begin and end and helps keep the team on track by watching the time allotted to different agenda items.

Remember this . . .
When evaluating how well a team collaborates, the critical measure is not that the team feels they worked well together but that they can affirm that student outcomes were achieved.

4. The *jargon buster* makes sure language or information discussed is understood by all team members and calls out or rings a bell whenever professional jargon or unfamiliar terms are used. Some teams charge members
a quarter when jargon is used (Thousand & Villa, 2000).

5. The *reflector* may be a core or extended team member who reviews team
interaction, assists others in analyzing their own interactions, and gives
feedback to individual team members. Did they stay true to their purpose,
respect each other, accomplish their identified tasks, follow their rules for
engagement for communication, and efficiently conduct their business?

Thousand and Villa (2000) suggested that some teams may use other task roles
such as a harmonizer, a conflict recognizer, an encourager, or a praiser. As a group,
team members need to consider their purpose and operations to determine which
roles are needed to facilitate effective interaction.

One approach to facilitating an informed discussion among team members
about collaborative occupational therapy is to objectively review how therapists
currently use their knowledge and skills to provide team and system supports and
hands-on services. Worksheet 3.4A (located in the Appendix) can help occupational therapists identify their hands-on services and team supports for a sampling
of students. Space is also provided on the worksheet to identify the system supports provided to a school district or districts.

Team Collaboration Through Mentoring or Coaching

Therapist Voices: Help increase effectiveness

Therapists practicing in public schools need wise people who can help them
to see their roles differently and who can teach them new skills that will enable them to be increasingly effective in these new roles. (Niehues, Bundy,
Mattingly, & Lawlor, 1991, p. 209)

Table 3.4. Rules of Engagement for Team Interaction

Does Your Team Explicitly Have Rules on These Items?		Suggested Items for Consideration
Yes	No	Goals or vision of the team stated each week
Yes	No	Attendance expectations
Yes	No	Punctuality regarding when team meeting begins and ends
Yes	No	Participation of all members
Yes	No	Confidentiality
Yes	No	How each meeting will begin and end (process)
Yes	No	Sharing of responsibilities: facilitator, recorder, time keeper, agenda maker, team process observer, or similar
Yes	No	Communication and team process (expected interpersonal skills, documentation, decision making, feedback, conflict management)
Yes	No	Action plan or task assignment and follow-up

Mentoring and coaching are collaborative partnerships between two people with different levels of expertise who agree to share experiences and learn from each other (Brockbank & McGill, 2006; Hanft et al., 2004). Both partnerships are based on voluntary engagement in a relationship that involves guiding another person to acquire new or refine current skills, knowledge, and experiences. Coaches focus primarily on reflection and self-discovery as the means to enhance a *partner's* performance and learning, and mentors share their knowledge and wisdom with a *protégé* through counseling and networking as well as coaching (Clutterbuck, 1991; Megginson & Clutterbuck, 2004).

Both mentoring and coaching are effective approaches to providing team and system supports in education settings, and they typically individualize information and resources to address the goals, learning style, and role of each protégé or partner. Although coaches and mentors transfer knowledge and information similar to a teacher, they usually share their expertise through individual relationships rather than presenting a course, in-service, or workshop to a group, whose members must then apply the new information to their own situation. This individualized guidance and support is a critical feature of both coaching and mentoring.

Another important function is to orient a new, or assist a seasoned, team member in understanding the influence of a school's culture on team roles and interactions. For example, how is a principal or school superintendent addressed? Are team meetings usually formal or informal? Are all team members expected to participate in the parent–teacher association or supervise extracurricular activities? What are the unspoken rules for team interaction? Their mutually beneficial relationship helps both the mentor–coach and the protégé–partner reframe events from another point of view. Professional growth is encouraged through observation, modeling, demonstration, sharing print and Internet resources, building professional and support networks, and perhaps pursuing further education. Mentoring and coaching promote the development of professional and personal skills through a focus on a protégé's or partner's self-concept, motivation, knowledge, performance, and competence. Table 3.5 identifies typical roles and effective characteristics of mentors–coaches and protégés–partners. Refer to Reflection 3.4 and consider which of those characteristics are most important to you.

Reflection 3.4

What Do You Want in a Mentor or Coach?

Consider the characteristics of mentors–coaches and protégés–partners identified in Table 3.5. If you were to choose or become a mentor or a coach, which characteristics would be most important to you as a mentor–coach or as a protégé–partner?

Table 3.5. Characteristics of Effective Mentors–Coaches and Protégés–Partners

Relationship or Role	Personal Qualities
Mentors emphasize advising and counseling. *Coaches* emphasize facilitating and reflecting. Both are guides, supporters, communicators, and role models. Neither are supervisors.	• Excellent interpersonal and communication skills • Motivate others to refine knowledge and experience • Willing to share expertise, resources, and networks • Respect individual learning styles and cultural backgrounds • Caring • Honest
Protégés or *partners* are learners, advocates, colleagues, and team members.	• Observe and ask questions • Receptive to feedback • Willing to assess ideas and actions through reflection • Articulate goals and action steps • Elaborates or clarifies ideas

In schools, mentoring and coaching may occur between occupational therapists, formally or informally, and often help perpetuate the culture of the team as informal or unstated rules, values, or expectations are shared. Mentoring and coaching may also occur across professions, teams, or schools. An occupational therapist and another team member such as a parent, special education teacher, general education teacher, a physical therapist, a speech–language pathologist, an administrator, or a guidance counselor may collaborate to mentor or coach one another. The following vignette illustrates how an occupational therapist increased the skills and confidence of a special education teacher.

Therapist Voices: Coaching confidence

I remember the first day Nettie came to our class. Every part of her body was strapped to the wheelchair, and she could not talk or move by herself. Her gorgeous smile engaged me, but I was scared to death that I would break this frail child. I didn't understand her noises or why she moved so much while she was sitting in the wheelchair. Thank goodness Tammy, an OT, and Nancy, an SLP, supported me in my classroom. They observed Nettie, listened to my fears, and helped me and the classroom aide learn transfers and interpret and use Nettie's movements or sounds as communication. Tammy coached us every week on different things to do with Nettie and was supportive of our attempts. About 2 months into the year, both the aide and I were totally comfortable with having Nettie as part of our class.

—Jayne Shepherd, former special educator
and occupational therapist, Virginia

Promotion of Communication Through Coaching

Therapist Voices: Encouraging reflection

I try to be flexible and stay involved with the team by asking reflective questions. This allows team members to experience their own self-discovery about what works, and then they too are invested in being part of the team.

—Rebecca Argabrite Grove, administrator, occupational therapist,
and assistive technology specialist, Virginia

Prompting reflection is a unique element of coaching and assists a protégé or partner who works in a school setting to assess and refine practices and behaviors to improve students' academic and functional performance. A coach must learn to ask the right questions, at the right time, and in the right way (Kinlaw, 1999). Table 3.6 provides examples of three kinds of reflective questions: objective, comparative, and interpretive. Reflective questions typically begin with *wh*—for example, *who, what, when,* and *where*—or *how*. Beginning a question with *why* tends to place blame or imply something was done incorrectly and should be avoided. In addition to their content expertise in school-based practice, coaches and mentors are experienced in the art of collaboration, specifically, in promoting another person's development through observing, listening, responding, and planning, as described below (Hanft et al., 2004).

Table 3.6. Asking Reflective Questions

Information Elicited	Examples
Objective questions elicit information.	What did you want to happen? What are you doing now? What have you tried? When does this behavior occur? Who is involved? What evidence is there to support a specific intervention?
Comparative questions prompt reflection on situations.	How does this [intervention, student, environment] compare to . . .? How have you worked previously with a similar student [colleague]? On the basis of what you know now (from reading, discussion, observation), what would you do differently next time?
Interpretive questions solicit hypotheses about actions and interactions.	What does it mean when she . . . ? What would you do if . . . ? When would be a good time to . . . ?

Observation occurs in four patterns:

1. A coach–mentor observes a partner–protégé interact with a student or team member.
2. A partner–protégé observes a coach–mentor model an intervention or interaction.
3. A partner–protégé engages in self-observation via reflection or reviewing an audio- or videotape with a coach–mentor.
4. Both parties observe a student in a school place or space (an ecological assessment) and reflect together on their observations.

Listening objectively and respectfully to a partner–protégé is essential for prompting his or her reflection about assumptions, perceptions, knowledge, and hypotheses related to student (and team member) behavior, interaction, and performance. Listening depends on attending fully to another person's words, meanings, and feelings without passing judgment; acknowledging the person's message with verbal and nonverbal responses; and associating the message to evidence-based practices, a school's mission, and the mutually agreed-on goals.

Responding refers to sharing information and feedback in just the right amounts at selected times to support and build the partner–protégé's knowledge and skills. Coaches and mentors respond to learners by

- Asking questions that clarify a partner's–protégé's statements or request further information (e.g., *Partner:* "Teachers prefer me to take students out of the classroom"; *Coach:* Tell me about the teachers who request this");
- Summarizing discussion and planning future directions;
- Sharing feedback, information, resources, and support; and
- Engaging a partner–protégé in deciding how to cope with specific concerns and issues.

Planning can involve actions or strategies for a partner–protégé to initiate before the next coaching meeting (e.g., visit an online site, read an article, collect data about a student's behavior, try a different strategy with a student, observe a colleague using the suggested strategy). In the following scenario, Kathleen, a special education resource teacher, describes how Pam, the occupational therapist, observed, listened, and responded to her concerns about Benjamin, and together they planned the next step:

Teacher Voices: Building skills together

Pam, the OT, sees things that I sometimes miss when I'm co-teaching in a general education classroom. For example, Benjamin had trouble copying sentences from the board and was getting frustrated with his in-class work. Together, Pam and I observed him during fourth-grade social studies. Pam immediately saw that his seat placement was obstructing his view of the blackboard/screen and his seat was too big for him! Together, we considered other seating options and discussed how each change would affect his vision, his ability to attend, and his socialization with peers. During a classroom break, we shared our observations with Jana, the classroom teacher, and she agreed to try a different seat placement for Benjamin.

A week after Benjamin's seat was changed, Pam checked back with me to see if his on-task behaviors and copying from the board had improved. We had expected more improvement than our data demonstrated, so we brainstormed some other ideas, and an air cushion, [elastic band] stretched on the bottom of the chair, and scheduled movement breaks were then incorporated into Benjamin's daily routine. Voila. . . . We had the right combination of environmental adaptations to engage Benjamin in learning! My understanding of possible physical adaptations in the general education classroom as well as the use of sensory breaks has expanded. Now, thanks to Pam's coaching, Benjamin is progressing but so are my observation skills and ability to problem solve when I enter a classroom.

—Kathleen Morra-Sloan, special education resource teacher, Virginia

Informal Models for Mentoring and Coaching New Professionals

When a therapist is a recent graduate or new to school-based practice, a call or visit to another school-based therapist, former fieldwork supervisor, or college professor can provide a practical orientation to working in education settings. Therapists may ask, "What assessments do you use and why?" "Can I observe your work with students in the assistive technology lab?" or "How do you share information with your special education supervisor?" These conversations help clarify a therapist's professional identity and role on a team. This informal interaction occurs when a new-to-school practitioner chooses a team member (or effective practitioner elsewhere in the school district) to emulate or discuss concerns and ideas. Occasionally, this person is not even aware that he or she has been placed in a mentor or coach role. Fieldwork I or II supervisors and their coworkers who have established collegial relationships with students often offer informal coaching or mentoring experiences to them, especially after they are no longer in a supervisory role (Nolinski, 1995).

In Wisconsin, Judie Sage (personal communication, January 3, 2007) arranges for teachers to mentor occupational therapy students. Early in their school fieldwork experience, the occupational therapy students spend a few days shadowing various teachers during the day and compare roles and responsibilities across the education curriculum and in different grades. The teachers informally mentor the occupational therapy students about communicating with them and other team members and how to provide meaningful supports within the classroom. Sometimes an occupational therapy student continues a relationship with a specific teacher if a personal connection was made during their observation and dialogue. Refer to Reflection 3.5, and consider your experiences and preferences as a protégé, mentor, or coach.

Formal Mentoring–Coaching Programs

In some school systems and in some states, new teachers and related services personnel are supported by a formal mentoring–coaching program. Mentoring or coaching is often used as a retention strategy to avoid high therapist turnover. Sometimes a state department of education initiates a program to mentor or coach new employees. Some recent graduates or therapists new to schools prefer mentors or coaches who are not on their school team or even in their school system. This approach creates opportunities to ask questions, admit mistakes, or solve challenging team situations without losing face with current team members. However, an external mentor or coach may not understand all the expectations or policies of a protégé's or partner's school. As protégés or partners gain confidence, they may ask their own team members to mentor or coach them.

A formal mentor–coach program orients all participants to the process and pairs them based on expertise and desired goals, personal characteristics, and responses to a preliminary questionnaire. An agreement about the roles and responsibilities of the mentor–coach and protégé–partner is formalized in writing, and there is always an option to end the relationship if it is not working for either party. Some formal programs have guidelines regarding how often and how long a mentor and protégé will work together and how they will record their experience. Figure 3.2 illustrates how to establish a formal mentoring–coaching program and facilitate effective relationships between mentors–coaches and protégés–partners.

University Mentoring Program

A formal mentorship program was developed by Virginia Commonwealth University's Department of Occupational Therapy and the Virginia Department of Education when they collaborated on submitting an interdisciplinary grant to prepare occupational and physical therapists to work in the public schools. Funding from the Department of Education covered tuition for entry-level and postprofessional students to complete three or four school-related courses and to participate in a mentorship experience. The mentorship program provided in-services for both the mentors and the protégés about how to use mentoring to promote professional and personal growth, and it arranged a communication network for mentors and protégés for the year after graduation. At the end of the mentoring program, 64% of protégés ($n = 16$) agreed that their mentor relationship influenced their decision to continue working in schools (others commented that they had already planned to work in the schools). The top four topics discussed between mentors and protégés were intervention strategies, evaluation and assessment, educationally relevant objectives and activities, and school politics (Shannon & Shepherd, 1999).

Reflection 3.5

What Is Your Experience as a Protégé–Partner or Mentor–Coach?

- Have you ever engaged in mentoring–coaching? Who was your mentor–coach?

- How did you find this person?

- What characteristics of your mentor–coach did you find helpful?

- Do you mentor–coach another person in your school district?

Step 1: Develop a Mentoring–Coaching Program

- Articulate vision and goals of program.
- Clarify procedures (e.g., selecting mentors–coaches, orientation training, roles and responsibilities, confidentiality).
- Obtain funding, if possible, for training materials, meetings, and networking.
- Solicit participants using separate questionnaires for the mentor–coach and partner–protégé (e.g., identify availability, expertise, goals).
- Orient participants to the mentoring–coaching program.

Step 2: Establish a Relationship

- Match mentor–protégé or coach–partner.
- Share professional backgrounds.
- Discuss expectations and availability of both parties.
- Identify areas of need, and develop a written plan specifying protégés'–partners' goals with criteria for success.

Step 3: Implement the Mentoring–Coaching Program

- Observe, listen, and share concerns and reactions.
- Provide continuous feedback to each other.
- Reinforce positive and effective achievements.
- Offer support to protégé–partner via phone, e-mail, and in-person meetings.
- Discuss the culture and organization of the educational environment.

Step 4: Cultivate Collegial Relationships Among Mentoring–Coaching Pairs

- Share stories and support each other.
- Encourage continual participation in challenging developmental activities.
- Promote relationships with other educational personnel and networks.

Step 5: Evaluate Relationship and Program

- Collect feedback via surveys (e.g., focus groups, phone interviews) about the mentor–coach program.
- Incorporate changes for future programs.

Figure 3.2. Steps for establishing a mentoring–coaching program.

State Department of Education Mentoring Program

The Colorado State Department of Education requires all occupational therapists to obtain a special service providers license and participate in a state-mandated induction program if they are recent graduates, therapists entering school-based practice from a medical model, or therapists from other states or districts who have already worked in school-based practice. The structure of Colorado's mentoring program is described below:

Administrator Voices: Support through mentorship

Mentor induction is the responsibility of the local hiring agent and is implemented differently by each school district. Induction criteria for mentors and protégés may include activities, such as protégés submitting portfolios that document professional growth, mandatory attendance at district-sponsored workshops, mandatory ongoing meetings between mentors and protégés, and logs or journals kept by mentors and protégés to validate the partnership.

Mentors and protégés usually communicate through e-mail or phone, but meeting in person is always the first choice and a top priority.

In Poudre School District, Colorado, every new certified employee (e.g., teachers, counselors, school psychologists, OTs, PTs [physical therapists], social workers, nurses) is given a paid one-on-one mentor to provide supports in professional practice during their first year. A new OT would have the support of a fellow OT. The mentor and protégé define their focus and set up their own meeting schedule. This information is made formal in an action plan given to me [the mentor coordinator]. Along with great professional advice, new folks also receive wonderful emotional support. I love my work!

—Mary Hasl, Poudre School District mentor coordinator, Colorado

The district's mentoring program document (Poudre School District, 2006) has identified a mission, vision, values and a variety of strategies to provide professional development opportunities and supports for mentor–protégé relationships. This school district also recognizes mentoring as a recruitment and retention strategy for keeping personnel. The program includes focus groups, a bank of expertise for training, book study groups, in-service presentations, an annual day-long academy, and quarterly assessments of the program. The collaborative practices of mentors and protégés are also highlighted on the district's educational channel. Resource 3.5 identifies additional online resources for developing mentoring or coaching programs.

Vignette: Will a Mentor Help?

In the following vignette, consider how the team could support Clarissa through a mentor or coaching program:

Collaboration in Action: Supporting team members

Clarissa, a registered occupational therapist, has joined the rural school district staff. She inherited the schools, teachers, and children from another therapist, who was well liked and had worked for 12 years with most of the staff. As the first month of school ends, you hear rumors that Clarissa feels very lonely and is contemplating changing jobs before the school year even ends.

Finding Clarissa a mentor or coach within the school district will build connectedness to the team and system. In small or rural school systems, it is imperative to remember that this person should not be Clarissa's supervisor. A fellow occupational therapy employee (with similar interests and, if possible, near her age) may serve as Clarissa's coach to learn how to provide team and hands-on services within her school district. By observing each other and by responding to objective, comparative, and interpretative prompts, Clarissa reflects on and delineates what she wants to be able to do. In addition, she may review the AOTA *Professional Development Tool* (2003) to focus her concerns.

A core team member from another profession may also coach or mentor Clarissa about the structure and

Resource 3.5. Mentoring and Coaching
- *The Mentoring Group:* www.mentoringgroup.com/
- *Mentoring Leadership and Resource Network:* www.mentors.net/index.html
- *Best practices resources:* www.teachermentors.com/
- *Coaching and mentoring:* www.coachingandmentoring.com/Articles/mentoring.html

operations of her team. Sharing resources across disciplines or school districts may aid in the implementation of a mentoring and coaching program in a rural setting and hopefully encourage and retain therapists to practice in the schools. As occupational therapists enter the schools or change jobs or roles within the schools, team structure and a support network (e.g., coach, mentor, team celebrations) become essential for collaboration.

Summary

This chapter has focused on the interactive team process that is the center of school-based collaboration. Six major characteristics of collaboration are key to building team structure: (1) voluntary participation, (2) equality among members, (3) common purpose, (4) joint responsibility for outcomes, (5) shared resources, and (6) collective decision making (DeBoer & Fister, 1995). Examples of decision-making models and strategies that have been highlighted are initiating collaboration, using effective communication techniques, giving and receiving feedback, and reviewing team interaction. In addition, mentoring and coaching strategies to support new graduates or therapists now working in the schools have been discussed. The following comment from a school therapist reinforces the basic message of this chapter—that teamwork is more satisfying and effective in promoting students' participation in school than is acting as a "Lone Therapist":

Therapist Voices: Teamwork in preschool

My best example of collaboration is when our school began a new preschool program. Immediately, the early childhood special education teacher wanted to collaborate and try a transdisciplinary program as was done at her previous job. All of the team members (OT, PT, teacher, SLP) agreed to co-teach lessons once a week while being coached by this teacher. We committed to meeting once a week to develop a week's worth of lessons, which we shared with each other. I was responsible for running circle time and center time on Tuesdays. As I taught the group, the teacher, the classroom aide, and the other related services personnel learned how to use my suggestions in everyday activities, and all of us learned from each other.

Remember this . . .
Teamwork is more satisfying and effective in promoting students' participation in school than acting as a "Lone Therapist."

It was strange at first, and some therapists became a little territorial. But once involved, we all realized that because you are an OT, it doesn't mean you don't speak or if you are a speech–language pathologist, it doesn't mean that you don't combine hand skills with activities to learn about sounds and letters. Soon, all the different lessons became such a blur that an outsider would not know who was what profession. We respected and shared knowledge with each other for the benefit of the children. Such teamwork!

—Patty Vesper, occupational therapist,
New Jersey

Acknowledgments

This chapter was produced in collaboration with Judith Schoonover, Marita Villegas, Judy Davis, Darcie Votipka, Rebecca Argabrite Grove, Maria Mendoza-Smith,

Mary Hasl, Patty Vesper, Judie Sage, Jan Emerick-Brothers, Ilene Banker, and Kathleen Morra-Sloan.

Thanks to all for being team players and not lone rangers!

Selected Resources

Giangreco, M. (www.uvm.edu/~mgiangre/)
> Michael Giangreco is an educator and professor at the University of Vermont. His numerous research projects involve assessment development of the Vermont Interdependent Services Team Approach (VISTA) and Choosing Outcomes and Accommodations for Children (COACH), related services personnel, paraprofessionals, making IEP decisions, and providing services to students with severe or multiple disabilities. This Web site includes articles to download and books to order.

Hanft, B. K., Rush, D. D., & Shelden, M. L. (2004). *Coaching families and colleagues in early childhood.* Baltimore: Paul H. Brookes.
> Written by an occupational therapist, a physical therapist, and a speech–language pathologist, seven chapters discuss the coaching process, evidence for coaching, and effective qualities of coaches. Specific strategies for coaching families, colleagues, and staff of early care and education programs are illustrated in numerous coaching stories, and the Coaching Skills Rating Scale, a self-assessment, is organized by four essential coaching skills: observing, listening, responding, and planning.

Hayden, P., Frederick, L., Smith, B., & Broudy, A. (2001). *Tasks, tips, and tools for promoting collaborative community teams: Collaborative Planning Project for Planning Comprehensive Early Childhood Systems.* Denver: University of Colorado. Retrieved January 7, 2007, from www.nectac.org/~pdfs/topics/inclusion/TasksTipsTools.pdf
> This collaborative project from the Denver area collated documents from a variety of programs and developed a manual to help teams begin the collaborative process. Tips include how to recruit and organize a team, sample ground rules and tracking forms, action plans, and a variety of activities to focus the team. Any of the forms or activities may be copied or changed without permission from the authors.

Villa, R., & Thousand, J. (Eds.). (2000). *Restructuring for caring and effective education* (2nd ed.). Baltimore: Paul H. Brookes.
> Villa and Thousand have collected works from educators and researchers throughout the country to describe practical ways to facilitate successful inclusion in educational settings. Sections in the book include the purpose of schooling, curriculum, instruction and assessment, emerging roles, examples in action, and future directions and reflections. Two chapters of particular interest to occupational therapists are "Collaborative Teaming" and "Related Services Personnel in Public Schools."

References

Accreditation Council for Occupational Therapy Education. (2006). *2006 ACOTE accreditation standards and interpretive guidelines.* Bethesda, MD: Author. Retrieved June 21, 2007, from www.aota.org/nonmembers/area13/links/LINK13.asp

American Occupational Therapy Association. (2003, May). *Professional development tool.* Bethesda, MD: Author. Retrieved September 3, 2006, from www.aota.org/pdf

American Occupational Therapy Association. (2004). *Guidelines for supervision, roles, and responsibilities during the delivery of occupational therapy services.* Bethesda, MD: Author. Retrieved September 4, 2006, from www.aota.org/Practitioners/Resources/Docs/Popular/36202.aspx

Block, M., & Chandler, B. (2005, January 24). Understanding the challenge: Occupational therapy and our schools [Continuing Education]. *OT Practice,* pp. CE1–CE8.

Brockbank, A., & McGill, I. (2006). *Facilitating reflective learning through mentoring and coaching.* Philadelphia: Kogan Page.

Case-Smith, J. (1997). Variables related to successful school-based practice. *Occupational Therapy Journal of Research, 17,* 133–153.

Chandler, B. (2007). Classroom clinic: IEP goals, but not an OT goal in sight. *Advance for Occupational Therapy Practitioners, 23*(20), 16.

Clutterbuck, D. (1991). *Everyone needs a mentor.* London: Institute of Personnel Development.

Comings, J., Garner, B., & Smith, C. (2007). *Review of adult learning and literacy, Volume 7: Connecting research, policy, and practice.* Boston: World Education.

DeBoer, A., & Fister, S. (1995). *Working together: Tools for collaborative teaching.* Longmont, CO: Sopris West.

Demchak, M., Alden, P., Bergin, C., Ting, S., & Lacey, S. (1995). Evaluating transdisciplinary teaming for student with disabilities. *Rural Special Education Quarterly, 14*(1), 24–32.

Dettmer, P., Thurston, L., & Sellberg, N. J. (2005). *Consultation, collaboration, and teamwork for students with special needs* (5th ed.). Boston: Allyn & Bacon.

Dillon, M., Flexman, C., & Probeck, L. (1996). *Examining the role of the occupational therapist and the educator in the transition planning process.* Unpublished master's research project, Virginia Commonwealth University, Richmond.

Dinnebeil, L. A., Hale, S., & Rule, S. (1996). A qualitative analysis of parents' and service coordinators' description of variables that influence collaborative relationships. *Topics in Early Childhood Special Education, 16,* 322–347.

Dunn, W. (2000). *Best practice occupational therapy: In community service with children and families.* Thorofare, NJ: Slack.

Falvey, M., Forest, J., Pearpoint, J., & Rosenbury, R. (2004). *All my life's a circle: Using the tools: Circles, MAPS, and PATHS.* Toronto: Inclusion Press.

Fishbaugh, M. S. (2000). *The collaboration guide for early career educators.* Baltimore: Paul H. Brookes.

Folio, M. R., & Fewell, R. R. (2000). *Peabody Developmental Motor Scale* (2nd ed.). Austin, TX: Pro-Ed.

Friend, M., & Cook, L. (2007). *Interactions: Collaboration skills for school professionals* (5th ed.). Boston: Allyn & Bacon.

Giangreco, M. F. (1995). Related services decision-making: A foundational component of effective education for students with disabilities. *Physical and Occupational Therapy in Pediatrics, 15*(2), 47–67.

Giangreco, M. (1996). *Vermont Interdependent Services Team Approach (VISTA).* Baltimore: Paul H. Brookes.

Giangreco, M. F. (2001). Interactions among program, placement, and services in educational planning for students with disabilities. *Mental Retardation, 39,* 341–350.

Giangreco, M. F., Cloninger, C. J., Dennis, R. G., & Edelman, S. W. (2000). Problem-solving methods to facilitate inclusive education. In R. A. Villa & J. A. Thousand (Eds.), *Restructuring for caring and effective education* (2nd ed., pp. 293–327). Baltimore: Paul H. Brookes.

Giangreco, M. F., Cloninger, C. J., Dennis, R., & Edelman, S. W. (2002). Problem-solving methods to facilitate inclusive education. In J. S. Thousand, R. A. Villa, & A. I. Nevin (Eds.), *Creativity and collaborative learning: The practical guide to empowering students, teachers, and families* (pp. 111–134). Baltimore: Paul H. Brookes.

Giangreco, M. F., Edelman, S., & Dennis, R. (1991). Common professional practices that interfere with the integrated delivery of related services. *Remedial and Special Education, 12*(2), 16–24.

Giangreco, M., Prelock, P. A., Reid, R. R., Dennis, R. E., & Edelman, S. W. (2000). Roles of related services personnel in inclusive schools. In R. Villa & J. Thousand (Eds.), *Restructuring for caring and effective education: Piecing the puzzle together* (2nd ed., pp. 360–388). Baltimore: Paul H. Brookes.

Giangreco, M., St. Denis, R., Cloninger, C., Edelman, S., & Schattman, R. (1993). "I've counted Jon": Transformational experiences of teachers educating students with disabilities. *Exceptional Children, 59,* 359–371.

Hanft, B., & Place, P. (1996). *The consulting therapist.* Austin, TX: Pro-Ed.

Hanft, B. K., Rush, D. D., & Shelden, M. L. (2004). *Coaching families and colleagues in early childhood.* Baltimore: Paul H. Brookes.

Hanft, B., Shepherd, J., & Read, J. (in press). Competence in numbers: Working on pediatric teams. In S. Lane & A. Bundy (Eds.), *Kids can be kids: Supporting the occupations and activities of childhood.* Philadelphia: F. A. Davis.

Hargreaves, A. (1994). *Changing teachers, changing times.* New York: Teachers College Press.

Jackson, L. L. (Ed.). (2007). *Occupational therapy services for children and youth under IDEA* (3rd ed.). Bethesda, MD: AOTA Press.

Johnson, D. W., & Johnson, R. T. (1999). *Learning together and alone: Cooperative, competitive and individualistic learning* (5th ed.). Needham Heights, MA: Allyn & Bacon.

Johnson, D. W. & Johnson, R. T. (2000). *Joining together: Group theory and group skills* (7th ed.). Boston: Allyn & Bacon.

Johnston, J., Knight, M., & Miller, L. (2007). Finding time for teams: Student achievement grows as district support boosts collaboration. *Journal of Staff Development, 28*(2), 14–18.

Khorsheed, K. (2007). Four places to dig deep: To find more time for teacher collaboration. *Journal of Staff Development, 28*(2), 43–45.

Kinlaw, D. C. (1999). *Coaching for commitment: Interpersonal strategies for obtaining superior performance from individuals and teams.* San Francisco: Jossey-Bass/Pfeiffer.

Knippenberg, C., & Hanft, B. (2004). The key to educational relevance: Occupation throughout the school day. *School System Special Interest Section Quarterly, 11*(4), 1–4.

Knowles, M., Holton, E., & Swanson, R. (2005). *The adult learner: The definitive class in adult education and human resource development* (6th ed.). Woburn, MA: Butterworth-Heinemann.

Megginson, D., & Clutterbuck, D. (2004). *Techniques for mentoring and coaching.* New York: Elsevier.

Niehues, A., Bundy, A., Mattingly, C., & Lawlor, M. (1991). Making a difference: Occupational therapy in the public schools. *Occupational Therapy Journal of Research, 11*(4), 195–212.

Nolinski, T. (1995). Multiple mentoring relationships facilitate learning during fieldwork. *American Journal of Occupational Therapy, 49*, 39–43.

Odom, S. L., Boyd, B., & Buysse, V. (2007). *Promising practices to support effective early childhood inclusion for Pre-K to Grade 3.* In V. Buysse & L. Aytch (Eds.), *Early school success: Equity and access for diverse learners* (Executive Summary, FirstSchool Diversity Symposium, pp. 14–17). Chapel Hill: University of North Carolina, FPG Child Development Institute. Retrieved November 2, 2007, from www.fpg.unc.edu/~firstschool/assets/FirstSchool_Symposium_ExectuiveSummary_2007.pdf

Pearpoint, J., O'Brien, J., & Forest, M. (1995). *PATH: A workbook for planning positive possible futures: Planning alternative tomorrows with hope for schools, organizations, businesses, families.* Toronto: Inclusion Press.

Polichino, J. (2004). Moving out of the "therapy room." In Y. Swinth (Ed.), *Occupational therapy in school-based practice: Contemporary issues and trends* (AOTA Online Course, Lesson 7). Bethesda, MD: American Occupational Therapy Association.

Polichino, J., Clark, G., & Chandler, B. (2005, February 21). Supporting students in the natural environment. *OT Practice*, pp. 11–15.

Poudre School District. (2006). *Poudre School District mentoring program, 2006–2007.* Unpublished manuscript, Fort Collins, CO.

Rafoth, M. A., & Foriska, T. (2006). Administrator participation in promoting effective problem solving teams. *Remedial and Special Education, 27*(3), 130–135.

Rainforth, B., & York-Barr, J. (1997). *Collaborative teams for students with severe disabilities* (2nd ed.). Baltimore: Paul H. Brookes.

Salisbury, C. L., & McGregor, G. (2002). The administrative climate and context of inclusive schools. *Exceptional Children, 68*(2), 259–274.

Shannon, P., & Shepherd, J. (1999). *Mentorship program results for the interdisciplinary school-based training program for occupational and physical therapists.* Richmond: Virginia Commonwealth University.

Snell, M., & Janney, R. (2005). *Collaborative teaming* (2nd ed.). Baltimore: Paul H. Brookes.

Stone, D., Patton, B., & Heen, S. (2004). *Difficult conversations: How to discuss what matters most.* Boston: Penguin.

Swinth, Y., Hanft, B., DiMatties, M., Handley-More, D., Hanson, P., Schoonover, J., et al. (2002, September 16). School-based practice: Moving beyond 1:1 service delivery. *OT Practice*, pp. 12–16.

Thousand, J., & Villa, R. (2000). Collaborative teaming: A powerful tool in school restructuring. In R. Villa & J. Thousand (Eds.), *Restructuring for caring and effective education* (2nd ed., pp. 254–291). Baltimore: Paul H. Brookes.

Villa, R., Thousand, J., Nevin, A., & Malgeri, C. (1996). Instilling collaboration for inclusive schooling as a way of doing business in public education. *Remedial and Special Education, 17*, 169–181.

Wiggins, K., & Damore, S. (2006). "Survivors" or "friends"? A framework for assessing effective collaboration. *Teaching Exceptional Children, 38*, 49–56.

CHAPTER 4

Getting Into a
Collaborative School Routine

Gloria Frolek Clark, MS, OTR/L, BCP, FAOTA

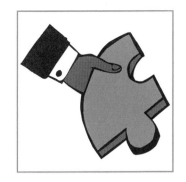

Collaboration needs to be on a regular and weekly basis, and involve co-working with children as well as time for mutual knowledge exchange.

—Priest & Waters, 2007, p. 146

As occupational therapists work with people across the life cycle, they have an incredibly important and challenging role in enhancing their clients' ability to engage and participate in meaningful activities and occupations. Activities are "a class of human actions that are goal directed" (American Occupational Therapy Association [AOTA], 2002, p. 630); those with meaning and value to the person are considered *occupations*. In an educational setting, occupational therapists focus on helping students participate in meaningful and purposeful daily occupations that make them successful and engaged in school life (Swinth, Chandler, Hanft, Jackson, & Shepherd, 2003).

After reading this material, readers will be able to

- Recognize the *Occupational Therapy Practice Framework: Domain and Process* (the *Framework;* AOTA, 2002) as a foundation for collaborating with team members to provide occupational therapy supports and services;

- Identify strategies for collaboration during evaluation, intervention, and ongoing assessment and reassessment;

- Recognize hands-on services and team and system supports in a variety of school places; and

- Choose a broad array of occupational therapy interventions in inclusive school environments.

Key Topics

- School-based occupational therapy

- Applying the *Occupational Therapy Practice Framework: Domain and Process* in education settings

- Early intervening services (EISs)

- Collaboration during evaluation, assessment, and intervention

Occupational Therapy's Role in Education Settings

Seven areas of occupation are described in the *Framework:* activities of daily living (ADLs), instrumental ADLs, education, work, play, leisure, and social participation (AOTA, 2002). Table 4.1 identifies the school-related outcomes of each area of occupation. In education settings, occupational therapists may address one or more areas of occupation as related to each student's academic achievement and functional

Table 4.1. School-Related Occupations Addressed During Occupational Therapy Assessment and Intervention

Areas of Occupation	Educational Outcomes
Activities of daily living	Cares for basic self-needs in school (e.g., eating, toileting, moving around building, managing shoes and coats).
Instrumental activities of daily living	Uses communication devices to interact with others, able to access bus for school, and recognizes unsafe environment.
Education	Participates in a learning environment including academic (e.g., math, reading), nonacademic (e.g., lunch, recess), prevocational, and vocational activities.
Work	Develops interests, habits, and skills necessary for engaging in work or volunteer activities for transition to community life on graduation from school.
Play	Identifies and engages in age-appropriate toys, games, and nonacademic experiences (e.g., sports).
Leisure	Identifies and engages in appropriate and intrinsically motivating activities (e.g., listening to music, exploring the Internet) during time not committed to other occupations.
Social participation	Develops appropriate school relationships with peers, teachers, and other educational personnel within classroom, extracurricular and preparation for work activities.

performance in school and his or her desired outcomes. Those outcomes are expressed as goals on an individualized education program (IEP).

The education area of occupation includes academic, nonacademic, extracurricular, and vocational participation. As identified in Figure 4.1, occupational therapists may address specific skills, such as attention to task, access to education (e.g., using computers, positioning devices, materials), literacy skills, routines and habits for initiation and continuation of tasks, interaction with peers, work completion, and following school rules. Educators are vitally interested in these skills because they form the foundation for how well a student performs in the school setting across academic, nonacademic, prevocational, and vocational areas. Within each area, therapists may view the activity demands, the student's performance skills and performance habits, and the client factors (e.g., body functions and structures) that affect performance for each student.

As discussed in Chapter 2, when therapists are present in school spaces (e.g., the classroom, cafeteria, gymnasium, playground), they are able to observe students' occupations or activities in context. Information such as a teacher's instructional style and expectations, the school curriculum, and peer performance are available to therapists as they observe or work with the student in the natural routine of the classroom and other school contexts. Table 4.2 illustrates the physical environments in which students engage in school occupations each day.

Although therapists frequently manipulate the physical environment to enhance performance, they may overlook the social environment and temporal context. School buildings and classrooms have their own unique environments that

Tasks	Routines and Habits	Socialization, Play, and Leisure
• Completes classroom lessons. • Completes school chores (e.g., line leader, feed the pets, office errand, other jobs). • Participates in school, community, and work activities (e.g., recess, assemblies, extracurricular activities, school sports events). • Follows classroom rules.	• Develops routines and organizes self to participate in the school environment. • Organizes school or work materials. • Uses appropriate work habits. • Manages free-choice time. • Listens or records directions given. • Finishes what is started.	• Engages in play and leisure activities. • Socializes with peers and makes friends. • Interacts with teachers and other adults. • Respects other people, their belongings, and school property. • Participates in group activities without interrupting others. • Uses self-control to manage frustrations and other emotions. • Transitions between classes and when there is a change in tasks.

Figure 4.1. Skills and behaviors that support a student's role in school.

From Shepherd, J., Peters, S., Weise, C., Lowman, D. K., & Hatcher, B. (1999). *Therapy activities for the classroom.* Richmond: Virginia Commonwealth University. Copyright © 1999 by Virginia Commonwealth University. Adapted with permission.

have specific social and cultural expectations, typically set by the principal. Understanding the rules, whether written or unwritten, enables therapists to help students blend into the routines or pace of their school day more easily. Social expectations are evident in the classroom as students interact with peers and adults and attempt to follow routines while fulfilling the student role. The number of students and their personal characteristics (e.g., whether the students are verbal, aggressive, friendly, competitive, or fearful) may influence the type and number of social interactions within the classroom. As discussed in Chapter 3, the temporal context (i.e., the time of day) can be very important for therapists to consider when providing hands-on services and team supports. For instance,

Reflection
4.1

What Supports Have You Provided?

Select a student and think about the team and system supports that you have provided to assist him or her to participate successfully in the physical contexts identified in Table 4.2.

- Is the student more alert and ready for learning in the morning or afternoon?
- Are there more instances of inappropriate behavior just before lunch, when the student is hungry?
- Does the student perform better on handwriting tasks after he or she has been playing on the playground?
- If the student takes medication, do the effects wear off at a certain time?

Occupational therapists should collaborate with educational staff and parents to modify and adapt the temporal environment to enhance student performance. Reflection 4.1 provides an opportunity to consider how team and system supports help students participate in school environments.

Collaboration Through Data Collection

Occupational therapists working in public educational settings must know and adhere to AOTA professional standards (AOTA, 2005), state regulatory laws, and Individuals With Disabilities Education Improvement Act (IDEA) laws and regulations regarding data collection for evaluation and assessment. Therapists choose assessment strategies and tools that will gather information about the student's functional, developmental, and academic skills. Those strategies and tools should be part of the review of the student's ability to meet the academic, nonacademic, extracurricular,

Remember this. . . .
Occupational therapists should collaborate with educational staff and parents to modify and adapt the temporal environment to enhance student performance.

Table 4.2. Key Physical Contexts in an Education Setting

Academic	Nonacademic	Extracurricular	Vocational
Classroom	Hallway	School trips	Grocery store
Computer lab	Lunchroom	Sports arena	Restaurant
Prevocational class	Playground	Concert hall	Business office
Study hall	Bathroom	Track field	Nursing home
Library	School bus	Museum	Child care center
Science labs	Gymnasium, art or music rooms	Recreation center	Retail store

and vocational expectations in the school. For example, comparing student writing samples with those of his or her peers will provide more information about the student's performance in the general education setting than will administering standardized tools in a formal evaluation. Multiple methods of data collection are used to obtain reliable and valid information (Stewart, 2005).

Therapist Voices: How do you know?

When making recommendations to the team, I always let them know what factual or research-based information is the foundation for my suggestions. I go back to the literature to support what I am doing, and as a team, we collect and monitor data and identify regular times to review student progress based on the data. All decisions about the intervention are then dependent on what data and progress the student has made.

—Rebecca Argabrite Grove, administrator, occupational therapist, assistive technology specialist, Virginia

Conducting Interviews

Using the *Framework* as a basis for evaluation, the occupational therapist gathers information (called the occupational profile) to guide the decision-making process. This process begins with an interview to determine a student's strengths, interests, and challenges related to school performance and participation. Interviews are conducted to determine team member concerns, priorities, and resources. Therapists may interview key people such as the student, the parent, the general educator (e.g., classroom, art, physical education, or music teachers), paraprofessionals, special education teacher, and others in the school and community environment who may be part of a student's extended team (e.g., principal, lunchroom staff, librarian, bus driver, job coach or supervisor, or private therapists). Figure 4.2 provides important questions to ask when gathering information for a student's occupational profile.

One important outcome of interviewing is that the occupational therapists, educators, and parents collaborate to identify and develop a realistic picture of a student's strengths, concerns, and frequency of behaviors. Additional evaluation data may be obtained through methods such as record reviews, observation, and testing. Record reviews may include school records, medical records, or classroom portfolios. In the

- Who made the initial request for occupational therapy services (e.g., parents, general education teacher, recess monitor, student)?
- What is the primary concern for which you are seeking occupational therapy services?
- Describe the student's current educational program (e.g., obtain a feel for the student's daily routine and key adults in the day).
- How does this concern interfere (affect) the student's current educational program (e.g., establish an educational relationship)? (What is the student's current performance in this area?)
- What is the student's expected performance in that area (e.g., peer performance, school standards)?
- What attempts have been made to make the student more successful (e.g., instruction, curriculum, environmental modifications)? What was the outcome of these attempts? (How long did you try this?)
- Is there any medical or educational history that would be significant to this concern (e.g., vision screening, hearing screening, medical diagnosis, absences from school)?
- What activities does the student successfully perform during the school day? What activities are difficult?
- Are there certain times of the day or environments when the student appears more successful? Are there certain times of the day when or environments in which the student appears to have more difficulty?
- What are your priorities and targeted outcomes for this student?

Figure 4.2. Occupational profile—Key questions to ask teachers.

following vignette, June, the occupational therapist, was consulted to assess whether hands-on or team supports could help a student participate in an elementary school classroom.

Collaboration in Action: Interpreting history

Lisba, an elementary school teacher, was concerned about Marina, a third-grade student who was very bright but was having difficulty reading and writing fluently. The occupational therapist, June, interviewed Lisba and observed Marina as she worked in her classroom. Marina had had a head injury as an infant and consequently had paralysis in her right arm and leg. As she worked, Marina seemed to tilt her head and did not scan smoothly across the page. Review of her current IEP did not reveal any visual concerns.

40% TS
60% HO

The occupational therapist contacted Marina's parents, who remembered that she had had some medical evaluations when she was a baby. June conferred with Eva, the school nurse, who reviewed all past medical reports for Marina. It was discovered that as a toddler, Marina had been diagnosed with cortical-blindness in one eye and a visual field loss in the other. Marina had modified her performance to participate in educational activities so well that key people in her life had overlooked the possibility of visual system problems as a cause for her problems with speed and fluency in reading and writing.

June worked with Marina to determine which compensatory techniques were most helpful in improving her reading and writing performance. Hands-on and team supports were provided when June taught Marina and Lisba compensatory techniques. For example, Marina used a color strip over the sentence she was reading to allow her eyes to focus on the appropriate sentence and move more quickly across the page. Marina was more accurate with the red strip than either the yellow or green. When writing, Marina was able to write faster if her paper was highlighted with a middle line. The teacher incorporated those suggestions into Marina's school routine when reading and writing.

Remember this. . . .
The therapist collaborates with key team members to identify which school activity to observe, as well as when, where, and how long the observation should occur.

Observations

As discussed in Chapter 2, observing a student's actual performance within a specific school context allows the occupational therapist to view student behavior as it occurs in the natural environment with the usual materials, distractions, or people present. If an academic problem exists, the occupational therapist is also able to observe the instruction, curriculum, and other student behaviors. Before scheduling an observation, the occupational therapist begins collecting information for the occupational profile. In addition, the therapist collaborates with the key team members to identify which school activity to observe as well as when, where, and how long the observation should occur. It is also important that the occupational therapist understand what student behaviors are deemed appropriate by the teacher for the students within the lesson or activity.

Observations may be set up to yield qualitative data, quantitative data, or both. Qualitative data (e.g., how the child puts on his or her coat) may be obtained by structuring the observation to observe the target student and one or two peers (Figure 4.3). When quantitative data are desired (e.g., number of prompts needed for the child to put on his or her coat), the therapist will need to develop some sort of tally sheet (Figure 4.4) to use during the observation. Sometimes the occupational therapist may want to collect a mixture of qualitative and quantitative data. Using a systematic method of observation, a therapist can make inferences about a student's performance when compared with predetermined peer performance data (Linder & Clark, 2000). During a systematic observation, an occupational therapist remains a neutral party gathering quantitative data, whereas during a structured observation the therapist may interact with the student or other team member to gather qualitative data. Both methods of data collection are used in the following vignette about Amos.

Collaboration in Action: Multiple sources of data

Amos was not able to put his coat on independently and line up with the rest of the first-grade students. General and special education teachers Lyla and Michael contacted Alex, the occupational therapist, because some days Amos can put on his coat and other days he cannot. Their question was, Is Amos's poor performance the result of his physical disability?

80% TS
20% HO

To answer this question, Alex decided to collect both quantitative and qualitative data. He worked with Lyla and Michael to define acceptable and unacceptable behaviors. They agreed on the following definitions:

- *Acceptable behavior:* First-grade students go into the hallway to get their coats, put them on independently, and line up against the wall.
- *Unacceptable behavior:* Touching other people or someone else's belongings, not putting on the coat, not securing the fasteners, not lining up against the wall, loud talking, and not being ready when the classmates are ready.

After defining the behaviors, Alex, Lyla, and Michael identified a convenient time for Alex to observe Amos putting on his coat. They also agreed to record data on a data collection sheet over the next week.

METHOD: Structured Observation *(yields qualitative information)*

Before the observation, the occupational therapist and teacher discussed what the teacher had tried. The teacher felt Amos should be able to do this task independently.

Findings: The occupational therapist observed Amos during recess break as he struggled to put on his coat. Peers were also putting on their coats in the hallway around Amos. Amos could pull the coat partially up his arms, but getting it over his shirt sleeves was difficult. The sleeve kept getting caught because the coat appeared to be too small. Amos then lost interest and began engaging in off-task behavior, that is, talking or fooling around with other children. The occupational therapist shared her observation of the small coat size with the teacher. The teacher suggested trying a coat from the lost and found. When the teacher returned with a larger coat, Amos was immediately able to put it on.

Hypothesis: The current coat is too small. Amos becomes distracted if he has to struggle. If the coat fit properly, Amos could complete the activity without frustration and off-task behaviors.

Plan: Teacher to talk with parent about the size of Amos's coat. Try a different coat. Teacher to collect data three times in the next week. Teacher will e-mail the information to the occupational therapist. Then they will discuss the next steps.

Figure 4.3. Example of structured student observation that yields qualitative information.

METHOD: Systematic Observation *(yields quantitative information)*

Prior to the observation, the occupational therapist and the teacher picked out three average students (A, B, and C) to serve as the peers for comparison to Amos. The therapist used a tally sheet to keep track of the number of times the peers and Amos demonstrated unacceptable behaviors (by making a check in the corresponding column for each occurrence). The therapist also documented the time elapsed for the peer to put on his or her coat and stand against the wall. The occupational therapist and teacher collected data over 3 days in a week. Then they analyzed the data.

Findings:

Day 1—Amos was the 8th student ready, with 4 unacceptable behaviors, out of 18 students (unacceptable behavior of peers ranged from 0 to 1).

Day 2—Amos did not complete the task. He demonstrated 12 unacceptable behaviors (peers ranged from 0 to 2).

Day 3—Amos did not complete the task. He demonstrated 10 unacceptable behaviors (peers ranged from 0 to 1).

Hypothesis: Amos is easily frustrated. He seemed distracted by his surroundings and had difficulty pulling on his coat if he was wearing a bulky sweatshirt.

Plan: Try a different coat; move him to an area where there are fewer distractions. Teacher to collect data three times in the next week. Teacher will e-mail the information to the occupational therapist.

Figure 4.4. Example of systematic student observation and data collection.

More information about the therapist's observation and hypothesis is included in Figures 4.3 and 4.4. Refer to Reflection 4.2 to consider how the team shared information about Amos.

Assessment Tools

Therapists should choose assessment tools and methods that are designed to answer the question they seek to answer. Those tools may include classroom or district assessments as well as diagnostic or curriculum-based program assessments (Coster, Deeney, Haltiwanger, & Haley, 1998). For example, if a therapist is trying to determine whether a student's social interaction skills are discrepant from those of peers, observing the student in various settings and interviewing the significant adult in each of those settings, rather than administering tools specific to occupational therapy, may provide the information needed. Common collaborative assessments to evaluate student performance and develop IEP goals are presented

Reflection 4.2

What Is Possible for Collaboration?

Track how Alex, the occupational therapist, and Amos's teachers, Lyla and Michael, collaborated.

- What information would be helpful for Alex to know from Lyla and Michael?

- What information could Alex share with the teachers?

Resource 4.1. Review of Occupational Therapy Assessments
A review of specific assessments used by occupational therapists is given in Jackson, L. L. (Ed.). (2007). *Occupational therapy services for children and youth under IDEA* (3rd ed.). Bethesda, MD: AOTA Press.

***Remember this.* . . .**
Therapists should choose assessment tools and methods that are designed to answer the question they are seeking to answer.

in Chapter 2 and in Exhibit 2.1A in the Appendix. Additional skill-level assessments (e.g., the School Assessment of Motor and Process Skills; Fisher, Bryze, Hume, & Griswold, 2005) may be administered to augment observations. See Resource 4.1 for more about occupational therapy assessments.

Developing IEP Goals

Family Voices: Focus on the positive

The occupational therapist provided a validating perspective of Matt that was positive, instead of focusing on the negative. That is why I think the OT is vital to the IEP team!

—Betty Thompson, parent of Matt, Virginia

When an occupational therapist gathers information about a student, the information must be shared with the IEP team. The information gathered by all team members will assist them in making collective decisions about the student's strengths in functional, developmental, and academic skills; it also will help with decisions about the areas in which the student is discrepant from peers and needs additional hands-on services or team supports (e.g., modifications, accommodations). The team uses all evaluation information to determine whether the student requires special education and related services.

The occupational therapist, with the parent, educational staff, and student, as appropriate, develops a student's IEP. There must be baseline data (e.g., present level of academic achievement and functional performance) and documentation of how to conduct ongoing assessment to determine progress toward meeting the student goal. Developing a measurable goal and determining the methods for data collection should be discussed and agreed to by parents, educators, therapists and, when possible, the student. Four simple steps (Clark, 2005) produce student goals (note that IEPs do not include occupational therapy goals, only student goals):

1. *Collect data* to determine a student's current level of academic and functional performance, strengths, and needs. The occupational therapist can analyze occupational performance and contribute to developing a hypothesis.
2. *Define the desired behavior for the student.* This item is an emerging skill or, in the case of negative behaviors, one that is decreasing. The behavior or skill can be academic ("will complete written assignments"), functional ("will play with peers"), or developmental ("will drink 4 oz. of water from a cup").
3. *Identify the conditions necessary for the student to meet the goal.* This item may include a time of day ("during snack time"), certain materials ("with a computerized writing program"), specific prompts ("when told to write his name"), or even specify the area ("when seated at his desk").
4. *Establish the criterion for goal mastery.* The standard for this behavior or skill is typically defined by key people in the student's environment (e.g., peer, teacher, principal, school board, school district).

Goals to which occupational therapists contribute are developed jointly with a teacher and parents through ongoing conversations. Respecting that a teacher or parents know a student and are actively involved on a daily basis, the occupational therapist identifies and records the behavior, conditions, and criteria that they desire. This approach increases daily carry-over because the parent's and teacher's "voice" is echoed in the goal and the data collection process. Consider the following scenario:

Remember this. . . .
There are no occupational therapy goals on an IEP, only student goals.

Collaboration in Action: Communicating for feeding success

Jamald is a third grader who was diagnosed with autism and developmental disability. He is in general education classes for at least 80% of his school day. To keep him hydrated, his parents offered Jamald a sippy cup to drink liquids at home. His mother Sabrina and his teacher Bonita agreed he needed a more appropriate method for drinking at school. Wynn, the occupational therapist, conducted a structured observation of Jamald during noon lunch and tried various adaptations of drinking cups. After multiple attempts, Jamald was able to purse his lips and initiate one suck from a straw. Wynn shared this information with his mother, who agreed to try straw drinking at home, too. This life skill is critical for Jamald because he was not otherwise getting fluids at school, so the team agreed they wanted it listed as an IEP goal.

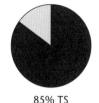

85% TS
15% HO

At Jamald's IEP meeting, Wynn outlined various methods and strategies to develop straw drinking and recommended that the school and family purchase the same type of straw and cup for consistency. They were listed as equipment on the IEP. Together they developed Jamald's goal (Figure 4.5) and worked with him to achieve it. Wynn provided hands-on intervention for Jamald with team supports for his teacher every 2 weeks to help her follow through with daily oral–motor exercises. Bonita and Sabrina communicated with each other weekly. After several months, Jamald was able to hold the cup and make several independent sips from the straw!

Occupational therapists are encouraged to use their district's template for goal writing. If there is none, they are encouraged to use the sample IEP template in Figure 4.5, which includes conditions, learner, behavior, and criteria. (Chapter 5 discusses technology aids for developing IEPs.)

Conditions	Learner	Behavior	Criteria
By September 15, 2007, during school lunch in the cafeteria,	Jamald	will drink from a straw	emptying his glass (6 oz.) without any prompting, for a week.
By May 15, 2007, during noon recess,	Natasha	will play with peers	for 15 consecutive minutes, without screaming or swearing, 3 days a week.

Figure 4.5. Sample individualized education program template.

Collaboration and Intervention

As discussed in Chapter 1, occupational therapists should blend their services and supports to students, teams, and school systems. This section illustrates how to link hands-on services with team and system supports to the *Framework's* intervention approaches and types of interventions (AOTA, 2002).

Collaborative Role: Hands-on Services With Team Supports

Doreen and Maureen are occupational therapists who work in two different schools. Although Doreen provides hands-on services in a separate therapy place, Maureen's school has been providing staff training on collaborative strategies in the classroom and has made it a priority for the past several years. Compare the similarities and differences in how they provide occupational therapy services and supports to students and teams. Think about the outcomes and effectiveness of services for the students and for the educational staff when occupational therapy services and supports are provided in or out of context (places and spaces) within students'·naturally occurring routines and activities (paces).

Collaboration in Action: Handwriting in and out of context

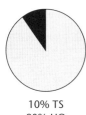

10% TS
90% HO

Out-of-context intervention. Doreen, an occupational therapist, arrives at 10:30 every Wednesday to take 6-year-old Daniel from his first-grade classroom. They work in a small room practicing writing and cutting. After 30 minutes, Doreen walks Daniel back to the room where the rest of the class is listening to the teacher, Mrs. Willow, read a story aloud. Today Doreen has some suggestions that she has written down for the teacher to try to enhance Daniel's classroom performance. Doreen leaves the note on Mrs. Willow's desk, and then she is off to another classroom to work with another child.

In the meantime, Daniel reenters the classroom and tries to figure out what the class is doing. He is unable to join in the group discussion because he missed the story. When the class works on a project involving cutting and writing, Daniel is frustrated and confused. He remembers how he could cut in the "OT Room" with the special scissors and construction paper. Ms. Doreen told him he was getting to be a good cutter, but now he cannot do it at all! He does not remember how to hold the scissors and tears his project. He hates coming to school.

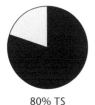

80% TS
20% HO

In-context intervention. Maureen, an occupational therapist, has met with Galiana's teacher, Virginia, to discuss Galiana's IEP goal related to her writing and cutting skills during first-grade classroom activities. They decided that Maureen should come to the classroom when Galiana is in language arts between 10:20 and 10:45. Maureen arrives in the classroom and sits at the table with Galiana and three other students. While Virginia presents the lesson, Maureen observes Galiana and the other students' attentiveness, ability to follow directions, and position at the table. As Galiana begins to work on the task, Maureen provides verbal cues to assist Galiana's performance and offers guidance to other students, as needed. This interaction occurs naturally as Maureen interacts with Galiana and the other students at the table.

Maureen observes that Galiana is having difficulty remembering how to hold her scissors. Maureen draws a picture of a hand and marks which fingers hold the scissors. She tapes it into Galiana's pencil box. Before she leaves, Maureen writes a quick note to her family and Virginia, documenting her intervention and sharing some observations. Later Maureen e-mails Virginia, and they discuss Galiana's current performance. Virginia remarks that she saw Galiana refer to the picture when she took her scissors out of her box in the afternoon.

Both Maureen and Doreen provided hands-on services to students to assist them in meeting their IEP goals. Each therapist's method, however, was different. Daniel was seen out of context in a separate room that had materials and distracters different from those in his classroom. He had to generalize what he learned during his occupational therapy session to his classroom without any supports from the therapist. In contrast, because Galiana was seen in context and was given hands-on services with team supports, she could use her own materials and apply the strategies she used with her occupational therapist in the classroom. She was able to immediately practice those skills as the materials and distracters were familiar to her.

As noted in Chapter 1, providing hands-on services to individual students and small groups in separate therapy spaces has been a traditional practice of occupational therapists in the schools. This out-of-context therapy, however, does not support the least restrictive environment mandate of IDEA and should never be the only way occupational therapy intervention is provided to students. Instead, the least restrictive environment is defined in the law as students with disabilities participating in the same contexts as students without disabilities to the maximum extent appropriate; only those students with the most severe disabilities are expected to be educated in separate classes away from their peers (IDEA 2004, 20 U.S.C. § 1412(a)(5) and § 300.114). Refer to Chapter 1 for more discussion about least restrictive environment and inclusion and to Exhibit 1.1A.

When hands-on services are provided, they should always be paired with team supports, system supports, or both. Together, team members try to answer the question, What does this student need to do or learn to be successful in school? While helping students engage in occupations appropriate to their student role, the therapist brainstorms with other team members about what is working for the student and how to continue to support the student's progress throughout the school day. In the example above, Maureen combined hands-on services for Galiana in the context of classroom lessons with team supports (e.g., sharing knowledge useful for a teacher to facilitate a student's successful performance in school activities; recommending strategies and then conferring together about their effectiveness in reaching a specific goal). Maureen's collaboration in the classroom with Galiana's teacher enabled Galiana to practice the strategies that Maureen and the teacher agreed were most helpful every day, not just once per week with Maureen.

Remember this. . . .
Out-of-context therapy does not support the least restrictive environment mandate of IDEA and should never be the only way occupational therapy intervention is provided to students.

Collaborative Role: Team Supports

Occupational therapists provide team supports through a variety of methods, including collaborative consultation, co-teaching, progress monitoring, mentoring team members, providing in-services, and participating in developing and implementing IEPs. As part of a collaborative process, team supports are often provided instead of or in addition to hands-on services so that families, education personnel, and therapists can share their knowledge and experience to ensure that all children participate successfully in the general education curriculum to the extent possible. An example of how Remy, an occupational therapist, responded to a team request for collaborative consultation is illustrated in the following vignette about Huang, a high school student whose educational program included two afternoons of community work experience training.

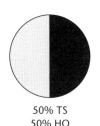

50% TS
50% HO

Collaboration in Action: Adaptations for the work environment

Huang's community job training included washing dishes at a local pizzeria. Because of a genetic disorder that caused decreased strength and musculature in the shoulder girdle and neck area, Huang could not pick up the heavy pans and kettles to move them into the washing area. After discussing his concerns with the IEP team, Huang's vocational teacher, Will, contacted Remy, an occupational therapist, for assistance so that Huang could successfully perform his job.

Remy met Huang, Will, and Mr. D'Angelo, the onsite supervisor at the restaurant, and discussed Huang's job performance and what they had already tried. Huang and Remy went into the small kitchen area where the sink and dishwasher were located, and Will checked on another student. Deciding to use a structured observation, Remy asked Huang to demonstrate filling the commercial dishwasher with trays of glasses, plates, and silverware. Huang could slide the trays along the counter without needing to lift them. His other task was washing the large kettles and pans. The counter area by the sink was small, so the large items had to be placed on another counter behind and to the side of the sink. Transporting these items to the sink was problematic because of Huang's genetic condition. The dishwashing area was very narrow, so a cart could not be moved around.

Observing Huang performing his dishwashing tasks enabled the occupational therapist to provide the core team (i.e., vocational teacher, job coach, onsite supervisor, special education teacher) with several modifications and adaptations to the environment so that Huang could successfully perform an occupation that was meaningful to him and valued by him and his teachers. For example:

- The cart was set alongside the sink, a position that allowed Huang to use it as a bridge to slide items from the counter area to the sink.
- A small platform to stand on helped Huang to lift the kettles higher to move them from the sink into the rinsing area.
- Huang was taught how to stabilize his body during lifting.

Remy made a follow-up visit to observe Huang with the modifications and adaptations in place and to confer with Mr. D'Angelo, Huang, and Will about her recommended modifications. Huang was excited about his independence! The team valued Remy's input and agreed to call in the future if additional assistance was needed. Resource 4.2 provides more examples for monitoring student progress.

Collaborative Role: Systems Supports

Occupational therapists also provide supports to a school system by participating on a variety of committees and task forces and presenting in-services to educational staff. This participation benefits students beyond those on an individual occupational therapist's workload. The vignette below continues the previous story of occupational therapist Maureen and illustrates how she provided both system and team supports.

Collaboration in Action:
System supports for self-regulation

Maureen noticed that she was receiving numerous referrals about students with poor attending skills. Some of the complaints from the teachers included that students were wiggling in their seats, playing with items in their desks, and chewing on their pencils or shirt sleeves. The therapist met with the principal to discuss using a systems approach to these referrals. They agreed that the upcoming school in-service would be a good place for Maureen to train the staff in self-regulation strategies using the "How Does Your Engine Run?" program (Williams & Shellenberger, 1996).

During the in-service, Maureen modeled language the teachers could use when talking with students about their attention and behavior, provided observation sheets for the teachers to document the types of sensory input individual students sought, and suggested more appropriate strategies the students could use to regulate their behavior during the school day. The principal had the "Engine Sheets" printed on colored paper and laminated for all classrooms, including art, music, computer lab, and physical education. As a result, Maureen saw a big dip in her referrals for poor attention as the teachers began to manage the more simple wiggles and off-task behavior. The teachers also noticed the change in student behavior and commented to Maureen about the results they observed. Maureen always answered the teachers' e-mails and the notes left in her school mailbox.

Maureen shared their outcomes with two other school building principals, highlighting the teachers' success in managing their students' behavior. They also requested an in-service. Before the year was through, Maureen had presented this in-service to seven schools, co-teaching with three of her occupational therapy colleagues in their buildings. Students were getting many of their sensory needs met within the classroom as the teachers incorporated the strategies schoolwide. Maureen and her colleagues focused their hands-on services and team supports on students who had more complex needs.

Resource 4.2. Progress Monitoring

The following resources provide more ideas for monitoring student progress:

Barnett, D. W., Daly E. J., III, Jones, K. M., & Lentz, F. E. (2004). Response to intervention: Empirically based special service decisions from single-case designs of increasing and decreasing intensity. *Journal of Special Education, 38,* 66–79.

Clark, G. F., & Miller, L. E. (1996). Providing effective occupational therapy services: Data-based decision making in school-based practice. *American Journal of Occupational Therapy, 50,* 701–708.

Linder, J., & Clark, G. F. (2000). Best practice in documentation. In W. Dunn (Ed.), *Best practice occupational therapy* (pp. 135–146). Thorofare, NJ: Slack.

Student Progress: www.studentprogress.org (Office of Special Education Programs Web site)

Progress Monitoring: www.progressmonitoring.net (Office of Special Education Programs Web site)

Collaboration Through Early Intervening Services

Collaborative practice blends hands-on student services with team and system supports. Several recent general education initiatives combine all three collaborative roles to enhance outcomes for students. IDEA (2004) uses the term *early intervening services (EIS)* to describe how local education agencies (LEAs) may use Part B funds (federal funding to provide special education services for children ages 3 through 21) to develop and provide EIS for all students in kindergarten through 12th grade. EIS include providing professional development or educational and behavioral evaluations, services, and supports to assist students before they are identified as needing special education or related services (20 USCS 1413(f)(2)). LEAs with disproportionality issues (i.e., overidentification by race and ethnicity of children as children with disabilities) must use these EIS federal monies to correct these issues (20 U.S.C. 1418(d)(2)(B)).

The following vignette illustrates the instrumental role of occupational therapist Michelle Cullen and her school team in bringing EIS to promote literacy in the kindergarten classes in an urban school district in New York State. As the district occupational and physical therapy supervisor, Michelle recognized an opportunity to advocate for the role of occupational therapy in a proposed plan for EIS for young children in her school district. When the assistant superintendent of schools decided to initiate EIS, he set aside 15% of IDEA federal funds for preventive intervention to promote phoneme awareness as part of a literacy program for kindergartners. The previous relationships and team experiences of the related services providers and supervisors provided Michelle and her colleagues with the essential foundation for building on trust and respect to develop a comprehensive literacy program. The program included contributions from occupational therapists to facilitate handwriting skills.

Collaboration in Action: EIS for handwriting and early literacy

System supports. As a supervisor on a collaborative team, Michelle learned about the preliminary plans for EIS from her colleague, a speech–language pathology supervisor, who was developing the proposal emphasizing speech therapy services. Handwriting was not formally taught in the team's school district, and occupational therapists received many referrals from kindergarten and first-grade teachers to address handwriting and tool use. Michelle wondered how occupational therapists could help improve student performance in the early years of school. She poked her head into her colleague's office at various points and suggested, "Wouldn't it be great to include motor intervention and handwriting in your proposal?" After many informal meetings and comments, the proposal was finalized; it included occupational therapy, speech, and special education services for students as well as team supports for the classroom teachers.

The Great Beginnings Program was subsequently launched, and it funded additional staff positions to serve all 230 kindergarten and first-grade classes in the city by the second year of the project. In every class, an occupational therapist, speech–language pathologist, and special educator each provided

30 to 60 minutes of intervention per week, primarily through co-teaching with general educators during the half to 1 day per week they devoted to the Great Beginnings curriculum. The activities focused on phoneme awareness, preacademic skills, and handwriting and were planned jointly by the speech–language pathologist, occupational therapist, special educator, and classroom teacher.

As a baseline for occupational therapy intervention, the Minnesota Handwriting Assessment was administered to a cohort control group of 2,500 first graders before the launch of the Great Beginnings Program. At the end of their first-grade year, five student protocols were randomly selected and scored from each classroom; those students typically scored two or more standard deviations below the test means. After the first year of the Great Beginnings program, participating first-grade students scored, on average, less than 1 standard deviation below the test means. Preliminary data from the second year of the program revealed similar results. During both years of the program, the percentage of students achieving mastery of the skills evaluated increased for all students who participated in the program. The team continues to collect data to analyze student outcomes for intervention.

Team supports. Each team (occupational therapist, speech–language pathologist, special education teacher, and kindergarten teacher) planned activities they could implement together in the classroom. The related services personnel attended grade-level team meetings and met informally with the classroom teachers (or asked for copies of their lesson plans) so they could coordinate lesson themes and intervention activities. For example, one activity involved reading a story with a transportation theme. The speech–language pathologist read the book to the students and asked them questions about the story plot and characters. The occupational therapist transitioned the children, helping them move like the vehicles in the story, to tabletop activities at a fine motor station. At other stations, the special education teacher facilitated letter recognition and prereading, and the speech–language pathologist worked on phoneme awareness. Throughout the joint planning and co-teaching, the classroom teacher learned how to use the techniques modeled so she could incorporate them at other times.

The success of the Great Beginnings program hinged on team members embracing collaboration as a two-way street.

Therapist Voices: Supporting teachers

Collaboration is a dialogue, not a monologue. If you want teachers to carry out your recommendations, you must reinforce their strategies also. Always ask to see what they are doing, and how you can reinforce the concepts they are trying to teach. Soliciting input from teachers helps build a relationship with them.

—Michelle Cullen, occupational therapist, New York

Response to Intervention

The National Association of State Directors of Special Education (NASDSE) has developed a model for EIS for general education students supported by a grant from the U.S. Department of Education Office of Special Education Programs. This process, called *response to intervention (RtI),* is defined as "the practice of providing high-quality instruction and interventions matched to student need, monitoring progress frequently to make decisions about changes in instruction or goals, and applying child response data to important educational decisions" (NASDSE, 2006, p. 3).

Many states use a three-tier model for RtI to illustrate a continuum of instruction to ensure that *all* students learn the expected material (see Figure 4.6). The first tier of the RtI model provides scientifically based core instruction to all students. It is expected that 80% of students will respond to universal core instruction and learn the expected curriculum. Using a schoolwide model, students are screened and at-risk students are identified. The second tier provides targeted individual or group supplemental instruction to students who are at risk (approximately 15% of students). This level of instruction generally repeats what was taught in the core instruction but provides additional practice and review of the information. The third tier is an intensive intervention generally focusing on individual students (about 5% of students). Resource 4.3 provides resources to learn more about RtI and EIS.

Once occupational therapy services and supports are initiated, the occupational therapist and other team members must track the effectiveness of their intervention. Ongoing data collection to assess progress can be shared among team members working with a student. Charting the data in a visual format allows the data to be easily followed and analyzed by everyone (Clark & Miller, 1996; Linder & Clark, 2000). The following scenario about Charlie demonstrates how an occupational therapist collaborated with a general education teacher to enhance a student's ability to complete his written work under the auspices of an EIS program in a school district in Iowa. In some states, this student would be served through a program such as RtI, and an occupational therapist could work with general education teachers and students before a formal referral for special education and related services. In other states, because of local education agency or state regulatory laws not implementing RtI, occupational therapists may only be able to provide the teachers with nonspecific student information. It is strongly suggested that the reader check his or her state regulatory information and education agency policies to determine practice guidelines.

Resource 4.3. Early Intervening Services and Response to Intervention Resources

Find out whether your state department of education and occupational therapy regulatory procedures (e.g., licensure) allow you to use prereferral activities or problem-solving or response to intervention strategies to work with general education students. Read more about this new innovative approach from the following sources:

- Early Intervening Services Fact Sheet (U.S. Department of Education, Office of Special Education and Rehabilitative Services, n.d.): www.ed.gov/policy/speced/guid/idea/tb-early-intervent.doc

- *FAQ on Response to Intervention for School-Based Occupational Therapists and Occupational Therapy Assistants* (AOTA, 2007): www.aota.org/Practitioners/PracticeAreas/Pediatrics/Highlights/FAQonRtI.aspx

- *Responsiveness to Intervention (RTI): How to Do It* (Johnson, Mellard, Fuchs, & McKnight, 2006): www.nrcld.org/rti_manual

- Responsiveness to intervention in the SLD determination process (U.S. Department of Education, Office of Special Education Programs, 2006): www.osepideasthatwork.org/toolkit/ta_responsiveness_intervention.asp

Collaboration in Action: RtI for handwriting

Charlie could not complete his written work in first grade. Anne, his general education teacher, contacted Charlie's parents about his difficulty, and they offered to work more with him at home. Anne provided daily lessons to the class on letter formation, yet Charlie's performance was very slow and

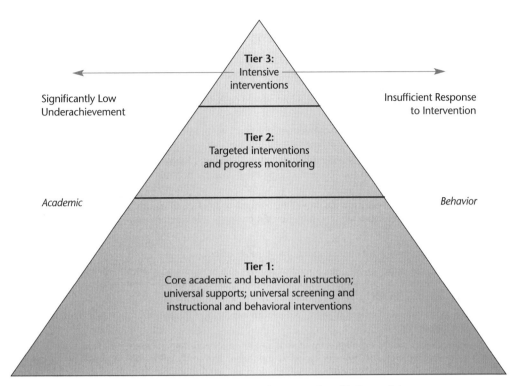

Figure 4.6. An example of a tiered response-to-intervention (RtI) model.

From Batsche, G., Elliott, J., Graden, J. L, Grimes, J., Kovaleski, J., Prasse, D., et al. (2005). *Response to intervention: Policy considerations and implementation.* Alexandria, VA: National Association of State Directors of Special Education. Copyright © 2005 by the National Association of State Directors of Special Education. Used with permission.

difficult when forming letters. Even after providing additional instruction and practice, Charlie's improvements were minimal.

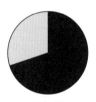

70% TS
30% HO

Rhonda, an occupational therapist, met with Charlie's parents; his teacher, Anne; and Brock, the first-grade aide, to review his work and discuss his needs. They all agreed on the hypothesis "If Charlie's letter formation were more automatic, then he could form letters quickly and correctly." As part of the screening activities, Rhonda gathered baseline data for Charlie's performance. During dictation, peers were able to write any lowercase letter within 3 seconds. Charlie could not form any letters within this timeframe. Initially, he required up to 10 seconds to form letters such as *f, q,* and *y* (his present academic achievement level). It was determined that Charlie did not have the skills to complete the task of writing the alphabet independently.

The Building-Level Team (e.g., parents; representatives from the teaching staff; and Rhonda, the occupational therapist) set the following goal for Charlie: "In 6 weeks and within 3 seconds after each letter is dictated, Charlie will write the 26 lowercase alphabet letters, forming them correctly and placing them properly between the lines on the paper."

Charlie's EIS plan (Figure 4.7) outlined the who, what, where, and why of helping him reach his team-identified goal. Data were collected each week on Monday. The teacher worked with Charlie daily on writing specific lowercase letters. Once a

---

Early Intervening Services Plan

Student: _____Charlie Blackfoot_____   Birth Date: _____   School District: _____

Concern: Charlie is unable to form letters correctly and place them on the lines.

Current Level of Academic Achievement: Charlie could not write any lowercase letters within 3 seconds after each letter was dictated.

Expected/Peer Level of Academic Achievement: Peers are able to write 26:26 lowercase letters within 3 seconds and place them correctly on lined paper.

Goal: In 6 weeks and within 3 seconds after each letter is dictated, Charlie will write the lowercase alphabet letters, forming them correctly and placing them properly between the lines, 26:26 letters (100%).

Method of Monitoring Performance: Anne (the teacher) or Brock (the first-grade aide) will collect data once a week using an alphabet tally and plot it on the chart.

Planned Activities:

1. Charlie will have extra practice on forming the alphabet letters.

2. Rhonda (occupational therapist) will provide team supports to Anne and Brock about which letters to focus on, how to use a multisensory approach to writing, and how to collect data to determine progress. Information will be communicated to parents each week.

3. In addition to daily writing lessons, Anne will provide supplemental assistance for Charlie for 10 minutes each day.

4. A home program will be developed by Rhonda and Anne with the family. Parents will work with Charlie each evening for 10 minutes. Ongoing supports to the family will be provided by a phone call every 2 weeks from Anne or Rhonda.

5. Data will be collected once a week by Anne or Brock using an alphabet tally sheet.

6. Rhonda will meet with Anne every 2 weeks to review the chart and give new suggestions for enhancing Charlie's performance.

7. Data will be reviewed in 6 weeks by Charlie's core team (e.g., teacher, classroom aide, parents, and occupational therapist).

Figure 4.7. Charlie's early intervening services plan.

Note. Occupational therapists must follow their state's regulatory laws. These activities all occurred before a referral for special education was made, so they are considered screening activities in some states.

Reflection 4.3

How Do I Explain Student Performance to Others?

Think about explaining a student's progress (or lack of progress) to parents using a visual graph. The software used to create the graph used for Charlie was Excel. If you are unfamiliar with Excel, consider taking a computer course to learn how to chart student IEP goals.

week, he was given a probe (quiz) regarding his knowledge of the letters. Brock, the first-grade aide, would name a letter of the alphabet for Charlie to write. If he wrote the correct letter within 3 seconds, formed it correctly, and placed it correctly between the lines, the teacher put a "+" on the tally sheet. If he did not, a "–" was placed on the tally sheet (Figure 4.8). This approach allowed Anne and Rhonda to jointly analyze which letters had been mastered. Charlie's intervention was effective, as depicted in Figure 4.9. For Charlie to meet his goal (remember he started at 0 letters and had to write 26 letters by the end of 6 weeks), he needed to progress at a rate similar to that shown by the diagonal black line, or *goal line,* in Figure 4.9. In Reflection 4.3, consider how you would explain student progress to a parent.

After 2 weeks, the occupational therapist and teacher reviewed the data in Figure 4.8. Charlie was making progress, but not at a rate at which he would meet the goal in 6 weeks. Analysis of the data indicated that forming diagonal lines for the letters was difficult for Charlie. Rhonda, his occupational therapist, suggested additional daily activities to incorporate practice time that focused on making diagonals. Two weeks later, when the teacher and occupational therapist met to collaborate on Charlie's work, they noticed that he had

Goal: In 6 weeks and within 3 seconds after each letter is dictated, Charlie will write the lowercase alphabet letters, forming them correctly and placing them properly between the lines, 26:26 letters (100%).

Letter	March 4	March 11	March 18	March 25	April 1	April 8
a	–	+	+	+	+	+
b	–	–	–	–	+	+
c	–	+	+	+	+	+
d	–	–	–	+	+	+
e	–	–	–	–	+	+
f	–	–	–	–	+	+
g	–	–	–	–	+	+
h	–	–	–	+	+	+
i	–	+	–	+	+	+
j	–	–	–	+	+	+
k	–	–	–	–	–	+
l	–	-	+	+	+	+
m	–	–	+	+	+	+
n	–	–	+	+	+	+
o	–	+	+	+	+	+
p	–	–	+	+	+	+
q	–	–	–	–	–	+
r	–	–	–	+	+	+
s	–	–	–	+	+	+
t	–	–	+	+	+	+
u	–	–	–	+	+	+
v	–	–	–	–	+	+
w	–	–	–	–	+	+
x	–	–	–	–	–	+
y	–	–	–	–	–	+
z	–	–	–	–	–	+
Totals	**0**	**4**	**8**	**15**	**21**	**26**

Figure 4.8. Tally sheet for Charlie's handwriting progress.

Note. + = correctly writes letter within 3 seconds of hearing it, forming it correctly within the lines of his paper; – = incorrectly writes letter after 3 seconds of hearing it or did not form it correctly with the lines of his paper.

made significant improvements. However, he was unable to place the letters correctly between the lines.

The occupational therapist, teacher, and parent agreed to highlight the bottom line of the paper to help Charlie distinguish where letters belonged (this was only done during the practice; during the probe, he had to use typical classroom paper). Daily work and once-a-week data collection continued, and the team met to review progress. Charlie met the goal after 6 weeks

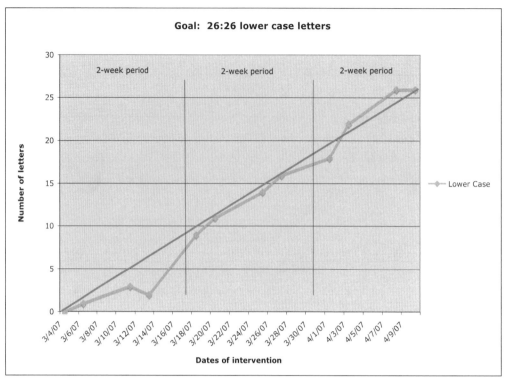

Figure 4.9.   Charlie's progress in learning to write lowercase letters.

***Remember this.* . . .**
Once occupational therapy services and supports are initiated, the occupational therapist and other team members must track the effectiveness of their intervention.

of targeted instruction. The teacher noticed a marked improvement in Charlie's ability to complete his class work and in the legibility of his written work. Charlie now had the skill to write the alphabet and was also able to perform the tasks he was required to do. No further work in handwriting was needed by the team, and Charlie was able to apply his new knowledge within his classroom routine.

Charlie is a general education student whose school district used the RtI model to deliver EIS. After initial intervening services were not as effective as expected, Charlie received short-term occupational therapy (team supports) at the third-tier level of the RtI model (see Figure 4.6) to improve the legibility of his handwriting.

Each state determines its own state regulatory language and district procedures for RtI (AOTA, 2007). In some states, such as Iowa, a student like Charlie would be served through a program such as RtI, and an occupational therapist could work with general education teachers and students before a formal referral for special education and related services. In other states, that is not an option; an occupational therapist's participation in EIS for an individual student like Charlie could not be provided without an evaluation. In some states, occupational therapists can participate in EIS but must keep recommendations general to avoid breaking state regulatory laws.

Administrator Voices: Valuing early collaboration

I recognize the value of having the team (OT, speech, PT, [special education] personnel) involved in meetings from the beginning. I ask related services staff to attend Child Study Team meetings and to be available to the Teacher Assistance Teams (for informal supports) whenever their schedule permits. By brainstorming together, other resources and ideas to help the student are exchanged [Team Supports]. These often benefit all students (RtI, EIS) and may avoid an unnecessary referral to the Child Study Team.

—Ilene Banker, assistant principal, Virginia

As an occupational therapist, think about how to support RtI by collaborating with educational staff at each of these tiers. For example, at Tier 1, consider suggestions for general education teachers who are concerned about social interactions among peers. An occupational therapist could suggest general classroom strategies (based on peer-reviewed evidence) to enhance appropriate social interactions on the playground, in the classroom, in the lunchroom, or in extracurricular activities. At Tier 2, an occupational therapist may provide more specific suggestions to team members concerned about one particular student (e.g., a student pushes peers who are too close to him), so strategies for dealing with conflicts are shared with the teacher. At Tier 3, the occupational therapist may be part of a team to evaluate this student's behavioral needs. Throughout the RtI process, collaboration among parents, educators, and therapists (e.g., sharing information, screening results, collectively identifying goals, targeting intervention) is critical to achieving positive outcomes for students. Refer to Reflection 4.4 to consider what recommendations are appropriate for Charlie (in the previous case study).

Using the *Framework* to Support Collaboration

Using the *Framework* as a foundation for occupational therapy evaluation and intervention provides therapists with consistent guidelines to review and discuss their collaborative roles in a school setting. When providing services or supports to students, teams, and school systems, occupational therapists may use different approaches and types of interventions (AOTA, 2002).

Approaches to Intervention

The *Framework* defines *intervention approaches* as "specific strategies selected to direct the process of intervention that are based on the client's desired outcome, evaluation data, and evidence" (AOTA, 2002, p. 627). Five approaches are identified (see Table 4.3 for examples of collaboration for each approach). When using the *create* approach, an occupational therapist does not assume a disability; rather, the therapist enriches the context or activity to enhance a student's performance. The *establish* approach is commonly used by occupational therapists to restore or develop new skills for a student. *Maintain*ing is important to preserve a student's current performance and assumes that the performance would decrease if follow-up intervention were not provided. *Modify*ing the context or activity allows a student to participate in a school task or interaction. The *prevent* approach is important for students at risk for performance problems and eliminates, as much as possible, any barriers to full participation in the school environment.

Reflection 4.4

What Early Intervening Services Would Be Appropriate for Charlie in My State?

If your state regulations do not allow occupational therapists to make recommendations for individual students without a referral including parent notice and consent, what could you do to provide team supports for Charlie, as part of the school's EIS team?

- Consider giving verbal ideas.
- Educate teacher with a handout or handwriting tips.
- Give an in-service to all school staff about possible solutions to handwriting problems.

Table 4.3. Occupational Therapy Intervention Approaches

Intervention Approach[a]	Example of Collaboration	Collaborative Role
Create, promote	Promote or encourage peer relationships during field days by identifying games that any elementary student can play, even if from a wheelchair.	System supports
	Together with the life skills teacher, develop or create a weekly restaurant program in which students gain knowledge about planning, preparing, and serving meals.	System supports
Establish, restore	Establish or develop a functional method of written communication for a student who uses a computer.	Hands-on services and team supports
	Restore eating routines for a student who refuses to eat by working with the student and training the teachers in specific strategies to use.	Hands-on services and team supports
Maintain	Maintain self-feeding skills of a student by identifying a list of foods the kindergarten teacher can use during daily snack times.	Team supports
	Assist the physical education teacher in developing an exercise program for a high school student in a wheelchair to maintain his flexibility and strength.	Team supports
Modify	Consult with a teacher and student to modify a locker so that a student can be independent in opening the locker and hanging up his items.	Team supports
	Attend home economics or life skills class with a student who has a hemiplegia and modify the activities to enable her to participate in the sewing, cooking, and housekeeping units.	Team supports and hands-on services
Prevent	Provide an in-service to teachers regarding lifting and carrying students to prevent back injuries.	System supports
	Collaborate with the school nurse to complete monthly weights on students with individualized education programs to prevent weight loss or gain.	System supports, team supports

[a]From AOTA, 2002.

Types of Intervention

The five approaches for occupational therapy intervention described above are supplemented by selecting types of interventions. Four types of occupational therapy interventions are identified in the *Framework* (AOTA, 2002) for practitioners as they work with teams, systems, or individual students: (1) consultation, (2) educating others, (3) therapeutic use of self, and (4) therapeutic use of occupations and activities (see Table 4.4 for examples of school-based collaboration for each type of intervention). Consultation and education of others are two primary methods for providing collaborative supports and services in school settings. Several types of interventions may be used together to address a student's goal. For example, an occupational therapist may combine collaborative consultation (e.g., sharing knowledge and expertise, as appropriate, with other team members) with hands-on services with a student (e.g., helping a student with a visual impairment and wants to brush his teeth). Thus, an occupational therapist works with a student (hands-on role) and shares the responsibility for achieving the student's outcome with the teaching staff (team supports role).

The following scenario illustrates how an occupational therapist combined several approaches and types of intervention for a middle-school student who receives special education and related services in her general education class.

Collaboration in Action: Support prevocational activities

The IEP team recommended occupational therapy services to assist Kekoa's teacher, Charlotte, with community prevocational activities. The occupational therapist, Cheryl, met with Charlotte to determine appropriate community

Table 4.4. Types of Occupational Therapy Interventions

Type of Intervention[a]	Example of School Collaboration	Collaborative Role
Consultation	Talk with a teacher to determine the most efficient method for a student to develop turn-taking social skills.	Team supports
	Participate on a school committee to modify the building to accommodate students in wheelchairs.	System supports
Education (of others)	Provide an in-service on in-hand manipulation skills of classroom materials as a key component of writing for all kindergarten teachers.	System supports
	Provide materials to an individualized education program team regarding the specific mental health diagnoses, with implications for school performance, and suggest intervention strategies.	System supports and team supports
Therapeutic use of self	Use a playful personality to engage a student to join peers at the sensory table while co-leading a classroom lesson related to literacy.	Hands-on services and team supports
	Use insight about a student's interests and preferences to teach others how to encourage and reinforce a middle-school student with a severe behavior disorder to complete difficult work.	Hands-on services and team supports
Therapeutic use of occupations and activities	Use the natural routine of getting ready for recess to practice toileting and putting on a coat and hat.	Hands-on services and team supports
	Find jobs within the classroom and school office to enable students to gain prevocational skills in a supportive environment.	Hands-on services and team supports

[a]From AOTA, 2002.

job experiences for Kekoa. Kekoa has autism, and her behavior is sometimes very aggressive. She interacts more successfully with adults than with young children or adolescents. Intensive or unexpected sensory input would trigger screaming or aggression.

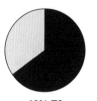

65% TS
35% HO

Cheryl used several intervention approaches during her collaboration with Charlotte and the paraprofessional, Jonathan:

- *Prevent:* Reviewed lists of school and community places where Kekoa participates and identified routines and activities that could trigger aggressive behavior to prevent problems from occurring

- *Create:* Discussed ways to create activities or experiences in various school and community places to promote successful participation for Kekoa

- *Establish:* Identified the work skills that Kekoa needed to learn and suggested strategies to establish or develop these skills.

Cheryl then considered what type of intervention to use as she provided team supports as well as hands-on services for Kekoa. Two types of interventions were chosen:

1. *Consultation:* Cheryl translated specific information about self-regulation and attention to help Kekoa's teachers, paraprofessionals, and parents fulfill their role responsibilities

2. *Therapeutic use of occupations and activities:* Cheryl observed Kekoa in her community-based job experience to identify opportunities for her to

work on social skills (e.g., greeting others, requesting assistance) and work skills (e.g., showing up to work on time, performing the task as trained).

Choosing from a variety of approaches and types of interventions helps occupational therapists work collaboratively with school teams to achieve desired student outcomes. Individualizing intervention strategies meets students' needs and enhances team members' skills.

Tying It All Together: Collaborative Routine Vignettes

Therapist Voices: Routines support intervention

Working within classroom routines supports my intervention by allowing me to have a realistic perspective of the contexts in which the child is performing, giving me more opportunities to consult with teachers, increasing the chances of repetition and practice, and providing extra sources of motivation for the child to participate in whatever play and self-care routines have been identified.

—Linn Wakeford, occupational therapist in preschool, North Carolina (Wakeford, 2003, p. 3)

School places and spaces provide a context are specific occupations that are meaningful to and valued by students, parents, and educational staff. These daily school routines and learning activities set the pace for students to interact with peers and adults and participate in the general curriculum. They provide excellent opportunities for occupational therapists to collaborate with teachers, classroom aides, physical therapists, speech–language pathologists, and other school personnel.

Preschool Collaboration

Preschools are often structured by the self-care and social needs of the children. Figure 4.10 lists the various activities established by a preschool teacher for her preschool morning program. This 4-day-per-week preschool program is run by a school district for preschoolers in Iowa who are 3 to 5 years old. Preschoolers with and without special education programming attend this program (generally, 75% of students have typical development, and 25% of students are in special education programming). Understanding the daily schedule provides the occupational therapist with information about the places and spaces (physical and social environments) in which a student will interact and how he or she is expected to keep up with the pace or temporal context of the routine. Reviewing schedules and observing a student in context opens the door to collaborating with the teacher. The natural routines and activities of the school day form the basis for helping the preschoolers engage and participate in school and in classroom activities.

Reflection 4.5

How to Integrate Occupational Therapy Into the Classroom Schedule?

Review the preschool classroom schedule in Figure 4.10. Identify when

- An occupational therapist could integrate self-help activities into the current classroom routine;

- Literacy activities (e.g., prewriting and prereading) could be integrated into the current routine (see Resource 4.4); and

- The teacher and occupational therapist may choose to have a student practice using an assistive technology switch to make choices.

Resource 4.4. Web Sites of Interest Related to Technology and Preliteracy

- University of Connecticut (research about effective literacy instruction): www.literacy.uconn.edu/resart.htm

- Center for Improvement of Early Reading Achievement: www.ciera.org/library/index.html

- National Center to Improve Practice in Special Education Through Technology, Media, and Materials (NCIP): www2.edc.org/NCIP/

- National Association of Education of Young Children Position Statement about literacy and assistive technology: www.naeyc.org/about/positions/PSTECH98.asp

- National Institute for Literacy (numerous evidence-based publications available related to lifespan literacy): www.nifl.gov/nifl/publications.html

Times	Activities	Curriculum Objectives
8:30–8:40	Students arrive (hang up coats, bags, check in names)	Self-help, greetings, and social time with adults and peers
8:40–9:00	Bathroom/free choice	Self-help and independence
9:00–9:20	Table work	Work on peer interaction to reinforce content and IEP skills, to embed IEP work into the daily activities, and to foster independence
9:20–9:40	Learning centers (one-on-one work)	Increase social skills, build peer interaction, increase independence, and embed IEP work into daily activities and to foster independence
9:45–10:00	Calendar time (hello song, attendance, calendar, weather, days in school, show 'n' tell)	Increase social skills, build peer interaction, increase independence, and embed IEP work into daily activities and to foster independence
10:05–10:20	Recess	Increase gross motor and fine motor skills, increase turn taking and wait time, build social skills, and increase independence
10:20–10:40	Snack and milk	Increase life skills, social skills, and independence
10:40–11:05	Language activity	Attending to a story, sitting in body basics, listening to directions, and following and complete tasks
11:05–11:10	Ready to go home (pass out daily reports, sing song, check mailbox, papers in folder, line up and walk to front)	Transition to home
11:15	Go home	

Figure 4.10. Sample preschool classroom schedule.

Reprinted with permission from Lisa Brickman, special education teacher, Van Meter Elementary Schools, Van Meter, IA. IEP = individualized education program.

Using the *Occupational Therapy Practice Framework* (AOTA, 2002) as a guide, this preschool schedule can be categorized into occupations with opportunities for team collaboration. Examples of how occupational therapists can provide hands-on services and team supports for students in this preschool are identified in Figure 4.11. Refer to Reflection 4.5 to consider when occupational therapy might be integrated into this preschool classroom schedule. For instance, several opportunities arise during table work or learning centers to facilitate social interactions for students who also need to work on fine motor skills for literacy (e.g., hold pencil correctly, make prewriting strokes). During snack, the teacher might choose two students to work together to pass out the napkins, straws, drinks, and food; the occupational therapist might develop visual supports or design a system to carry items from place to place. During free play, the teacher might design areas that encourage interactions (e.g., grocery store, school bus, post office); the occupational therapist considers the sensory aspects of the different centers. Resource 4.4 lists Web sites related to technology and preliteracy.

In the following vignette, review how collaborative goals were written and implemented for Sakina:

Collaboration in Action: Implementing collaborative goals for feeding

Sakina is 3½ years old and attends the district's preschool program 4 mornings a week. Because of prematurity (i.e., born at 26 weeks' gestation), Sakina has a medical diagnosis of cerebral palsy. Her spasticity interferes with her ability to perform fine motor and self-care tasks during her classroom

Classroom Activity From Teacher's Schedule	ADLs	Social Participation	Education– Academic	Play– Leisure	IADLs	How Occupational Therapist Might Provide HO and TS
Students arrive (hang up coats, bags, and check in names)	x	x				*TS:* Suggest cubby placement and type of hook for hanging up coat.
Bathroom/free choice	x	x		x		*HO/TS:* Practice transfers to toilet with paraprofessional helping and using provided adaptive equipment.
Table work	x	x	x			*HO/TS:* Co-teach and provide manipulatives for one of the activities.
Learning centers (one-on-one work)	x	x	x			*TS:* Develop independent activities for center time that incorporate prewriting, sensory exploration of objects, and so on.
Calendar time (hello song, attendance, calendar, weather, days in school, show-and-tell)	x	x	x			*HO/TS:* Provide positioning or hand-over-hand assistance to gesture to the song or hit a switch to sing the "hello song."
Recess		x		x		*HO/TS:* Teach the child and teacher different ways to get on the swing or climb the jungle gym.
Snack and milk	x	x				*HO/TS:* Work with student on oral–motor skills and using a straw. *TS:* Provide and educate teacher about how to use a special cup and straw for drinking.
Language activity	x	x	x		x	*HO/TS:* Provide special markers or pencils and show aide how to use them. *TS:* Develop a "talking book" for the teacher to use.
Ready to go home (pass out daily reports, sing song, check mailbox, papers in folder, line up and walk to front)	x					*HO/TS:* Assist student with learning how to put on his or her coat with input from teacher.

Figure 4.11. Example of integrating occupational therapy into a preschool schedule.

Note. ADLs = activities of daily living; IADLs = instrumental activities of daily living; HO = hands on; TS = team supports.

program. Sakina's IEP includes one goal focused on independent eating that the teacher, classroom aide, and occupational therapy assistant will work on together. The goal is, "By May 15, 2007, during snack, Sakina will finger feed or use a spoon (as appropriate), drink her milk from a straw, and will wash/dry her hands independently, for 4 out of 5 consecutive days."

Figure 4.12 shows how the team collaborated to ensure Sakina reached her goal.

Team Collaboration in High School: What Helps Leo Succeed?

When students with moderate to severe needs attend high school, the special education program combines life skills and academic instruction. Students can be placed in

Area	Description
IEP collaborative goal	By May 15, 2007, during snack, Sakina will feed herself by finger feeding or using a spoon (as appropriate), drink her milk from a straw, and will wash and dry her hands independently for 4 out of 5 consecutive days.
Context and environments	*Temporal:* The occupational therapy assistant will provide hands-on services and team supports during the routine snack time in the preschool classroom for 30 minutes. *Social/cultural:* During snack, there are other adults (e.g., parent helpers, paraprofessionals, peer helpers) in the room to assist the other students with snack. Students are expected to wash their hands before snack and clean up after themselves. At the table, Sakina will sit with Sheama, who is talkative and friendly. *Physical:* Sakina will wheel her chair to the table and will be transferred into her adaptive chair (for trunk support). She will use a thick commercial straw that is bent to fit her mouth while sitting up to drink. A built-up handle spoon and a scoop plate with nonskid backing on the bottom will be used as needed.
Therapeutic approaches: Promote, establish, and modify	An *establish* approach was used to help Sakina learn the skills needed to self-feed. When not participating in feeding, the occupational therapy assistant gave the preschool teacher scooping activities for the class learning centers so Sakina and her classmates could practice this skill. The occupational therapy assistant also collaborates with the classroom aide about what Sakina likes to eat and what is difficult for her. She demonstrates how to use hand-over-hand methods and verbal cuing to help Sakina initiate self-feeding. She also helps the aide practice the technique.
Hands-on services with team supports	When doing a round-robin co-teaching activity, the occupational therapist brought in an art project using straws to blow the paint to reinforce lip and tongue mobility. The environment and objects with it were modified as described above. During snack the occupational therapy assistant provides verbal or physical prompts to initiate or sustain Sakina's self-feeding and drinking from the straw. As the team tweaked their intervention with Sakina, they used a home communication notebook to keep her parents informed of Sakina's progress. The occupational therapist also suggested that Mom volunteer to be a snack helper one day so she could observe Sakina. Following snack, Sakina's mother, the occupational therapy assistant, the classroom aide, and the teacher discussed Sakina's strengths and needs. Another concern emerged: Sakina splashes water everywhere when washing her hands before snack. After a discussion, the team discussed some options to try the next day.

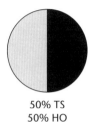

50% TS
50% HO

Figure 4.12. Team collaboration for Sakina's individualized education program (IEP) goals.

both general and special education classrooms with prevocational or vocational community experiences, as determined by the IEP teams. Students' daily school routines are based on their needs and can be structured in small groups or individually. Unlike preschool classrooms, high school schedules can change from day to day, often causing confusion and frustration for students with moderate to severe needs. Even if the schedule changes from day to day, such as longer classes that meet every other day (block schedules), routines are essential. The students know that whatever happens in the day, their routine is the same. Visual supports, such as color codes and picture symbols for schedules and colored folders, help promote more independence in following the schedule and organizing class materials.

In the following scenario, Leo has just entered high school after receiving occupational therapy services for several years. The therapist and core team members have developed an intervention plan for Leo, who has moderate to severe disabilities. Leo participates in general education classes for homeroom, lunch, physical education, and special school events.

Collaboration in Action: Using routines for vocational success

In reviewing Leo's schedule, Raab, a registered occupational therapist, identified at least three places within the daily contexts where she could work with Leo on his desired educational outcomes and provide team supports. Raab used naturally occurring routines in Leo's life skills class, during physical education, and at break times or when he completed school jobs. Review Figure 4.13 and consider when and how occupational therapy could provide hands-on services and supports for Leo and his team members.

Raab provided the following hands-on services and team supports on Leo's behalf:

- By providing hands-on services during life skills class, Raab could help the teacher assess what type of chores Leo could do in the classroom and possibly learn to do as a beginning vocational placement. Realizing that Leo was fascinated with the computer, the team brainstormed the types of computer jobs that might work for Leo. Some ideas included keeping simple school inventories or attendance records, printing mailing labels, and typing short lists or assignments for teachers. Because Leo did well with routines and visual supports, the team decided he could do simple school inventories using just a number pad. This routine is structured, it uses Leo's math skills and his interest in computers, and it reinforces sight vocabulary. One example of team support Raab provided was a visual schedule incorporating suggestions from the speech–language pathologist, paraprofessional, and teacher. She also highlighted suggestions for sensory breaks on Leo's schedule (see Figure 4.14).

- Collaboratively with Leo's input, the team decided to teach Leo to act more maturely in his school job. His buddies, homeroom classmates, and the education staff were enlisted to deter his constant hugging and crashing into objects with his wheelchair. During gym class, Raab and the physical education teacher identified some warm-up activities for Leo that required heavy work and strengthening. They talked about how hugging or high fives were okay for sports but not for interactions in his school job. With Leo's permission, the team enlisted his peers to help remind him to shake hands or say "Okay" instead of hugging.

- For showering and using deodorant, Raab provided hands-on services for Leo with team supports for Leo's parents and the classroom aide working with him. Scheduling Leo for physical education the last period of the day meant that he could take his time, receive assistance from the classroom aide, and use the accessible shower with more privacy during these initial stages. Raab taught the classroom aide how to assist Leo in his transfers and to follow the same steps of showering every time they came to the gym. Pairing his school job with expectations for cleanliness also helped motivate Leo to maintain his grooming skills. Education, checklists, and follow-up with a home program helped Leo obtain those skills at school and home.

Student: ___Leo___   *Grade:* ___11th___   *Date:* ___9–20–06___

1. FACES (core team members)	
• Leo, student • Leon and Angelica, parents • Jada, special education teacher • Barney, general education teacher	• Raab, occupational therapist • Zeke, paraprofessional • Chestina, speech–language pathologist

2. Listen to key team members and record their words below.

Student's Strengths and Interests	*Student's Challenges*
• Writes in his journal and draws pictures (writes at about a third-grade level) • Completes two-digit addition • Communicates in two-word sentences • Outgoing and friendly with people he knows. Has a great smile! • Learns new tasks easily • Likes the computer and is fascinated with mechanical things • Goes to the bathroom by himself • Works like a fiend to get a treat or a special privilege • Beginning to show an interest in doing a "job" at school	• Getting around the school environment, runs into objects with his wheelchair. Is his vision OK? • Tries to take apart anything mechanical (including everyone's cell phone!) • More communication options would be great for him, especially when he is frustrated • Refuses to take a shower in gym class • Forgets deodorant and to recomb hair after gym class • Hugs others when excited, "Sometimes too hard or at the wrong time"

Desired Educational Outcomes

1. To read better (learn more sight-reading words)

2. To have a chore or job that includes his interests in mechanical objects

3. In gym class, take care of personal hygiene independently (e.g., take a shower, use deodorant)

4. Learn to greet others in an age-appropriate manner (no hugging!)

3. PLACES and SPACES in which student was observed in the school environment:
(a) General and special education classes   (b) Physical education   (c) Life skills class

What's working for this student in this environment?	*What challenges are present in this environment?*
• Likes routines and can follow them with visual supports • Visual supports used in special education and history class keep Leo organized (schedules and Social Stories) • Classroom space and classroom materials are accessible • Peers in history talk to Leo in class and in gym class • Leo likes to model the behaviors of his friend Robert • Leo responds well to redirection and often asks to do jobs in the classroom	• Doesn't seem to know what to do or how to participate in the shower portion of gym class and then just refuses to do anything. No visual supports or assigned peer buddies • Gym is loud, smelly, and filled with fluorescent lights • Bumps into others or trash cans in the hallways when he has audience or when it's crowded near lunch time • Peers laugh with or at him when he crashes and tell him "Give me a big hug"

4. PACES: Describe how the student meets role expectations and keeps up with the pace of school life (e.g., schedule, study habits, homework, time use, hygiene and health habits).

What is expected of this student?	*How do the student's routines and habits influence his or her performance?*
• Come to school neatly groomed and ready to work • Follow the schedule with few verbal prompts • Bring papers, permission slips, and books and materials to school • Respect others, ask before borrowing items from others • Teacher's motto is "do your best work"	• Leo's routines that use visual supports help him complete class tasks • Leo dislikes changes in the schedule and occasionally tantrums if he is "caught off guard." • Leo has never taken a shower independently at home • Habit of taking everything apart gets Leo in trouble with peers and teachers • Hugging is his "social" routine to get people to respond to him

Figure 4.13. Identifying faces, spaces, and paces for Leo.

School day: (time in/out) Start of the day: 7:55–8:20		
To Do/Done	Activity	Purpose
	Homeroom in general education	To build social relationships with general education peers and teachers
	Direct review	Students review what had been worked on during previous lessons (15–20 minutes)
	Break time	Sensory break; that is, pushes library cart to library after gathering returned library books, washes the board or table, does chair push ups, or gets a drink of water.
	Reading/language arts	In general education with classroom aide
	Math	In general education with classroom aide
	Break time	Sensory break; that is, pushes library cart to library after gathering returned library books, washes the board or table, does chair push ups, or gets a drink of water
	Daily living skills	Alternates each month around a theme (e.g., cooking, money, measurement, laundry, cleaning)
	Lunch	Always in school cafeteria with general education class
	Social studies/science	Alternate days in general education with an aide
	School jobs, assemblies, or other special events	In school environment or general education classroom with classroom aide assistance when needed
	Journaling	Special education room at the end of the day. Special education teacher or classroom aide reviews positive behavior support plan and progress and writes notes home with Leo's input

Figure 4.14. Leo's high school schedule.

Reprinted with permission from Marilee Mapes, special education consultant, Heartland Area Education Agency, Johnston, IA.

- Symbols for visual supports were decided by working with the speech–language therapist and the team, and Raab suggested different ways to mount the symbols for efficient access in different settings. Simple words with symbols were used to increase some of Leo's sight vocabulary, and they were kept in a small, organized notebook that easily fit into Leo's side wheelchair pocket for easy access by all team members.

Raab was committed to providing collaborative services and supports to help Leo succeed in learning new skills. She knew that practicing skills daily in naturally occurring contexts would help his success. By establishing the habits and routines for appropriate social greetings and grooming, she helped Leo's team create and adapt a school job to meet his interests and functional needs. Progress monitoring was used to modify supports as needed, and all team members, especially Leo, contributed input into these discussions.

Summary

Occupational therapists collaborate in many varied and creative ways with school teams; there is no one way to collaborate effectively. The *Occupational Therapy Practice Framework: Domain and Process* (AOTA, 2002) and *The Guide to Occupational Therapy Practice* (Moyers & Dale, 2007) provides foundational information for occupational therapists to focus on promoting student participation in educationally relevant occupations. Therapists use a variety of strategies for collaboration during evaluation, intervention, and ongoing assessment, using the routines and activities of a student's day. Practitioners can provide hands-on services and team supports within the context of school routines, lessons, and activities. They can be an integral part of system supports, such as EIS and RtI programs (as allowed by state licensure and department of education regulations).

When principals, parents, teachers, paraprofessionals, related services providers, and other education personnel collaborate, they dramatically expand the opportunities for all children to participate in and experience success in school. Consider the following quote from a parent who recognizes how team collaboration benefits her child, the entire school, and team members during IEP meetings:

Parent Voices: Administrator support

The principal in my daughter's elementary school allowed the occupational therapist to present some OT exercises during our televised morning announcements for the whole school! Teachers [in general and special education] found that doing the exercises helped the whole class to focus, relax, and be more warmed up and prepared for their day! In addition, we often start our IEP team meetings with these same exercises: This makes the team start the session working together and brings us all in focus with each other and the plan in hand. My hat goes off to [the OT and the principal] for supporting better learning for all children in our school.

—Joni Kilgore, parent of Ally-Jane, Maryland

Acknowledgments

This chapter was a collaborative effort among the author and Barbara Hanft and Jayne Shepherd, the editors; Lisa Brickman, teacher; Marilee Mapes, teacher; Michelle Cullen, occupational therapist; Joni Kilgore and Betty Thompson, parents; Ilene Banker, administrator; and the children, families, and teachers with whom I have been blessed to work over the years.

Selected Resources

American Occupational Therapy Association. (2002). Occupational therapy practice framework: Domain and process. *American Journal of Occupational Therapy, 56,* 609–639.
This AOTA document replaces the previous document (*Uniform Terminology*) and has a twofold purpose: "(a) to describe the domain that centers and ground the profession's focus and actions and (b) [to outline] the process of occupational therapy evaluation and intervention that is dynamic and linked to the profession's focus on and use of occupation" (p. 609).

IDEA Partnerships: www.ideapartnerships.org
This Web site is a partnership between the Office of Special Education Programs and 55 national organizations, technical assistance providers, and state and local organizations and agencies. New information on No Child Left Behind and Individuals With Disability Education Improvement Act statutes and regulations can be found here, as well as information about RtI, EIS, and transition. The following book is especially helpful:

National Association of State Directors of Special Education. (2006). *Response to intervention: Policy considerations and implementation.* Alexandria, VA: Author.

Intervention Central: http://interventioncentral.org
> This site presents free tools and resources to promote positive behaviors and learning for all children. The home page lists multiple topics that include academic and behavioral strategies. Information about progress monitoring and response to intervention are also included.

National Resource Center for Learning Disabilities: www.nrcld.org/resource_kit/#rti
> This kit of materials was developed for professionals to learn about response to intervention and particularly how it relates to students with specific learning disabilities. General information, tools for change, the manual, a PowerPoint presentation, and parent pages are available on the Web site and are in the public domain.

References

American Occupational Therapy Association. (2002). Occupational therapy practice framework: Domain and process. *American Journal of Occupational Therapy, 56,* 609–639.

American Occupational Therapy Association. (2005). Standards of practice for occupational therapy. *American Journal of Occupational Therapy, 59,* 663–665.

American Occupational Therapy Association. (2007). *Frequently asked questions on response to intervention for school-based occupational therapists and occupational therapy assistants.* Retrieved October 20, 2007, from www.aota.org/Practitioners/PracticeAreas/Pediatrics/Highlights/FAQonRtI.aspx

Barnett, D. W., Daly, E. J., III, Jones, K. M., & Lentz, F. E. (2004). Response to intervention: Empirically based special service decisions from single-case designs of increasing and decreasing intensity. *Journal of Special Education, 38,* 66–79.

Clark, G. F. (2005). Developing appropriate student IEP goals. *OT Practice, 10*(14), 12–15.

Clark, G. F., & Miller, L. E. (1996). Providing effective occupational therapy services: Data-based decision making in school-based practice. *American Journal of Occupational Therapy, 50,* 701–708.

Coster, W., Deeney, T., Haltiwanger, J., & Haley, S. (1998). *School function assessment (SFA).* San Antonio, TX: Psychological Corporation.

Fisher, A. G., Bryze, K., Hume, V., & Griswold, L. A. (2005). *School AMPS: School Version of the Assessment of Motor and Process Skills* (2nd ed.). Ft. Collins, CO: Three Star Press.

Individuals With Disabilities Education Improvement Act of 2004, Pub. L. 108-446, 20 U.S.C. § 1400 et seq. (2004).

Jackson, L. L. (Ed.). (2007). *Occupational therapy services for children and youth under IDEA* (3rd ed.). Bethesda, MD: AOTA Press.

Johnson, E., Mellard, D. F., Fuchs, D., & McKnight, M. A. (2006). *Responsiveness to intervention (RTI): How to do it.* Lawrence, KS: National Resource Center for Learning Disabilities. Retrieved November 27, 2007, from www.nrcld.org/rti_manual/

Linder, J., & Clark, G. F. (2000). Best practice in documentation. In W. Dunn (Ed.), *Best practice occupational therapy* (pp. 135–146). Thorofare, NJ: Slack.

Moyers, P., & Dale, L. (2007). *Guide to occupational therapy practice* (2nd ed.). Bethesda, MD: AOTA Press.

National Association of State Directors of Special Education. (2006). *Response to intervention: Policy considerations and implementation.* Alexandria, VA: Author

Priest, N., & Waters, E. (2007). "Motor magic": An evaluation of a community capacity-building approach to supporting the development of preschool children (Part 2). *Australian Occupational Therapy Journal, 54,* 140–148.

Shepherd, J., Peters, S., Weise, C., Lowman, D. K., & Hatcher, B. (1999). *Therapy activities for the classroom.* Richmond: Virginia Commonwealth University.

Stewart, K. B. (2005). Purposes, processes, and methods of evaluation. In J. Case-Smith (Ed.), *Occupational therapy for children* (5th ed., pp. 218–245). St. Louis: Elsevier.

Swinth, Y. (Ed.), Chandler, B., Hanft, B., Jackson, L., & Shepherd, J. (2003). *Personnel issues in school-based occupational therapy: Supply and demand, preparation, and certification and licensure.* Gainesville: Center on Personnel Studies in Special Education, University of Florida. Available at www.coe.ufl.edu/copsse/docs/IB-1/1/IB-1.pdf

U.S. Department of Education, Office of Special Education and Rehabilitative Services. (n.d.). *Early intervening services fact sheet.* Retrieved February 9, 2007, from www.ed.gov/policy/speced/guid/idea/tb-early-intervent.doc

U.S. Department of Education, Office of Special Education Programs. (2006). Responsiveness to intervention in the SLD determination process. In *Tool Kit on Teaching and Assessing Students With Disabilities.* Retrieved January 3, 2007, from www.osepideasthatwork.org/ toolkit/ta_responsiveness_intervention.asp

Wakeford, L. (August, 2003). Integrating occupational therapy. In National Individualizing Preschool Inclusion Project, *Integrating therapy into the classroom* (p. 3.). Nashville, TN: Vanderbilt University Medical Center, Center for Child Development. Retrieved September 1, 2007, from www.collaboratingpartners.com/docs/R_Mcwilliam/Integrated%20 Services%20-%20April.pdf

Williams, M., & Shellenberger, S. (1996). *How does your engine run?* Albuquerque, NM: Therapy Works.

CHAPTER 5

Collaboration in Action: The Nitty Gritty

Yvonne Swinth, PhD, OTR/L, FAOTA

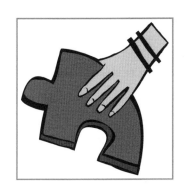

*W*e've seen OT working with children. She's seen how we work with children, and I think we have the respect for each other, and because we all believe in doing the best for the children, we respect any new ideas, they're not new ideas now. . . . We've internalized it because we believe in it. . . . Now we understand all the little nitty gritties of why things happen or why we're doing things.

—Kindergarten staff about collaboration with an occupational therapist (as quoted in Priest & Waters, 2007, p. 143)

The purpose of this chapter is to illustrate the principles presented throughout this book through vignettes depicting the steps therapists have taken to work toward and provide collaborative supports and services in education settings. The chapter discusses issues affecting the "nitty gritty" of collaboration (e.g., workload, communication, documentation, and administrative support) and suggests strategies in the text and the vignettes. Examples from different states are included to illustrate the various ways in which the Individuals With Disabilities Education Improvement Act of 2004 (IDEA) requirements have been implemented in the states to educate students with disabilities. Readers are strongly urged to align their current—and any planned— changes in practice with federal and state laws and regulations and their occupational therapy regulatory boards. Chapter 5 concludes with an extended case study emphasizing how an occupational therapist and her teammates collaborated to share information and observations to guide their decision making to help a student participate in general education with her peers.

After reading this material, readers will be able to

- Identify three strategies to encourage support moving toward a collaborative approach to service delivery in school environments;
- Recognize the demands (e.g., scheduling, time, communication) that collaboration may have on an occupational therapist's workload;
- Identify IDEA terminology for documenting occupational therapy team and system supports as well as hands-on services on student individualized education programs (IEPs);
- Recognize how assistive technology can support the development of collaborative IEPs; and
- Identify strategies occupational therapists can use to collaborate successfully with team members to promote a student's academic achievement and functional performance.

Key Topics

- Communicating about occupational therapy
- Managing workload
- Administrative support for flexible services
- Documenting collaborative services and supports

The "Nitty Gritty" of Collaboration

A variety of issues may affect an occupational therapist's successful implementation of collaborative services and supports in the schools. Some of the topics and strategies addressed in this chapter are practical and simply require therapists to rethink how they have traditionally approached services in the schools. Others require more thought about how professional philosophy and personal beliefs affect school-based practice. All depend on teacher and family acceptance and support from school administrators. The first part of this chapter is divided into four sections:

1. Communicating collaboratively
2. Collaboration and occupational therapy workloads
3. Administrative support for flexible services and supports
4. Documenting collaborative occupational therapy services.

Communicating Collaboratively

Occupational therapists must communicate effectively about their collaborative services using language that is easily understood by families and education personnel, as suggested in Table 5.1. Professional jargon and discipline-specific terms can isolate occupational therapists from other team members rather than facilitate a shared understanding of student performance and desired outcomes (Swinth, 2003).

Occupational therapists often use terminology such as "Johnny *qualifies* for 30 min/week of occupational therapy" in their reports and discussions with families and educators. IDEA does not identify "qualification criteria" specific to occupational therapy or other related services. If a student is eligible for special education, then that student has access to occupational therapy, as a related service, if the skills and expertise of an occupational therapist are needed to ensure that the student receives a free appropriate education in the least restrictive environment. (Note that each state may decide whether to include occupational therapy in early intervening services identified in IDEA 2004 and discussed in Chapter 4.) Additionally, some professional terms may be unfamiliar to families and education personnel, including terms such as *areas of occupational performance* and *analysis of occupational performance.*

Table 5.1. Occupational Therapy Jargon Regarding Services and Supports

Traditional Term or Phrase	Term or Phrase Supporting Collaboration
Qualify for occupational therapy services	Recommend occupational therapy supports and service
Push-in	Hands-on or team supports In-context or integrated therapy
Pull-out	Out-of-context[a] services and supports to support skill acquisition
Therapy or teacher goals	Student goals, focused outcomes
Discharge from occupational therapy	No longer requires the skills and expertise of an occupational therapist to meet student's educational needs
Motor, hand, or sensory integration therapy	Occupational therapy services and supports

[a]The goal is to move to in-context services and supports as soon as possible.

Therapists need to translate professional terms in ways that still convey the unique contribution of occupational therapy, as illustrated in the vignette below.

Collaboration in Action: *Translating professional jargon*

Sue Ann is a new graduate who recently started work in a small school district. Before sharing results from her first student observation and evaluation with her team, she shared a draft of her report with her mentor, Connie. After reading it, Connie encouraged Sue Ann to consider how to communicate *Occupational Therapy Practice Framework: Domain and Process* (American Occupational Therapy Association [AOTA], 2002) terms in teacher-friendly language. She also encouraged Sue Ann to be careful about using terms such as *performance,* which already have specific meanings in an education setting. Because a description of a student's academic achievement and functional performance is a required part of IEP planning, Connie suggested that Sue Ann refer to *school and play performance* rather than to *occupational performance areas.* Connie also suggested that Sue Ann use *role* instead of *performance role* and *habit* instead of *performance habit* to avoid introducing too many meanings for the word *performance.*

Identifying Services and Supports in IEPs

One critical communication challenge faced by school-based occupational therapists and occupational therapy assistants is how to describe their intervention, particularly on IEPs (Swinth, 2004). As discussed in Chapter 1, during the late 1970s and through the 1980s, the literature on school-based occupational therapy used the terms *direct, consult,* and *monitor* to describe options for providing occupational therapy services to students with disabilities who were typically taught in self-contained classrooms (Dunn, 1985, 1988). We have used the descriptive terms *hands-on services, team supports,* and *system supports* to emphasize the need for blending traditional service models in school settings. Professional occupational therapy documents use language consistent with the *Occupational Therapy Practice Framework* to describe school-based practice (for further discussion, see Chapter 4).

In education settings, school administrators prefer, or may require, that related services such as occupational and physical therapy be recorded on students' IEPs using specific IDEA terms such as *related services* (see Resource 5.1 for the IDEA definition of *related*). Although some school districts consider the team and systems supports discussed in this book to be included in related services, many school districts do not.

Some school districts differentiate team and system supports from hands-on services by using IDEA terms (i.e., *accommodations, modifications, supplementary aids and services, services on behalf of a child, assistive technology,* and *transition services;* for definitions, see Table 5.2). *Modifications* and *accommodations* refer to special education and related services but are not formally defined in the IDEA regulations. Nolet and McLaughlin (2000)

Remember this. . . .
IDEA 2004 does not identify qualification criteria specific to occupational therapy. Decisions about when and how to provide related services are made by IEP teams in collaboration with the occupational therapist.

Resource 5.1. IDEA Definition of *Related Services*

IDEA defines *related services* as

> Transportation and such developmental, corrective, and other supportive services as are required to assist a child with a disability to benefit from special education, and includes speech–language pathology and audiology services, interpreting services, psychological services, physical and occupational therapy, recreation, including therapeutic recreation, early identification and assessment of disabilities in children, counseling services, including rehabilitation counseling, orientation and mobility services, and medical services for diagnostic or evaluation purposes. (§ 300.34[a])

Table 5.2. IDEA Terms Regarding Team and System Supports

IDEA Term	Definition
Supplementary aids and services	Aids, services, and other supports that are provided in regular education classes, other education-related settings, and extracurricular and nonacademic settings to enable children with disabilities to be educated with nondisabled children to the maximum extent appropriate in accordance with §§ 300.114 through 300.11 (§ 300.42).
Services on behalf of the child	This term is mentioned in § 300.320(4) but is not specifically defined. However, an interpretation has been provided by the U.S. Department of Education, Office of Special Education Programs (2000): The term "on behalf of the child" includes, among other things, services that are provided to the parents or teacher of the child with a disability to help them to more effectively work with the child. . . . Supports for school personnel could also include special training for a child's teacher. However, for the training to meet the requirements of § 300.347(a)(3), it would normally be targeted directly to assisting the teacher to meet a unique and specific need of the child and not simply to participate in an in-service training program that is generally available in a public agency.
Accommodations or adaptations	No technical IDEA definition.
Modifications	No technical IDEA definition.
Assistive technology	Any item, piece of equipment, or product system, whether acquired commercially off the shelf, modified, or customized, that is used to increase, maintain, or improve the functional capabilities of a child with a disability. The term does not include a medical device that is surgically implanted or the replacement of such device (§ 300.5).
Assistive technology services	Any service that directly assists a child with a disability in the selection, acquisition, or use of an assistive technology device (§ 300.6).

Transition services	(a) A coordinated set of activities for a child with a disability that—
	
	(1) Is designed to be within a results-oriented process, that is focused on improving the academic and functional achievement of the child with a disability to facilitate the child's movement from school to post-school activities, including postsecondary education, vocational education, integrated employment (including supported employment), continuing and adult education, adult services, independent living, or community participation;
	
	(2) Is based on the individual child's needs, taking into account the child's strengths, preferences, and interests; and includes—
	
	   (i) Instruction;
	   (ii) Related services;
	   (iii) Community experiences;
	   (iv) The development of employment and other post-school adult living objectives; and
	   (v) If appropriate, acquisition of daily living skills and provision of a functional vocational evaluation.
	
	(b) *Transition services* for children with disabilities may be special education, if provided as specially designed instruction, or a related service, if required to assist a child with a disability to benefit from special education. (§ 300.43).

Note: Citations are from the Code of Federal Regulations (CFR), Assistance to the States for the Education of Children With Disabilities, *34 CFR Parts 300,* issued August 3, 2006.

defined modifications as alterations to the subject content or expectations of child performance; accommodations, or adaptations, are the services and supports that improve student access to subject matter and allow them to demonstrate what they know with the same learning outcomes required as for other students (unlike modifications, which allow for a different learning outcome).

Note that IDEA requires that related services and supports such as occupational therapy be identified on students' IEPs but does not mandate the terminology to describe how to provide them. IEPs must contain

a statement of the special education and related services and supplementary aids and services, based on peer-reviewed research to the extent practicable,

Table 5.3. Evolution of Terminology and Collaboration in the Schools

Descriptors of Collaboration	IDEA 2004 Terms[a]	Traditional Occupational Therapy Terms[b]
Hands-on services with team supports (group and individual)	Related services[c] Assistive technology services	Direct service (in and out of context)
Team supports System supports	Supplementary aids and services Services on behalf of the child Accommodations, adaptations Modifications Assistive technology services	Consult, monitoring

[a]See Exhibit 1.1A and Table 5.2 for Individuals With Disabilities Education Improvement Act (IDEA) definitions.

[b]Discussed for school practice in Dunn (1985, 1988).

[c]In a few states, occupational therapy can be specially designed instruction and is then provided as hands-on or team supports, individual or group.

to be provided to the child, or on behalf of the child, and a statement of the program modifications or supports for school personnel that will be provided to enable the child—

(i) To advance appropriately toward attaining the annual goals;

(ii) To be involved and progress in the general curriculum in accordance with paragraph (a)(1) of this section and to participate in extracurricular and other nonacademic activities; and

(iii) To be educated and participate with other children with disabilities and nondisabled children in the activities described in this section.

(34 CFR § 300.320[4])

Exhibit 1.1A in the Appendix identifies other IDEA requirements for students' IEPs.

Historically, occupational therapists have tended to only document hands-on services on the IEP. But, regardless of the terminology used, it is important that therapists be acknowledged for their work and advocate for documenting *all* occupational therapy supports and services on students' IEPs. The IDEA terms can be linked to the descriptive terms the authors of this book have used to emphasize the collaborative roles therapists play in education settings by blending hands-on services with team and system supports. Table 5.3 provides an overview of the evolution of the various terms used to describe occupational therapy in education settings.

The essential point for collaborative teams to remember about documenting occupational therapy services and supports on students' IEPs is that the communication skills and expertise of an occupational therapist is key to achieving student success, not *how* the service is labeled. Team members who value collaboration, and know how to engage in it, make sure it happens whatever the format is for developing the IEP document. As one school-based therapist observes,

Therapist Voices: Emphasize collaboration, not documentation

I find the IEP collaboration process is a *totally* separate issue from the documentation format. Unfortunately, we still have related service providers who write their own discipline-specific goals and objectives. They come to an IEP meeting with everything written and without having spoken to anyone else on the team. The teachers I work with have gotten used to having me stop by to talk about the child's program before the IEP.

—Dottie Handley-More, occupational therapist, Washington

Collaboration and Occupational Therapy Workloads

The challenge of scheduling related services and special education for students with disabilities has increased with the legal mandates for educating students in the least restrictive environment and the focus on student achievement in the IDEA and the No Child Left Behind Act of 2001. For many therapists, this has not created a problem because they already work in the context of students' school environments. However, for therapists who have primarily provided services in therapy places and spaces, the dual emphasis on student inclusion and achievement has created new challenges. Occupational therapists must provide, and receive credit for, a range of services and supports that assist all students to access, benefit from, and participate in general education programs (AOTA, 2006).

Workload vs. Caseload

Over the years, many school-based occupational therapists have asked, "What is a reasonable caseload?" (AOTA, 2006, p. 1). Historically, caseloads have been based on the number of students receiving hands-on intervention and have neglected to account for essential occupational therapy services such as team and systems supports. In contrast, the concept of a workload recognizes the numerous ways in which therapists meet student, team, and system needs (AOTA, 2006).

Traditionally, the number of students receiving occupational therapy has been used to determine staffing positions as well as therapists' caseloads and schedules. Many administrators request that therapists document schedules that clearly indicate when students receive hands-on services. This allows administrators to easily ascertain whether therapists provide the frequency and intensity of occupational therapy services identified in students' IEPs. Thus, a traditional occupational therapy schedule focuses almost exclusively on assigning students to specific time slots on a weekly or monthly basis.

However, a schedule should accurately reflect a therapist's entire workload, which includes not only hands-on services but team and system supports as well. A schedule that is flexible and reflects a variety of services and supports may also facilitate collaboration, although it may not make it easy for administrators to track a specific day-to-day, predictable schedule for each therapist. A schedule that reflects a therapist's actual workload may help achieve student outcomes because student needs and contextual factors drive scheduling rather than convenience or preferences of therapists or teachers. Figure 5.1 illustrates 2 weeks in a 4-week rotation in the workload (including travel time) of a therapist whose clients include students, families, other professionals working with students, and the school system. Reflection 5.1 provides an opportunity for comparison with how this occupational therapist provided hands-on services and team and system supports.

Remember this. . . .
A schedule that is flexible and reflects a variety of occupational therapy services and supports also facilitates collaboration.

Reflection 5.1

Workloads vs. Caseloads

The workload depicted in Figure 5.1 reflects all the services and supports actually provided by an occupational therapist to 50 students, their teams, and the school system.

- *Hands-on and team supports* in school spaces and places is achieved by combining occupational therapy "slots" for 2 or more students in a classroom. Time is also set aside for evaluation and assessment.

- *Team supports* are provided through team meetings, prereferral activities, planning, and in-class assistance. Eating lunch with teaching staff three times a week builds team relationships.

- *System supports* are provided through participation on the district assistive technology team and literacy committee.

How does your schedule reflect your actual weekly or monthly workload?

Week 1 (of a 4-week rotation)

Time	Monday	Tuesday	Wednesday	Thursday	Friday
7:30	*Life Skills Team Meeting—Elementary #1*	Student documentation[a]	*Bimonthly therapy meetings with team*	*Meetings and prereferral activities at Elementary #1*	*High school team meeting—plan monthly program*
8:00		**AT consults/training across district**			
8:30	**Elementary school #1 (8 students)—Individual and group services in life skills**		**Preschool #1 group activities/center based**		**Prevocational/vocational training with high school students at Goodwill, Safeway, and crafts store**
9:00					
9:30	**In classroom to address fine motor, IADLs, eating,* and functional skills**			Travel to Elementary #3	
10:00				Heather K	
10:30				Social skills group	
11:00	***Eats with students**	Lunch			
11:30		Travel to Elementary #2		Handwriting club	
12:00		**Lunch/recess group**	Lunch	Lunch	Lunch/travel
12:30			OT evaluation and write-ups	**Sports club**	**Eurie K**
1:00		**Sarah K**		**Martin S**	**Mia L**
1:30		**Trisha G**		**Jeff R**	**Jose K**
2:00	Travel	**Henry C**		Travel and	**Horatio V**
2:30	Student documentation[a]	Student documentation[a]		***Literacy Committee (1x/month)***	Student documentation[a]
3:00					

Week 2 (of a 4-week rotation)

Time	Monday	Tuesday	Wednesday	Thursday	Friday
7:30	*Life skills meeting—Elementary school #1*	Student documentation[a]	*Preschool #1 team meeting*	***Elementary school #2 Team meetings Prereferral activities***	Monthly meeting with COTA/program planning
8:00		**OT evaluations and write-ups**			
8:30	**Elementary #1 Community access with life skills classroom**		**Johnny C**		Travel
9:00			**Candy S**		
9:30			**Mona K**	Travel to Elementary #3	**Intervention based on student need and on teacher request. Supervision of COTA**
10:00			**Eurie H**	**OT evaluations and write-ups**	
10:30			**Keith R**		
11:00		Lunch	**Mark L**		
11:30		Travel to Elementary #2	Lunch		
12:00		**Lunch/recess group**	**PM Preschool #1 group activities and centers**	Lunch	Lunch/travel
12:30				**Sports club**	**Eurie K**
1:00		**Sarah K**		**Martin S**	**Mia L**
1:30	***Lunch in the community**	**Trisha G**		Travel	**Jose K**
2:00		**Henry C**		**Jr. high 1x/month**	**Horatio V**
2:30		Paperwork and communication			*Teacher training*
3:00			Student documentation[a]		

Figure 5.1. Collaborative approach to scheduling an occupational therapist's caseload.

Key: **Bold—Hands-on Services**   *Italic—Team Supports*   ***Bold Italic—Systems Supports***

Note. AT = assistive technology; COTA = certified occupational therapy assistant; IADLs = instrumental activities of daily living; OT = occupational therapy.

[a]Student documentation includes attendance, performance data, data collection for progress monitoring, and Medicaid documentation.

Remember this. . . .
Occupational therapists should provide, and receive credit for, a range of services and supports that ensure that all students participate in general educational programs.

Communicating About Workloads

Therapists need to communicate with their special education administrator(s) and other team members regarding the numerous team and system supports that they provide as part of their workload. For example, Marnie, an occupational therapist, was feeling overwhelmed with the number of students to whom she provided services and supports. After talking with her mentor, Marnie decided to ask for a meeting with her special education administrator to discuss her actual workload (Resource 5.2 delineates Marnie's workload). As a result of their discussion, the administrator agreed that all identified services and supports were indeed part of Marnie's job and recognized that she needed to consider Marnie's entire workload when addressing therapy schedules and caseload issues throughout the district.

Part of the scheduling challenge in schools is *how* occupational therapists establish their schedules. Traditionally, therapists have developed their schedules on their own or by going from teacher to teacher to ask for their preferences. As a result, students are scheduled in a yearly time slot that may never change except if a student moves or when a school's schedule changes (e.g., semester change at a high school).

Scheduling should not be viewed as static, however. In fact, as student, team, or system needs wax and wane, therapists may need to modify parts of their schedule several times throughout the year. The following vignettes illustrate how occupational therapists can collaborate with their education partners to develop schedules that reflect their workload more accurately and highlight their hands-on services and team supports.

Resource 5.2. Marnie's Occupational Therapy Workload

Hands-On Services With Team Supports

- Provide hands-on (individual and group) services with team supports in school spaces and places for students who require them to benefit from their educational program
- Assist teaching staff to integrate adaptive equipment, positioning, sensory strategies, and other needs related to a student's ability to participate in the educational setting
- Develop home programs with families, as needed, to support student learning
- Participate in team meetings, individualized education program (IEP) meetings, and so on, related to specific students
- Complete student reevaluations.

System Supports

- Supervise the occupational therapy assistant per licensure requirements
- Participate on evaluation teams to help determine students' eligibility for special education and provide input regarding their needs for occupational therapy
- Document services and supports (e.g., IEPs, progress reports, time sheets)
- Communicate with community therapists and other health personnel, as appropriate
- Participate on district committees, as assigned
- Stay current regarding regulations, evidence, and current intervention strategies.

Collaboration in Action: Take it to the teachers

Kathryn was tired of working so hard to finalize a therapy schedule for the school year only to get to the last two students and have a teacher tell her that none of her available times were appropriate. So at the beginning of the new school year, she decided to rethink how she scheduled her students. First, Kathryn determined what blocks of time she could be at each school. Then, during the first week of school, she brought several "ooey, gooey" desserts to each school. She placed big sheets of paper on a wall in the teacher's lounge during lunch to indicate when she could work at that campus. Then she encouraged teachers to sign up for their occupational therapy times and negotiate schedule changes with each other while she served dessert.

Recognizing that building relationships is part of the art of collaboration, Kathryn offered desserts as a concrete way to show her appreciation for the teachers' hard work and willingness to figure out schedules with her. She discovered that facilitating these discussions resulted in more collaborative services and supports than ever because the teachers scheduled occupational therapy during the instructional periods when *they* wanted her support. In addition, the teachers worked together to group students across several classrooms on the basis of common curricular and IEP goals. Later that year, the teachers were much more accepting when Kathryn needed to change her schedule to meet student needs because the teachers were all more aware of each other's time constraints.

Collaboration in Action: *Make it a district effort*

Claire worked with her administrator to secure a room at the district office so she could schedule all occupational therapy services on one day. Claire and the other occupational therapists in her small school district (i.e., three elementary schools, one middle school, and one high school) sent out an announcement that they would host an "arena scheduling" day for all students receiving occupational therapy. All teachers (general education and special education) were invited to come before school, during their lunch, or after school to collaborate with the occupational therapists (and one another) to find the optimum schedule for their students. This was a time when staff were already going in and out of the district office to pick up notices and materials.

Claire and her colleagues found that their system helped everyone work through the conflicts that inevitably arise when scheduling services and supports. With teachers and therapists in the same room, they were able to address the various needs of all students and staff in one day, albeit a long one. The administration also appreciated this approach, and the following year suggested that other related services providers join the arena scheduling to expand the opportunities for collaboration. For example, the occupational therapist and speech–language therapist found three groups they could plan with the school counselor and classroom teachers to support social participation, fine motor skills, and language acquisition in the classroom.

Collaboration in Action: *"Block" it*

By making two procedural changes, Antoine "found" time to collaborate with teachers and other school staff while he worked with students in their classrooms. First, he secured his special education administrator's support to document occupational therapy on the IEP as minutes per month rather than minutes per week. Second, he allocated his time to specific classrooms and schools in "blocks" (see Figure 5.1 for an example).

Antoine talked with specific teachers to determine how to provide hands-on and team supports within the assigned blocks of time to two students, Karl and Sasha. For example, Karl's IEP designated 120 minutes per month of occupational therapy, and Sasha's designated 60 minutes. Depending on each student's progress and the team supports the teachers found helpful, Antoine varied the amount of weekly services and supports he provided. One week Karl needed 60 minutes of hands-on services while Sasha needed only 10 minutes of team supports to stay on track with her goals. The next week, Karl received 20 minutes of hands-on with team supports, while Sasha received 30 minutes of hands-on with team supports.

Antoine realized that although a one-size-fits-all intensity of hands-on services (30 minutes per week) was convenient for some teachers and administrators because of its predictability, this approach did not address the evolving needs of his students. If he could work with students and teachers within school places, spaces, and paces, he could model strategies (e.g., how to use adaptive equipment strategies) for the teaching staff to incorporate numerous times in curriculum activities and tasks between his scheduled class visits. Block scheduling also allowed Antoine to provide team supports during field trips.

These scenarios reinforce that schedules are not static and illustrate how to develop an initial schedule based on a team's priorities for addressing student goals (Reflection 5.2). The vignettes illustrate how the therapists

- *Used creative problem solving* to come up with a strategy to address scheduling challenges to combine hands-on services and team supports in typical school contexts (e.g., Antoine used block scheduling to find the time to work with students and teachers in the classroom);
- *Asked teachers and paraprofessionals* to help determine the unique needs of students and when they needed assistance in the classroom (e.g., Kathryn discovered that teachers were more willing to accommodate modifications to occupational therapy services and supports when they were involved in setting up the initial schedule); and
- *Recognized scheduling as a systems issue* and secured administrator assistance to find a successful solution for each school district (e.g., administrative approval for Claire's arena scheduling was essential in encouraging her education colleagues to respond to her invitation).

Rescheduling is often needed throughout the school year to enable occupational therapists to adapt services and supports in various school places and spaces to address students' progress toward reaching their goals. For example, a therapist may need to demonstrate certain intervention strategies to a language arts teacher to help a student with written expression, then work with the student and her aide in the cafeteria to learn to navigate the lunch line and cashier without losing control and, finally, figure out how to prompt the student to manage the hygiene process after toileting (Jean Polichino, personal communication, April 10, 2007).

Administrative Support for Flexible Services and Supports

Administrators, parents, educators, and therapists should always leave an IEP meeting understanding what occupational therapy services and supports will "look like." Although many school districts still require that therapists select a traditional service model (i.e., consult, direct, and monitor; Dunn, 1985, 1988, 1992), it is more helpful to blend hands-on services, as needed, with team and system supports (Jackson, 2007; Polcyn & Bissell, 2005; Shepherd, 1999; Swinth & Brodbeck, 2002). Hands-on services must always include team support via collaborative consultation, coaching, co-teaching, modeling, demonstrations, and so on. System supports can also benefit individual children as well as special populations or the entire school system. Examples

Reflection 5.2

Finding Time for Collaboration

If finding time for collaborative occupational therapy services and supports in your school district is a challenge, first look at whether you schedule students into available time slots or consider student need and block scheduling with teachers. How could you enlist teacher and administrator support to consider implementing one of the strategies highlighted in the vignettes (or others you know about) to address workload issues?

Remember this. . . .
Schedules are not static and should identify all the hands-on services and team and system supports on a therapist's workload.

include participating on a task force to develop a program for preschoolers with autism spectrum disorder or offering an in-service to teachers about how to help children with attention-deficit/hyperactivity disorder focus on classroom lessons and activities. As described below, therapists may use a variety of strategies to help administrators, parents, and others understand that occupational therapy is more than hands-on individual and group services (Chapter 7 provides numerous examples of how to do this).

Therapist Voices: Administrative support

I cover seven buildings and use block schedules to group kids and set aside half or 1 day a week as a flex day for child study, IEPs, new evals, or community-based instruction. One of my schools has a very supportive assistant principal, Ilene Banker. OT has the time to be part of team meetings since they are run efficiently. Ilene knows my schedule and tries to schedule meetings when I am in her building or have a flex day. She gives me advance notice and begins and ends the meeting on time, running an efficient meeting while still listening to the concerns of all team members. I know I won't be there for 4 hours plus.

In the long run, it saves me time and inappropriate referrals when team members know about OT and who they can borrow materials from. In my county, the OTs have developed a "Helping Hands" picture book to give teachers ideas for handwriting and fine motor activities; a prereferral instruction manual; and other materials. During OT month, I have a bucket of freebies to give away to teachers that I put next to a sign-in sheet. I've also written columns for the parent newsletter and the PTA newsletters and include seasonal ideas for children and parents to do together.

—Jan Emerick-Brother, occupational therapist, Virginia

Flexibility Throughout the School Year

It is not uncommon for a student to require differing amounts or proportions of hands-on services with team supports from September to June. However, it can be very challenging to document changes in occupational therapy intervention on most IEP forms. School districts and states have addressed the issue of frequency of related services differently. For example, one cooperative in Texas records minutes per grading period to reduce team misperceptions about what "per month" frequency means. School personnel assumed short months like August and December would be prorated for service and support time, and families wanted the same amount of services as in longer months (Jean Polichino, personal communication, April 10, 2007). Some school districts even record minutes per year. The Washington State Department of Education ruled that occupational therapy would be documented by minutes per month to reassure any parents concerned that their child might not receive the full amount of occupational therapy.

In the following examples, therapists and their teammates have developed creative strategies for documenting a range of anticipated services on students' IEPs. These strategies also illustrate the IDEA requirement that special education and related

Remember this. . . .
Blending hands-on services with team and system supports can meet the changing needs of a student and team members more efficiently than choosing only one approach for an entire year.

services be provided in the least restrictive environment to ensure a student receives a free appropriate public education. (Exhibit 1.1A in the Appendix defines *least restrictive environment* and *free appropriate public education*.)

Collaboration in Action: Intermittent services and supports

Inbal, an occupational therapist, worked in a rural school district with several high school students who needed hands-on services with team supports to adapt to new school activities and routines for only 3 weeks at the beginning of each semester. The remainder of the school year, Inbal provided team supports via collaborative consultation with the students' teachers and paraprofessionals. Inbal scheduled a meeting with her administrator to discuss her workload and emphasized that it was costly to provide 30 minutes of weekly occupational therapy throughout the school year when her students only needed services for 6 weeks.

Inbal and her administrator worked with the office assistant who tracked IEP data and came up with a plan. Inbal recorded each student's needs on the present levels of academic achievement and functional performance section of their IEPs. Then she and her teammates recorded their decisions about the frequency and duration of occupational therapy as shown in Table 5.4. Using IDEA terms, *hands-on services* were identified on the IEPs as "OT-related services" and *team supports* were identified as "OT supplementary aids and services"

Collaboration in Action: Changing intensity

Li wanted to provide Jenna with intensive hands-on and team supports at the start of the school year and then transition to *less* hands-on service and *more* team support as the year progressed. Jenna's team agreed but still encouraged Li to average his time on a weekly basis throughout the school year. He felt this approach locked him into "underserving" Jenna at the start of the school year and "overserving" her at the end of the year, which would not meet Jenna's needs.

Li and other occupational therapists in his district proposed a strategy to the special education administrator. Their teams had already been working to increase the number of IEPs with integrated related services goals. Finding a way to document team supports from therapists would be their next step. What did they do? First, they developed a strategy for documenting the

Table 5.4. Documenting Occupational Therapy Services and Supports on IEPs

Services (Using IDEA 2004 Terms)	Intensity	Start Date	End Date
OT-related services	30 min/week	Sept. 10, 2007	Sept. 28, 2007
OT-related services	30 min/week	Jan. 15, 2008	Feb. 15, 2008
OT supplementary aids and services	60 min/month	Sept. 10, 2007	June 23, 2008

Note. IEP = individualized education program, IDEA = Individuals With Disabilities Education Improvement Act of 2004; OT = occupational therapy.

Occupational therapy as part of "Student's" educational program is recommended as

- Related services (to benefit from special education);
- Supplementary aids and services;
- Program modifications or support for school personnel (on behalf of the student); and
- Assistive technology devices and services.

It is anticipated that occupational therapy services for "Student" will proceed on a continuum. At the time of "Student's" annual Individualized Education Program or as part of a report card, the occupational therapy service may be adjusted to meet the student's educational needs, based on present levels of academic achievement and functional performance in the least restrictive environment. As the data indicates that "Student" is able to _____, it is anticipated that occupational therapy services will be discontinued unless additional needs are identified by the team on the basis of "Student's" current educational program.

Figure 5.2. Recommendations for occupational therapy services and supports in evaluation reports.

Source. University Place School District, University Place, Washington.

range of occupational therapy services and supports recommended in a student's occupational therapy evaluation report so that it would not be viewed as a change in placement by their state monitors (see Figure 5.2 for an example using IDEA terminology from the state of Washington). Team representatives met with their special education administrators and reviewed how this report language was consistent with preliminary research indicating that parents are more accepting of discontinuing services and supports if criteria for achieving goals are discussed from the beginning (Effgen, 2000).

Next, Li and the other team representatives clearly documented the recommended occupational therapy services and supports as part of a student's present level of academic achievement and functional performance on the IEP. They also attached a narrative describing different intensities of intervention, based on student needs. Plan A specified the initial intensity of occupational therapy intervention (hands-on services with team supports and systems support) a student would receive and described the proficiency the student was expected to reach for each IEP goal (documented with progress monitoring). Once achieved, the student would move to Plan B (decreasing services and supports). If sufficient progress was not made toward achieving goals, Plan C was initiated (reassessing the goal and intensity of intervention).

Collaboration in Action: Identifying an actual workload

After attending a workshop on best practice and collaborative services, Eduardo recognized that he usually recommended hands-on services for a student's IEP as "related services" for either 30 or 60 minutes per week. However, the team or system supports vital to his students' success were not recorded; no wonder his supervisor and teaching partners did not understand why he felt overwhelmed and could not add more students to his workload.

Eduardo asked his administrator how he could document his team supports on an IEP (e.g., demonstrating a specific strategy for a teacher, adapting the school environment to benefit all students). After much discussion, they agreed that Eduardo could document the occupational therapy supports and services actually needed for a student to receive a free appropriate public education in the least restrictive environment. In addition to "related services" minutes, he added team supports by using IDEA terminology (e.g., "supplementary aids and services," "services on behalf of the child") as appropriate.

After further discussion, the administrator worked with Eduardo and the secretarial staff to build an Excel database to track all the occupational therapy services and supports Eduardo provided. After a year, Eduardo found that for some students he significantly decreased his hands-on services and increased support to the staff and teachers. He continued to keep outcome data and documented that he could achieve the educational goals for some students by providing only team and system supports.

These scenarios represent real strategies that three therapists have implemented to provide and document flexible services and supports. They also illustrate how the therapists recognized that there was more than one way to meet a challenge and how, by respectfully engaging in collaborative (and sometimes challenging) conversations, solutions can be realized. Consider how these therapists

- *Enlisted their administrators* (e.g., therapy supervisors or special education coordinator) in the process of finding workable strategies to combine hands-on services and team support (e.g., Inbal convinced her administrator that providing flexible occupational therapy services over the course of a semester was cost effective);

- *Used creative problem solving* to come up with a strategy to document all occupational therapy services and support (e.g., Li documented hands-on services, team support, and system support in evaluations and on student IEPs using IDEA terminology); and

- *Engaged in and documented the collaborative process* (e.g., Eduardo worked with school administrators to track occupational therapy service minutes in an Excel database with the help of secretarial staff).

Another strategy that some therapists have used to transition from solely providing hands-on services in therapy places and spaces to combining hands-on supports with team supports in typical school contexts is the 3:1 model. In a 3:1 schedule, therapists provide traditional one-on-one service to individual students and small groups for the first 3 weeks of each month. The 4th week is devoted to providing team or system supports within the classroom and other school environments. During this "collaboration week," therapists observe and work with children in various school contexts and assist them in generalizing emerging skills; consult with teachers, parents, and other education personnel; order and adapt equipment for the classroom; modify classroom materials; address curricular issues; and develop in-class programs. Therapists document the team supports provided on behalf of each student in the 4th week.

The 3:1 transition model, like the previous strategies described, requires administrative support to initiate and sustain collaboration among all team members. Although administrators can assist school personnel with transitioning to collaborative services and supports by setting aside 1 week to highlight teamwork, blending hands-on services with team and system supports throughout each week of the school year may meet the changing needs of a student and team members more efficiently. When the 3:1 transition model separates hands-on service from team and system support, therapists may become "stuck" providing traditional direct service for 3 weeks, thus limiting classroom or system collaboration to only 1 week per month. Or it may be difficult to effectively meet a student's need if one has to "wait" 2 weeks to provide team or systems support (e.g., the student need arises during Week 2, and the 3:1 model does not allow for the flexibility to adjust the therapist's schedule until Week 4).

The team and system supports for a specific student should be documented regardless of whether they are provided throughout the month or only during Week 4. A concise form to document the hands-on services and team supports provided to a student over an entire school year is offered in Figure 5.3. This type of documentation can also help therapists track the needs of a specific student and team and revise intervention as appropriate adjustments. As described in Table 5.2, IDEA recognizes team supports "on behalf of the child," such as special training for parents and educators that "meet a unique and specific need of the child" (U.S. Department of Education, 2000, p. 32). System supports that are not student specific (e.g., providing an in-service to all teachers) are not identified on a student's IEP but should be documented as part of a therapist's workload in other formats (for an example, see "Collaboration in Action: Identifying an actual workload").

The 3:1 transition model may be a good first step in providing collaborative hands-on services with team supports in typical school contexts. However, it is important not to stop there and to continue to refine service options, document outcomes, and ensure that occupational therapy services and supports promote student achievement and functional performance as communicated in the IEPs. Table 5.5 identifies additional strategies that team members can implement to find time in their busy schedules to meet, plan, and work with students together.

Documenting Collaborative Occupational Therapy Services

Increased accessibility to the Internet, e-mail, and computers has also increased the opportunities and options for collaboration. Although school districts have unique ways to maximize technology supports for developing IEPs, there appear to be some commonalities across districts. The term *electronic IEP* refers to both (a) using the Internet, e-mail, Web servers, and other electronic means to help facilitate collaboration and the IEP process and (b) electronic IEP programs designed to increase staff efficiency in completing paperwork uniformly and tracking services.

Software programs such as FileMaker Pro, Microsoft Word, and Microsoft Excel can be used to format IEP templates and support collaborative decision making and documentation. This can help decrease the number of face-to-face team meetings and facilitate the development of integrated IEP goals and objectives for each student. Occupational therapists can educate team members regarding how to best use their expertise to meet a student's outcome and also increase their own understanding of the overall education program and core curriculum.

In addition, some districts are hiring programmers to write their own IEP management software to facilitate teamwork among all stakeholders, including parents.

2007–2008
Occupational Therapy Service Delivery Record

Student:	Date of Birth:	School:	Grade/teacher:
Service Provider:	IEP Date:		3 Yr. Date:

2007-08	M	T	W	T	F	M	T	W	T	F	M	T	W	T	F	M	T	W	T	F	M	T	W	T	F
SEP	•	4	5	6	7	10	11	12	13	14	17	18	19	20	21	24	25	26	27	28					
CODE																									
TIME																									
OCT	1	2	3	4	5	8	9	10	11	12	15	16	17	18	19	22	23	24	25	26	29	30	31		
CODE																									
TIME																									
NOV				1	2	5	6	7	8	9	•	13	14	15	16	19	20	21	•	•	26	27	28	29	30
CODE																									
TIME																									
DEC	3	4	5	6	7	10	11	12	13	14	17	18	19	•	•	•	•	•	•	•	•	•			
CODE																									
TIME																									
JAN	•	•	•	3	4	7	8	9	10	11	14	15	16	17	18	•	22	23	24	25	28	29	30	31	
CODE																									
TIME																									
FEB					1	4	5	6	7	8	11	12	13	14	15	•	•	•	•	•	25	26	27	28	29
CODE																									
TIME																									
MAR	3	4	5	6	7	10	11	12	13	14	17	18	19	20	21	24	25	26	27	28	31				
CODE																									
TIME																									
APR		1	2	3	4	•	•	•	•	•	14	15	16	17	18	21	22	23	24	25	28	29	30		
CODE																									
TIME																									
MAY				1	2	5	6	7	8	9	12	13	14	15	16	19	20	21	22	23	•	27	28	29	30
CODE																									
TIME																									
JUN	2	3	4	5	6	9	10	11	12	13	16	17	18	19	20	23	24	25	26	27	30				
CODE																									
TIME																									

CODE:

Hands-On Services

SA	Student absent	X	Direct instruction/therapy
GT	Group therapy	TA	Therapist absent
B	Behavior interferes w/therapy	SA	School activities
CR	Chart review	EA	Equipment adaptation
FT	Field trip	R	Reports/record keeping
SN	Snow day		

Team Supports

CN	Staff/parent consultation	PC	Phone calls
SM	Staffings/IEP meetings	PSD	Professional staff development
SD	Spec. ed duties		

Last day of school 6/20

_____
Service Provider's Signature

_____
Date

Note: calendar dates need to be adjusted each year.

Figure 5.3. One-page form for documenting hands-on services and team supports.

Table 5.5. Finding Time to Collaborate With Team Members

Requires Team Collaboration	Requires Administrative Support
• Set aside a portion of each hands-on visit for team supports • Team teach or co-lead classroom lessons • Revise schedule mid-year to visit certain schools at end or beginning of day • Use e-mail or voice mail, school Intranet, or Internet bulletin boards • Solicit items and send out agendas before meetings • With occupational therapy colleagues, develop Frequently Asked Questions, fact sheets, newsletters, or Web articles to respond to common classroom issues • Present in-service for all teachers in one school or district	• Hire a floating substitute (or use administrative staff) to free class-room teachers for team meetings • Schedule all-grade events once per month, freeing some teachers to plan and meet with team members • Reimburse staff for attending early morning meetings and planning sessions • Use block scheduling to engage therapists in a wider variety of classroom lessons and activities

This software can then be used to *draft* suggestions before an IEP meeting, share ideas, and even shape some of the language before face-to-face meetings. These strategies allow teams to focus on discussing individual student needs and planning programs during their limited meeting time rather than finalizing the wording of the paper-work. The following vignettes illustrate how technology promoted collective decision making about the IEP process in three school districts.

Collaboration in Action: IEPs goals and objectives

The special education team at University Place School District (UPSD), a small suburban district, worked with their administrators to post forms on the district Web server to start the process of drafting goals for each student's IEP. Special education teachers set up a file for each of their students that was posted to the school Web server and available with a security code.

To begin the IEP process, team members, including parents, established priorities for a student's goals via an e-mail discussion. Then team members logged on to the server, accessed the student's file, and started the actual documentation. (Only one team member could work on a document at a time to help prevent duplication of effort.) The teams in this district are working toward developing collaborative IEPs, so each goal is developed and measured by two or more disciplines. Thus, one team member drafts a student goal, and others refine it (e.g., the occupational therapist suggests a social participation outcome for a student, and the teacher and speech–language pathologist edit it). Sometimes teams assigned different members to draft specific outcomes so one member (e.g., teacher) did not end up with the responsibility for writing a majority of the IEP goals.

Once a draft IEP document was completed, it was e-mailed to all team members (including parents) for review and editing before the actual IEP meeting. During the IEP meeting, the student's program was further discussed and clarified, and the document was finalized with the parent's consent.

The UPSD teams are moving from each professional having a separate goal page to viewing all goals and objectives as belonging to a student rather than a specific discipline. In addition to more than one service provider (e.g., occupational therapist

Remember this. . . .
All goals belong to a
student, not to a
discipline.

and teacher) working on a goal, progress reports are also written collaboratively via the server. At first this process took time, especially as team roles were established and as individuals learned to access the server, but after the first year, everyone felt that the IEP process was more efficient and that the IEP document better reflected a student's program needs.

Collaboration in Action: Generating IEP templates

In one school district, the special education team used FileMaker Pro software to generate the IEP. Once student information was entered in the system, many forms could be automatically completed with vital information (e.g., student name, school, disability, address). Team members raved about the amount of time this function saved them because they did not have to retype or cut and paste this key information on each form every year.

During IEP meetings, the draft IEP was projected on a screen via an LCD screen, and changes were made to the electronic document so all present could see them. The team could all look together to ensure priorities were represented in the goals and to add anything not previously considered. Small edits sometimes were needed after the meeting, but the document was basically complete.

Collaboration in Action: Contributing to IEP meetings

In the Really Rural School District (RRSD), the challenge was not only how to use technology to complete a collaborative IEP document but also how technology could support the involvement of the occupational therapist during IEP meetings. Some schools in the RRSD were more than 100 miles apart. This made it difficult for the occupational therapist to serve students at one school and then rush over to another school for a meeting. So the RRSD used a speaker phone so the occupational therapist could attend the meeting from a distant location.

The only concern from team members who collaborated via speaker phone was that it was difficult to read body language. As technology advanced, the RRSD transitioned to using a computer with a camera or an interactive video set-up (depending on which schools the occupational therapist and the team were in and the available technology) so that all team members could see and hear each other simultaneously.

Challenges Associated With Software IEP Packages

Many therapists are finding that software packages create challenges to documenting collaborative services on IEPs. Some software requires each service identified on the IEP to document discipline-specific goals and objectives, and other packages provide a limited structure for documenting services and supports. Also, some software does not allow additional information (beyond what has been programmed into the software structure) to be entered in the IEP. Although many of these commercial software pieces appear to have an inflexible format, with some creativity solutions can be found.

Therapist Voices: Addressing software challenges

We are slowly getting the programmers to make a few changes to allow more flexibility. We also explain services and supports under the narrative section "present levels of academic achievement and functional performance." One problem districts are having is that our software package only tracks the services that are listed under specially designed instruction. So, if a district wants to track related services or supplementary aids and services, they have to use another system. Our special education directors are very supportive and do not let the forms drive the process. They have a secretary who keeps track of related services and supplementary aids and services in an Excel document. Those services are counted as long as there are minutes attached (on the part of the IEP that describes the services, duration, location, etc.).

—Dottie Handley-More, occupational therapist, Washington

Making Collaboration Work: Evolution of an Interactive Team Process

The following case study summarizes 4 years of one student's education program and highlights an occupational therapist's efforts to increase collaboration among team members to address the student's needs. Susannah (not her real name) was diagnosed with Asperger syndrome and initially was fairly isolated in her education setting because of her team's inexperience with addressing her problems with communication and interpersonal interaction. Team members initially collaborated infrequently and expected the occupational therapist, Mina, to provide occupational therapy in a separate therapy space. Mina used her skills in the art of collaboration to prompt Susannah's team to work together to design a general education program for her that included in-context occupational therapy services and supports. Table 5.6 identifies the core and extended members on Susannah's team.

20% TS
80% HO

History of Team Interaction

Mina began working with second-grader Susannah for 90 minutes per week primarily in a therapy room to help her with self-care, handwriting and keyboarding, and behavior during transitions (note this is the most restrictive occupational therapy intervention strategy identified in Figure 1.3 in Chapter 1). Occasionally, Mina worked in

Table 5.6. Susannah's Team

Core Team Members	Extended Team Members
Susannah, student	Community occupational therapist
Sarah Hudson, mother	Building principal
Ryan Hudson, father	Guidance counselor
Mina, occupational therapist	Family counselor (community-based)
Felicia, paraprofessional	
Arleathia, special educator	
Rebekah, third-grade teacher	
Speech–language pathologist	
School psychologist	
Behavior specialist	

the classroom with Susannah but was often met with resistance from the general and special educators. Susannah was included in a second-grade classroom with a full-time paraprofessional, Felicia, for 2 hours per day and also worked with Arleathia, special educator, for 4 hours in the resource room daily.

Mina was frustrated with the discrepancy between Susannah's potential and her education program. Other team members commented that "if we push Susannah, we get hitting, spitting, scratching, yelling, and more." When Mina worked with Susannah in her classroom or the OT room, Felicia (paraprofessional) would take a break or sit in the corner and read a book. Mina realized that Felicia spent most of the time keeping a bubble around Susannah to minimize behavioral outbursts rather than support her participation in classroom lessons and activities with other children. It also became apparent at the annual IEP meeting that Mr. and Mrs. Hudson did not trust the school and that the team felt the parents had unrealistic expectations for Susannah (i.e., they wanted her time in general education increased).

First Attempt at Collaboration

At the beginning of the third grade, Mina met with Susannah's new teacher, Rebekah, and Arleathia (special educator) to share her concerns and hear Rebekah's point of view. Mina and Rebekah, with Arleathia's support, wanted to try decreasing Susannah's out-of-context activities with Felicia while increasing her participation in general education. Rebekah was willing to try this plan with the understanding that she would have Mina's support to adapt classroom "paces" and materials (e.g., decrease distractions, use a picture schedule, choose sensory strategies to modify Susannah's behavior and enable her to learn new skills). The Hudsons were thrilled with increasing Susannah's participation in the third-grade classroom but only cautiously agreed to decreasing Felicia's one-on-one assistance until a review at the end of the first quarter of school.

By her first report card, Susannah was increasingly successful in her third-grade classroom. Mina met monthly with her teachers to plan lessons and integrate occupational therapy strategies within the context of the classroom. For example, during a science unit when they were learning about the brain, Mina taught the Alert Program (Williams & Shellenberger, 1996) to the entire class. She also co-taught with Rebekah to help students write Sensory Stories during journal time. Susannah still had "meltdowns," but Rebekah wanted to continue to increase the expectations regarding Susannah's performance, and the team agreed. Felicia, the paraprofessional, was assigned other classroom duties but assisted Susannah during transitions, which often resulted in behavioral outbursts, especially during lunch, recess, and assemblies. Susannah's IEP was amended to increase her time in general education and decrease the direct paraprofessional support (the paraprofessional support was reassigned to the teacher/classroom). Rebekah, Arleathia, and Mina continued their planning and co-teaching.

By the third report period in third grade, Susannah was participating in general education for all curricular areas except math. Mina expanded her hands-on and team supports in the classroom (e.g., facilitating peer interaction in numerous environments) to almost 90% of her allotted time with Susannah. However, two extended team members, the speech–language pathologist and behavior specialist, were still less optimistic regarding Susannah's potential for learning and participating with her typical peers.

Collaboration—At Last!

Susannah's triennial evaluation was due at the end of third grade. Rebekah, Arleathia, and Mina remained concerned about the lack of buy-in from some team members for Susannah's education program as well as the parents' ongoing lack of trust. Mina discussed their concerns with the special education director and

> **Resource 5.3. Making Action Plans Questions (Forest & Lusthaus, 1990)**
> - What is the student's history?
> - What are your dreams for the student?
> - What are your nightmares for the student?
> - Who is this student?
> - What are the student's strengths, gifts, and abilities?
> - What are the student's needs?
> - What would the student's ideal day at school look like, and what must be done to make it happen?

suggested the team complete a Making Action Plans planning process (MAPS; Forest & Lusthaus, 1990; Pearpoint, Forest, & O'Brien, 1996) as a team assessment for Susannah's triennial reevaluation (see Resource 5.3 for a list of the MAPS questions discussed). After Mina shared more about the MAPS with the special education director, he agreed to hire an outside consultant to facilitate a MAPS team meeting. (Mina was the only one who was familiar with the process, and she wanted to participate in, not facilitate, the process as a team member.)

Susannah's MAPS meeting was attended by her core team members: Susannah (who provided input and answered questions like any other team member) and her parents, Rebekah, Arleathia, and Mina. Extended team members also participated in the discussion and included the community occupational therapist, school physical therapist, speech–language pathologist, psychologist, principal, and special education administrator. Susannah (with the support of her parents) and the other participants had reviewed the MAPS questions to prepare for their meeting. The facilitator posed each question, recorded team members' responses on large pieces of butcher paper, and posted them around the room. Figure 5.4 summarizes team members' answers to the question "Who is Susannah?" Figure 5.5 summarizes responses to the questions "What are Susannah's needs?" and "What would Susannah's ideal day look like?"

SUSANNAH IS . . .		
Developing	Sensitive	Tall
Fun	Adam's best friend	A good sister
Challenging	Complex	Adaptable at times
Lovable	Clever	Fast
Smart	Funny	Opinionated
Growing	Strong	Exhausting
Unique	Creative	Rigid
Empathetic	Caring	Willful
Imaginative	A reader	Insensitive
Cooperative	Sensitive	Complex
Easy to take out into the community	Articulate	Changing
Sharp	Intelligent	Stubborn

Figure 5.4. Team responses to MAPS question "Who is Susannah?"

WHAT ARE SUSANNAH'S NEEDS?

- Meet her new teachers and see her new classroom before school starts
- Choose a teacher carefully and prepare ahead of time
- Play with her friends
- A quiet classroom with rules
- No limits are set
- Limitless expectations
- A teacher who loves her and truly wants her in the class
- The same friends from year to year as well as new friends
- Adult support as appropriate
- Less reliance on adults
- Computer keyboarding skills and access
- Basic handwriting skills for signatures and functional writing

- Self-determination and self-advocacy skills
- Fill out a job application and understand the adaptations needed
- Growth to independence and independence without isolation
- Financial independence
- An integrated individualized education program
- Balance between academic and life-living skills
- Personal care training and help learning to cross the street
- Miranda, my cat
- More aggressive social management and modeling of appropriate behavior at recess
- Social Stories for recess
- The school to purchase the resources the family has loaned to them

WHAT WOULD SUSANNAH'S IDEAL DAY LOOK LIKE?

- As an occupational therapist, I would like for there to be a way to move in and out of her day, not to be locked into a 30-minute group time, but to work with the whole Susannah
- More fluidity to her schedule, to bring resources in as needed or to put back if not needed
- For the occupational therapist, physical therapist, and speech–language pathologist to be more effective, we need to go into the home with ideas
- A way for transitions to be easier for Susannah

- Continue the collaborative services
- Susannah can dictate what she needs, and who she needs, and when she needs them
- Susannah will get ready by taking the initiative with homework and morning routines
- She tells her parents about her school day
- She learns strategies to deal with everything that comes along, from the bus to anything that may challenge her
- To build on her strengths
- She needs to learn compensatory strategies

Figure 5.5. Team responses to "What are Susannah's needs?" and "What would Susannah's ideal day look like?"

Continuing Collaboration

When the MAPS session ended, Susannah's parents commented, "We didn't know everyone cared so much about our Susannah!" After the MAPS meeting, the responses to all the questions were typed up and distributed among team members. Additional assessment tools or strategies, if needed, were also completed by different team members. Each team member read through the MAPS responses and marked them as accommodations and adaptations, potential goals, and areas for environmental or systems changes. Mina collaborated with the MAPS facilitator to help the team integrate all the information into Susannah's IEP. Regarding the potential IEP goals generated during their discussion, team members indicated whether they should be included on the new IEP or addressed in a future year.

Recommendations for current goals were then discussed at Susannah's IEP meeting following a team worksheet summarized in Figure 5.6. The team also discussed

Student: ___Susannah___	Grade: ___end of 3rd grade___	Date: ___5–4–XX___

1. FACES (core team members)

Susannah (student)
Sarah and Ryan Hudson (parents)
Mina (occupational therapist)
Felicia (paraprofessional)
Arleathia (special educator)
Rebekah (third-grade teacher)
Speech–language pathologist, school psychologist, behavior specialist

2. Listen to key team members and record their words below.

Student's Strengths and Interests	*Student's Challenges*
• Uses skills once learned • Moves about environment safely • Communicates likes and dislikes • Able to run • Likes to swing • Able to throw a ball • Hyperlexic • Motivated to work on the computer • Wants to make friends • Independent in toileting, except for some fasteners	• Hesitant learning and trying new activities (e.g., jump rope, ball skills) • Sensitive to some noises and movements, especially if unfamiliar • Difficulty learning novel motor activities or following unfamiliar routines or rules • Bumps into objects and other students when moving in environment • Aggressive behaviors (e.g., spitting) limits peer interactions, especially outside of school • Difficulty with some clothing fasteners (e.g., pants after toileting; coats)

Desired Educational Outcomes

• Improved personal and social skills to develop friendships
• Participation in physical education and recess
• Legible written communication skills with and without assistive technology
• Independence in self-help skills

3. PLACES and SPACES in which student was observed in the school environment:
               (a) regular classroom   (b) playground   (c) lunchroom

What's working for this student in this environment?	*What challenges are present in this environment?*
Physical • Familiar with school environment • Likes reading corner in classroom • Can move about the classroom independently without bumping into objects, and so on • Can carry a tray during lunch • Prefers calm and predictable environments • Playground: Likes recess, motivated to participate • Follows peers cues *Social* • Has 2 to 3 peers who are particularly sensitive to her needs and willing to develop a friendship • Communicates well with adults • Follows classroom and school routines once learned	*Physical* • Recess is busy, noisy, and overwhelming. • Limited support to learn new activities during recess *Social* • Overwhelmed by number of students, noise, and distractions in the lunchroom, especially if she is last to arrive • Parents admit to being inconsistent in reinforcing appropriate behaviors at home.

4. PACES: Describe how the student meets role expectations and keeps up with the pace of school life (e.g., schedule, study habits, health habits, homework, time use).

What is expected of this student?	*How do the student's routines and habits influence his or her performance?*
• Follow classroom routines and schedules • Treat others with respect and courtesy; keep hands to herself; work quietly and not disturb others • Try new activities, even if they are difficult • Be part of the school: go to assemblies, recess, lunchroom, library, participate in fundraising, class projects, and so forth	• Responds well to routines • Difficulty learning or following new routines or rules • When unsure of what to do, she spits, hits, or yells.

Figure 5.6. Faces, spaces, and paces worksheet for Susannah.   *(continued)*

5. Collaborative Roles (suggestions for IEP/team meetings)	Who will do what?
☐ *Hands-on services/team supports (OT)*	
• Teach Susannah to use word processor and sign her name	• OT shows Susannah and team how to use a word processor, slant board, pencil grip.
• Try out playground equipment with Susannah (with and without peers present)	• OT models how to reinforce social skills during recess activities.
• Write a Social Story with Susannah about frustration in recess and physical education	• OT prompts Susannah during language arts.
	(*All activities are reinforced by classroom teacher, special educator, para-professional, speech–language pathologist, and parents.*)
☐ *Team supports (OT)*	
• Break down written assignments into small chunks that Susannah can do	• Occupational therapist, teachers, and special educator
• Work with paraprofessional, general education teacher, and special educator to promote self-advocacy (i.e., Susannah asks for what she wants or directs others when she needs help)	• Occupational therapist will teach the Alert Program with the guidance counselor in the general ed classroom during Oct./Nov. science unit.
• Use a social skills curriculum and reinforce concepts taught each week	• Behavior specialist will select social skills program; general education teacher, special educator, occupational therapist, psychologist will implement the activities.
• Integrate sensory strategies that support learning into Susannah's daily routine	• Occupational therapist will work with Susannah to identify sensory strategies; will recommend resources for teachers and parents.
☐ *System Supports (OT)*	
• Work with classroom teacher to integrate sensory into entire classroom/school routine.	• Occupational therapist will work with the teacher and other support staff.
• Other teachers, support staff, and paraprofessionals (e.g., recess monitor) will have a basic understanding of Asperger's and the unique needs of students with autism.	• Occupational therapist and other team members will develop a formal inservice for continuing education as well as provide ongoing, informal information and support.
• Playground will be redesigned to meet the needs of all students but in particular Susannah's sensory needs.	• Occupational therapist, teacher, and principal will meet to discuss needs and gather input from other teachers and support staff.
6. COMMENTS	

Note. A blank, reproducible worksheet is in the Appendix as Worksheet 2.4A.

Figure 5.6. Faces, spaces, and paces worksheet for Susannah. (*continued*)

how to use the MAPS data to write collective statements about present levels of academic achievement and functional performance. Additionally, goals for future years were highlighted in the present levels of academic achievement and functional performance section of the IEP so future teams could act on them. Mina contributed to four goals on Susannah's integrated IEP as identified below. Data were collected collaboratively by the designated team members working on each goal. Each person used a different color to record observations on one set of data sheets. At the end of the school year, Rebekah made copies for all team members.

Goal: Within a specified time frame and with modifications (e.g., shortened assignments, word prediction), Susannah will use legible handwriting or a word processor to complete classroom work, for a minimum of two assignments each of 3 consecutive days, by 3/2/2008. *This goal will be addressed by the classroom teacher, special education teacher, paraprofessional, and occupational therapist; data will be collected by the occupational therapist and paraprofessional.*

Goal: Susannah will participate, interact, and communicate in six fourth-grade activities (see attachment to IEP) with her peers 3 of 4 consecutive days by 3/2/2008. *This goal will be addressed by the classroom teacher, special education teacher, paraprofessional, occupational therapist, behavior specialist, and speech–language pathologist; data will be collected by the speech–language pathologist and behavior specialist.*

Goal: With her peers, Susannah will participate in fourth-grade physical education and recess activities for a minimum of 30 minutes of physical education, 3 consecutive days by 3/2/2008. *This goal will be addressed by the classroom teacher, physical education teacher, special education teacher, paraprofessional, and occupational therapist. Data will be collected by the physical education teacher and occupational therapist.*

Goal: Susannah will recognize the need for and take care of toileting and hygiene needs in school as is typical of her peers 5 consecutive days by 3/2/2008. *This goal will be addressed by the classroom teacher, paraprofessional, occupational therapist, and speech therapist. Data will be collected by the paraprofessional and occupational therapist.*

Rebekah moved up with her students for their fourth-grade year, so Susannah started the year with a teacher who already knew her interests, strengths, and learning challenges. When the core team met with the new special educator to review Susannah's program, he commented, "After reviewing the MAPS and Susannah's program, I have a very good picture of who she is and what her education plan focuses on." Specific strategies for helping Susannah achieve these goals are identified on her accommodation–adaptation plan (Figure 5.7).

On the basis of the MAPS and team collaboration, it was determined that occupational therapy hands-on services and team supports should be in context (with occasional out-of-context services if a specific skill could not be addressed within her typical routines and lessons) for 120 minutes per month. Services and supports emphasized social interactions, using a portable word processor in the classroom, and sensory strategies for staying on task (e.g., use of headphones to block noises, crunchy snacks after recess) to support her participation in the general education classroom. Progress toward achieving her integrated IEP goals was measured by a data collection system that involved all core team members (see goals above). Progress reports were also written collaboratively via e-mail and then finalized by the special education teacher. By the end of fourth grade, Susannah was fully integrated, and all related services, including speech, were provided in the classroom and other school places and spaces.

Long-Term Outcomes

At Susannah's next triennial evaluation (in sixth grade), the MAPS process was updated. This time Susannah's grandparents attended to contribute their viewpoints and see how much people cared about Susannah. Mina, who was not a member of Susannah's team at her middle school, facilitated the MAPS update.

80% TS
20% HO

Several strategies supported the success of this team's collaborative process:

- The team used a collaborative process, the MAPS, to facilitate discussion and information sharing and streamline the development of the current and future IEPs.

- Susannah and her parents were included as key decision makers in the process.

- School administrators hired an impartial outside facilitator to lead the initial MAPS process to help build trust between the family and school personnel.

- Everyone had copies of Susannah's MAPS responses and used a team discussion guide (see Figure 5.7) to focus their discussion when considering new ideas for her IEP.

- The collaborative process started with the team members who were most invested; as Susannah benefited from the collaborative efforts of Mina, Rebekah, and Arleathia, other team members engaged in the process (e.g., the speech–language pathologist).

- Mina provided leadership and support to her team over a period of 3 years. She recognized that collaboration is an art and considered how to engage

The following accommodations–adaptations will facilitate Susannah's success within her educational program. Some of the accommodations–adaptations may not be needed every day, but Susannah must have access to the accommodations–adaptations as needs arise.

Overall Accommodations–Adaptations

- Susannah and her family need to meet her new teachers and see her new classroom before school starts.

General Classroom Accommodations–Adaptations

- Concrete checklist of daily routines, set-up with Velcro pictures–words (so routine can be changed as needed)
- Decrease noise level in classroom during times Susannah needs to concentrate
- Provide a clearly articulated structure with concrete rules in Susannah's classroom
- Provide adult support as appropriate to ensure she understands the activity or task
- Provide a safe place (e.g., bean bag chair in a quiet corner, special ed room) for Susannah to go to when needed
- Use Touch Points (Innovative Learning Concepts, n.d.) to complete math problems. A Touch Point strip can be mounted on a foam pad or mouse pad to decrease the noise that the tapping can make.
- Use of a calculator to check math and a word processor for written work
- When Susannah is having a difficult day, allow her to choose between two activities
- During testing, use a scribe to ensure that the correct bubble is filled in
- Allow the option for a snack at 10 a.m. to help Susannah stay focused throughout the morning.
- Send a daily note home with quantitative feedback (not simply a narrative note) regarding Susannah's day.

Other Accommodations–Adaptations

- Supervision during playground and recess.

Figure 5.7. Susannah's accommodation plan.

Note. This plan was attached to Susannah's IEP and was based on the data gathered from Susannah's Making Action Plans team discussion.

reluctant team members in an interactive process to promote Susannah's successful participation in the general curriculum.

The ongoing challenge for Susannah, her family, and her school team will be how to continue the collaborative process as team members change and she continues in middle school. Although Susannah successfully participates in her academic program, her team will need to address new challenges related to socialization with peers and developing independent life skills as she advances to high school.

Summary

Each of the vignettes and Susannah's case study demonstrate collaboration in action. Some vignettes represent first steps in the process of providing collaborative supports and services to students, and others portray teams that are further along this path. Certain strategies, consistent across all vignettes, are key to effective team collaboration. Administrators were included in the initial decision making about how to provide occupational therapy services and supports. Occupational therapists assumed responsibility for learning about the educational system and for integrating occupational therapy services and supports into the school environment rather than work in separate therapy places and spaces. Education personnel and families were willing to work with therapists in new ways in familiar school spaces and places. Finally, all team members recognized that collaboration is both an art and a science and is a process that evolves over time.

Acknowledgments

This chapter was a collaborative effort among the author; the editors, Barbara Hanft and Jayne Shepherd; Brenda Brodbeck; Dottie Handley-More; Jan Galvin, physical therapist; Nancy Judge, speech–language pathologist; Jean Polichino; the many occupational therapists across the country who have shared their stories with me during various workshops; and the families and students I have had the privilege to serve.

Selected Resources

American Occupational Therapy Association. (2006). *Transforming caseload to workload in school-based and early intervention occupational therapy services.* Bethesda, MD: Author. Retrieved October 11, 2007, from www.aota.org/Practitioners/Resources/Docs/FactSheets/School/38519 .aspx

    Tips regarding school-based practice describe the difference between workload and caseload, explain the benefits of managing a workload, and suggest strategies for capturing all the occupational therapy services and supports provided.

Jackson, L. (Ed.). (2007). *Occupational therapy services for children and youth under IDEA* (3rd ed.). Bethesda, MD: AOTA Press.

    Provides occupational therapists and occupational therapy assistants working in schools with guidance regarding decision making and service delivery. An update of the second edition, the book contains information relevant to the 2004 reauthorization of IDEA and includes updated information on scientifically based practices in the schools.

Law, M., Baum, C., & Dunn, W. (2005). *Measuring occupational performance: Supporting best practice in occupational therapy* (2nd ed.). Thorofare, NJ: Slack.

    Resource for moving toward evaluation and assessment strategies that are performance based rather than centered on client factors. Emphasizes the need to address a "top-down" approach to assessment as well as considering the "bottom-up" in order to support effective decision-making and intervention.

Nolet, V., & McLaughlin, M. J. (2000). *Accessing the general curriculum: Including students with disabilities in standards-based reform.* Thousand Oaks, CA: Corwin Press.

> Strategies for helping all students not only access but participate in the general education curriculum. Although written for K–12 teachers, many of the strategies provide practical ideas that occupational therapists can use in order to support student participation in inclusive environments.

U.S. Department of Education. (August 3, 2006). *Code of Federal Regulations (CFR),* Assistance to the States for the Education of Children With Disabilities, *34 CFR Parts 300.* Retrieved October 10, 2007, from http://idea.ed.gov/explore/view/

> This site was created to provide a "one-stop shop" for resources related to IDEA and its implementing regulations. It is a "living" Web site and provides searchable versions of IDEA and its accompanying regulations, access to cross-referenced content from other laws (e.g., the No Child Left Behind Act (NCLB), the Family Education Rights and Privacy Act (FERPA), video clips on selected topics, topic briefs on selected regulations such as IEPs and early intervention services, links to Office of Special Education Program's Technical Assistance and Dissemination (TA&D) Network and a Q&A Corner where you can submit questions.

References

American Occupational Therapy Association. (2002). Occupational therapy practice framework: Domain and process. *American Journal of Occupational Therapy, 56,* 609–639.

American Occupational Therapy Association. (2006). *Transforming caseload to workload in school-based and early intervention occupational therapy services.* Bethesda, MD: Author.

Dunn, W. (1985). Therapists as consultants to educators. *Sensory Integration Special Interest Section Newsletter, 8*(1), 1–4.

Dunn, W. (1988). Models of occupational therapy service provision in the school system. *American Journal of Occupational Therapy, 42,* 718–723.

Dunn, W. (1992). Consultation as a process: How, when, and why? In C. Royeen (Ed.), *School-based practice for related services* (AOTA Self-Paced Clinical Course, Lesson 5). Bethesda, MD: American Occupational Therapy Association.

Effgen, S. K. (2000). Factors affecting the termination of physical therapy services for children in school settings. *Pediatric Physical Therapy, 12,* 121–126.

Forest, M., & Lusthaus, E. (1990). Promoting educational equality for all students: Circles and maps. In S. Stainback, W. Stainback, & M. Forest (Eds.), *Educating all students in the mainstream of regular education* (pp. 43–57). Baltimore: Paul H. Brookes.

Individuals With Disabilities Education Improvement Act of 2004, Pub. L. 108–446, 20 U.S.C. § 1400 *et seq.*

Innovative Learning Concepts. (n.d.). *About Touch Math.* Retrieved March 28, 2007, from www.touchmath.com/index.cfm?fuseaction=about.welcome

Jackson, L. (Ed.). (2007). *Occupational therapy services for children and youth under IDEA* (3rd ed.). Bethesda, MD: AOTA Press.

Nolet, V., & McLaughlin, M. J. (2000). *Accessing the general curriculum: Including students with disabilities in standards-based reform.* Thousand Oaks, CA: Corwin Press.

No Child Left Behind Act of 2001, Pub. L. 107–110, 115 Stat. 1425 (2002).

Pearpoint, J., Forest, M., & O'Brien, J. (1996). MAPS, Circle of Friends, and PATH: Powerful tools to help build caring communities. In S. Stainback & W. Stainback (Eds.), *Inclusion: A guide for educators* (pp. 67–86). Baltimore: Paul H. Brookes.

Polcyn, P., & Bissell, J. (2005). Flexible models of service using the sensory integration framework in school settings. *Sensory Integration Special Interest Section Quarterly, 28*(1), 1–4.

Priest, N., & Waters, E. (2007). "Motor magic": Evaluation of a community capacity-building approach to supporting the development of preschool children (Part 2). *Australian Occupational Therapy Journal, 54,* 140–148.

Shepherd, J. (1999). Commentary: Practitioners. *School System Special Interest Section Quarterly, 12*(4), 1–3.

Swinth, Y. L. (2003). Evaluation of areas of occupation: Educational activities. In E. B. Crepeau, E. S. Cohn, & B. A. B. Schell (Eds.), *Willard and Spackman's occupational therapy* (10th ed., pp. 347–354). Philadelphia: Lippincott Williams & Wilkins.

Swinth, Y. L. (2004). *Current issues and trends in school-based occupational therapy.* Unpublished research.

Swinth, Y., & Brodbeck, G. (2002). Intervention implementation: Considerations for effectiveness and efficiency. In Y. Swinth (Ed.), *Occupational therapy in school-based practice: Contemporary issues and trends* (AOTA Online Course, Lesson 6). Bethesda, MD: American Occupational Therapy Association.

U.S. Department of Education, Office of Special Education and Rehabilitation Services. (2000, July). *A guide to the individualized education program.* Washington, DC: Author.

Williams, M. S., & Shellenberger, S. (1996). *How does your engine run? A leader's guide to the Alert Program for Self-Regulation.* Albuquerque, NM: TherapyWorks.

CHAPTER 6

Conflict Happens: Negotiate, Collaborate, and Get Over It

*Jayne Shepherd, MS, OTR, FAOTA, and
Barbara Hanft, MA, OTR, FAOTA*

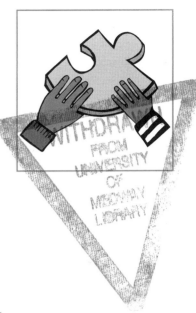

*W*hat I most appreciated from our occupational therapist was her willingness to "agree to disagree." Although I hadn't changed her mind about this issue [feeding], and she hadn't changed mine, we were able to move on and continue in our collaboration.

—Holzmueller, 2005, p. 584

Teams develop in predictable stages that are always evolving as membership changes (Miller, 2003; Tuckman, 1965). As a team works together, conflict often arises between team members. Recognizing potential sources for conflict, ways to defuse it before and when it occurs, and using negotiation strategies are important skills for teams to discuss and use.

After reading this material, readers will be able to

- Identify different stages and strategies for team building;

- Choose a coping strategy to defuse or address challenging team behaviors;

- Identify core concerns that may generate emotions during negotiations; and

- Apply negotiation strategies to resolve conflicts.

Recognizing the Impact of Stages of Teaming

Conflict on teams is inevitable, and when it arises several approaches can assist team members in addressing the challenges presented:

- Recognize the impact of the stages of teaming

- Defuse challenging communication

- Learn to negotiate.

It is helpful to look at models of team development to understand how occupational therapists, educators, families, and other school personnel become a team. One recognized model of teaming (Miller, 2003; Wheelan & Hochberger, 1996) is Tuckman's (1965) developmental stages of teaming.

As people begin to form a team and work together, they often follow predictable stages of development. Understanding those stages and possible areas of conflict guides team members as they consider how they want to interact with each other

Key Topics

- Stages of team development

- Problem-solving strategies

- Principles of negotiation

- Conflict resolution

and structure their team. Becoming a functioning, collaborative team involves four developmental stages: *forming, storming, norming,* and *performing.* A fifth stage, *adjourning,* was added by Tuckman and Jensen (1977) after they reviewed the research on group formation.

Forming Stage: Beginning

The forming stage covers the initial team evolution, when team members begin to work together instead of on their own. Members are usually optimistic and ready to "do something," yet may depend on a leader for direction. Open discussion about team goals, team structure (e.g., purpose, membership, organization, evaluation), and ground rules for operations (e.g., meetings, schedules, rules of engagement for interaction and communication; see Table 3.4 in Chapter 3), emerge, as do ideas about who should be included on the team as core and extended members. Teams form around a common purpose or vision and learn to respect one another as they share their backgrounds and knowledge in an open and honest discussion. Conflict may occur if members are reluctant to share their opinions or knowledge (indicating that some members may not embrace collaborative roles), if there is no agreement of purpose or ground rules, or if team members expect cohesiveness and direction right in the beginning.

Storming Stage: Competition and Conflict

The storming stage marks a period in which competition and conflict prevail among team members. It is often a time of disillusionment and, perhaps, high emotion if turf battles occur as team members try to establish their expertise or leadership within the team. It is essential that team members learn to negotiate with one another through coping and conflict resolution. Although this is a difficult, uncomfortable stage, it is typical and necessary for team development. If predictable conflict is handled and negotiated in a positive manner, the team will move forward in learning to be a productive and efficient team. Conflict may continue to occur if members are distracted by their own or another team member's emotional issues or difficult relationships or are unable to compromise on tasks and student services and supports.

Norming Stage: Learning to Negotiate

The norming stage occurs after the team has learned to manage and negotiate conflict and remains committed to the common purpose or vision of the group. Accepting that differences in opinions are necessary, team members now try different strategies to facilitate creative problem solving and collective decision making. Some decisions are made by the entire team, and others are delegated to smaller groups or committees. Team members' tasks and collaborative roles and responsibilities are solidified and accepted. Even though team members cooperate and even share leadership during this stage, they must continue to openly discuss underlying issues, refine team goals or visions, or address changes in team faces and paces. Conflicts may arise if these areas are not monitored.

Performing Stage: Productivity

In the performing stage, team members are now committed and loyal to the team and creatively functioning as a productive unit (Hanft, Shepherd, & Read, in press). Mem-

***Remember this.* . . .**
It is essential that team members learn to negotiate with one another through coping and conflict resolution. Although the storming stage is difficult and uncomfortable, it is typical and necessary for team development.

bers often refer to their team identity and celebrate accomplishments together. During the performing stage, teams work toward their goals, use agreed-on team structure and processing procedures, and are considerate of each others' knowledge, interpersonal style, and strengths. As a team, they resolve disagreements and value creative problem solving. Although teams are comfortable with their structure and processes, they still need to work together to maintain their commitment to collaborating with one another to promote student achievement and functional performance in school. This commitment is particularly true for occupational therapists and other related services providers, who usually work with the same students over numerous academic years (Hanft et al., in press) despite changes in other core team members.

Adjourning Stage: Our Work Is Complete for Specific Students

In the adjourning stage, team members achieve their purpose for coming together and no longer consider themselves as a formal group. Team members may meet socially and informally after a team has dissolved (Tuckman & Jensen, 1977). In school settings, the adjourning stage may be reached when a student no longer needs special education or related services or when he or she transitions to another program or school or graduates. Although a particular student's team may adjourn, the team usually remains operational for other students (e.g., preschool team, assistive technology). Membership on this mature team may change, sometimes dramatically, as the team continues to serve other students and families. Occupational therapists and other related services providers are often reassigned to other schools (and new teams) at the end of the school year, and other therapists then join the team.

The adjourning stage is an important point at which to celebrate accomplishments but also to understand that team members may feel threatened, insecure, or vulnerable. Teachers, paraprofessionals, students with disabilities, and their parents may feel abandoned when team membership changes and may desire to keep in touch. Whether to maintain contact with former team members varies according to personal preferences and the type of relationships developed during the teaming process (e.g., friendships, professional book club buddies). Students and families may present different issues when teams are adjourning (e.g., fears of not being understood or receiving the services they need in the future; not getting along with the new occupational therapist; losing an advocate during individualized education program [IEP] meetings). Be cognizant of different issues that may emerge when a team adjourns and be supportive during this time of change.

Most important, the team should be aware that they may once again cycle through earlier stages of the teaming process when new members join. Issues may be different, especially if only a small percentage of the team leaves. The new person is then joining a team that has already stormed and normed, and these stages may not be revisited. Resource 6.1 provides a link to an Internet site that illustrates how a preschool team experienced different stages of teaming when one member left the team and a new member joined.

As teams evolve through the stages of development, team members can use specific strategies to promote interaction by focusing their efforts on addressing the major tasks of each stage. When conflict occurs among team members, it is helpful to assess whether

Resource 6.1. Example of Team Development
Visit St. Benedict's Preschool and see how its team works together. The different stages of team development, creative problem solving, and good communication are evident in this scenario: http://circleofinclusion.org/english/demo/kckpreschool/team.html

Table 6.1. Strategies for Team Building at Different Stages of Team Development

Stage of Team Development	Strategies
Forming: Moving from individual to team status	• All members participate in open discussions. • Structure discussions to identify team's goals. • Focus discussion on team members' expectations and backgrounds. • Recognize that some members may be reluctant to participate at first. • Remember to view the team as an evolving unit.
Storming: Competition and conflict prevail	• Members must make an effort to see all sides of an issue. • Use active listening skills and encourage each other to do the same. • Confront conflicts in a positive manner, and adopt guidelines for conflict resolution and problem solving. • Encourage less active members to participate. • Remember that the discomfort of storming is a normal and necessary phase of development.
Norming: Cooperation and shared leadership emerge	• Risk taking during team decision making should be encouraged. • Acknowledge that disagreements are healthy and acceptable and often provide fertile ground for innovations. • Revisit the team's vision and goals frequently.
Performing: Team commitment, identity, and loyalty	• Be vigilant to prevent stagnation of ideas and activity. • Document and celebrate team accomplishments. • Facilitate creative problem solving by all team members. • Maintain high expectations for quality interactions among team members.
Adjourning: Completion of task, team satisfaction	• Celebrate team achievements. • Discuss feelings related to dissolution of the team. • Recognize and address concerns of abandonment. • Provide input to new teams that may be developing. • Consider ways to meet socially or informally to maintain relationships.

From Hanft, B., Shepherd, J., & Read, J. (in press). Competence in numbers: Working on pediatric teams. In S. Lane & A. Bundy (Eds.), *Kids can be kids: Supporting the occupations and activities of childhood.* Philadelphia: F. A. Davis. Copyright © F. A. Davis. Used with permission.

the conflict is related to storming or norming stages of team development or to inter-personal and communication issues. Table 6.1 summarizes key team-building strategies for the stages of forming, storming, norming, performing, and adjourning.

Creative Team Problem Solving

Creative problem solving is an important component of collective decision making (discussed in Chapter 3). Each team member brings his or her unique "lens" (Fisher & Shapiro, 2005) to the table for discussion to collectively determine what is best for the student. The team focuses first on the desired outcomes for a student and then brainstorms and identifies possible solutions. After brainstorming is complete, the team begins to evaluate the ideas so that premature decisions are not made. Decisions are then made collectively about how to proceed. According to Giangreco (1993) and Giangreco, Cloninger, Dennis, and Edelman (2002), effective problem solvers

- Expect that problems will be solved;
- Creatively solve problems;
- Bring a global point of view to the problem;
- Withhold judging ideas until hearing all team members' points;
- Approach problem solving in a playful and fun way;
- Generate many solutions;

- Weigh the strengths and weaknesses of the solutions;

- Focus on one solution after weighing the benefits of many ideas; and

- Act on their ideas.

In the following scenario, an IEP team uses creative problem solving to reach a collective decision to address the inappropriate behavior of Elaina, a student with autism in a special education classroom.

Collaboration in Action: Team problem solving

Elaina is in the second grade with supports from Mildred, her paraprofessional. She usually gets along fine with her classmates and works in her classroom twice weekly with Christy, her occupational therapist, to improve tool usage and independence in self-care skills. Underlying deficits in motor skills (strength, coordination, and grip) appear to be interfering with performance and her ability to keep up with the pace of the classroom. Elaina sometimes has difficulty transitioning between activities, and she will fall down and scream and kick if she doesn't want the activity to end. This behavior commonly occurs right before lunch and when the occupational therapist comes into the classroom.

Elaina's core team includes her parents; Shawn, the special education teacher; Christy, the occupational therapist; Mildred, the paraprofessional; and Lakshmi, the school psychologist. Together, they brainstormed what situations triggered Elaina's outbursts and possible solutions, and then agreed on a plan. Although Shawn thought Elaina's tantrums were triggered by transitions, such as Christy's arrival in the classroom for in-class occupational therapy, Shawn agreed to try visual supports with Elaina to help her anticipate transitions to different activities. Christy agreed to the back-up plan (i.e., change the OT schedule). Table 6.2 illustrates the creative problem-solving process used by Elaina's team to improve her behavior and participate in school lessons and interactions.

Consider the team's decisions about how to address Elaina's disruptive behavior. Would hands-on/team supports occupational therapy be necessary, or could Mildred and Shawn implement Christy's recommendations for Elaina? If Shawn as a special educator is well versed in task analysis and self-care skills, perhaps having an occupational therapist provide hands-on/team supports in the classroom to teach Elaina hand washing or putting on a coat is unnecessary. Christy could provide team supports to Shawn and Mildred (e.g., technical assistance through collaborative consultation) by suggesting a different method for putting on her coat or some adaptations for soap container or towel dispenser placement (note the *Occupational Therapy Practice Framework: Domain and Process* [AOTA, 2002] approach of adapt or modify).

By providing hands-on services with team supports, these adaptations are incorporated within the specific day-to-day paces of the class by a classroom teacher or paraprofessional on a routine basis. When occupational therapists and their colleagues consider the knowledge, skills, and experience of all team members and class routines and contextual variables, they use their expertise more efficiently to ensure student

Remember this. . . . **Each team member brings his or her unique "lens" to the table for discussion to collectively determine what is best for the student. The team focuses first on the desired outcomes for a student and then brainstorms and identifies possible solutions.**

70% TS
30% HO

Table 6.2. Examples of Problem Solving to Modify Elaina's Inappropriate Behavior During Transitions

Characteristics of Effective Problem Solvers	Examples of Problem-Solving Statements
Optimistic	• "Together, we can analyze what is setting Elaina off and how to modify it. It may take a few different hypotheses, but we can do it."
Global point of view on the problem	• "Maybe Elaina is asserting her preference for certain activities since this behavior doesn't occur during all transitions." • "I notice that Elaina's favorite activity, i.e., reading books by herself, is interrupted when someone new comes to the classroom." • "Elaina is playing with her friend Kira when I arrive, and she sits on the high-pile rug and rubs it with her hands. It's hard for her to switch to something else." • "In thinking about the schedule, Elaina may need some downtime between activities but especially after a group activity." • "Have we talked to Elaina's mother to see if she thinks this is a problem at home?"
Creative; numerous suggestions; playful, fun approach	• "Perhaps occupational therapy needs to occur at a different time of the day so Elaina is not interrupted during a favorite activity. Could you come during our motor group or when we eat snacks?" (teacher) • "Maybe Kira should sit next to Elaina when I work with her in class today." (occupational therapist) • "Replacement behaviors for kicking and screaming could include a visual schedule, a timer that graphically depicts elapsed time, reading a Social Story before transitions occur; using a peer buddy to help Elaina move to the next activity." (psychologist) • "What if she kicks a soccer ball on the playground—something she loves to do—before the biggest transition of the day...lunchtime?" (paraprofessional)
Embraces brainstorming; withholds judgment	• "What are your ideas?" • "Tell me how you think that might work." • "I want to hear what everyone else thinks."
Weighs the pros and cons to solutions; focuses on one solution	• "The easiest thing to try would be to introduce visual supports. Maybe if we cue her before and while we change activities, Elaina will do better." • "Let's use visual schedules and supports for the whole class, not just Elaina. I'll use them during my lessons and activities and make a set for the art teacher as well." • "If Elaina continues to kick and scream, maybe visual schedules alone won't work, and I'll have to rearrange my occupational therapy schedule."

Note. Based on the work of Giangreco, Cloninger, Dennis, and Edelman (2002).

progress without overlapping contributions and losing valuable time for learning (Giangreco et al., 2002; Rainforth & York-Barr, 1997).

Defusing Challenging Communications

Occasionally, one or more team members do not engage with their team because of their own interpersonal issues or ineffective communication. They can present challenging team behaviors (e.g., a monopolizer who dominates discussion, a know-it-all, a pessimist who never offers positive comments). Table 6.3 defines challenging team behaviors and identifies strategies to address them.

The following scenario illustrates how to use some of these strategies in team interactions along with good communication skills to promote collaboration (see also Table 3.2 in Chapter 3). Note how the faces of the team work together to meet Carmine's education needs, yet address Lena's teaching concerns through a brainstorming process (coping behaviors are in *italics,* and challenging behaviors are in **boldface**).

Table 6.3. Strategies for Coping With Challenging Team Behaviors

Challenge	Coping Strategies
Monopolizer—Takes over discussion; does not listen to others; preoccupied with own agenda or professional discipline	• Encourage a focus on the whole child rather than specific domains, so that everyone has an opportunity to contribute to intervention planning. • Provide team training on communication skills of active listening, paraphrasing, and summarizing
Voice of experience—Always knows better than anyone else what to do; unwilling to try out other ideas; blames others for any problems	• Acknowledge positive contributions of all team members in addressing situations and problems. • Supervisors can facilitate annual professional development goals for each team member and give feedback to this person regarding areas to work on.
Idea zapper—Negates strategies and ideas but never has any contributions of own	• Encourage brainstorming to emphasize generation of multiple strategies for consideration. • Break up into small groups with members who will speak up to limit the negativity of the idea zapper.
Pessimist—Tends to see only negative outcomes, problems instead of opportunities, deficits instead of delays	• Celebrate team and individual achievements. • In response to a concern or problem, asks "What opportunity is presented here to help this student/family. . . ?"
Whiner—First to complain about the workload but does not organize self or accept help from others	• Schedule periodic meetings to review all team operations and members' workloads. • Ask each member to suggest "what works" strategies in response to problem areas. • Solicit comments from all members about how team decisions will affect them and what will help.
Lone Ranger—Prefers to work alone, too busy to meet; doesn't back up team actions and decisions	• Assign projects or tasks that can be completed by one person but also contribute to team operations (e.g., solicit agenda items for meetings). • Encourage lifelong learning and opportunity to refine skills and knowledge through mentoring and peer coaching.
Tangent taker—Doesn't stay on task or follow discussion with pertinent contributions	• Post schedules and activities for everyone to see. • Review student intervention plans periodically, and publicize changes in meeting notes.

From Hanft, B., Shepherd, J., & Read, J. (in press). Competence in numbers: Working on pediatric teams. In S. Lane & A. Bundy (Eds.), *Kids can be kids: Supporting the occupations and activities of childhood*. Philadelphia: F. A. Davis. Copyright © F. A. Davis. Used with permission.

Collaboration in Action: Finding common ground

When Molly, an occupational therapy assistant, suggested sensory strategies for Carmine during a team discussion, the teacher, Lena, immediately stated, "That'll never work" [**idea zapper**]. In addition, Lena was skeptical about trusting Molly's judgment because "she is not the therapist I've worked with before, and I know more than she does about what will work in my classroom" [**voice of experience**].

Molly asked Lena to explain why the sensory strategies would not work in her classroom [*information seeking, clarifying*]. Lena explained, "I can see the rest of the class clamoring for their own fidget toy or throwing them at each other. And they'll all want to sit in that bean bag chair, and then you will have started the line to the principal's office for misbehavior" [**pessimist**].

Molly acknowledged Lena's concerns that all the students may want fidget toys and took the *initiative to elaborate* on Lena's statement while giving it a positive outcome. "Lena, that's a great idea to try and make it an activity for everyone. How could we do that without disrupting your class?" [*coordinating, information seeking*]. After Niaz, the special education teacher, reminds everyone of one of their team's rules of engagement, to accept all ideas without judgment, Lena, Molly, and Niaz *brainstormed* possible strategies [*orients*]:

- Molly shares the Alert Program manuals, activities (Williams & Shellenberger, 1996, 2001), and CDs (Williams & Shellenberger, 2006) with Lena and describes how she has used the program in other classrooms [*information giving, which demonstrates Molly's knowledge to Lena*].

- Before making a decision about the Alert Program, Lena will talk to or visit another teacher who uses fidget toys or a bean bag chair in their classroom [*initiating another way to learn about the program*].

- Molly gives a short talk about the Alert Program to Carmine's team and other interested special and general educators [*information giving*].

- Molly could work with the art teacher to encourage the students to design a "comfy corner" in the classroom and draw up "road rules" about earning the right to use it (e.g., use lightweight toys, only hold it in your hands, any distraction to others means automatic loss of the toys) [*coordinating*].

- Lena could try fidget toys for one class a day and see how it goes after Molly introduces the activities to the class and explains the purpose of using a fidget toy.

- If all goes well, Lena will let students pick or make their own toys by adding a gripper, tassel, piece of rubber, or stickers to a pencil that they keep in their desk.

- Forget the fidget toys and use quiet music, in-seat push-ups, or other activities (e.g., a movement group before reading) to help regulate students' sensory input.

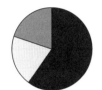

60% TS
20% HO
20% SS

Carmine's team developed trust and respect for each other by using several effective communication skills and strategies for coping with challenging team behaviors. To help balance the conversation with positives and defuse challenging communications, they involved other team members or a few of the idea zapper's colleagues who have successfully used a certain strategy. This approach takes the "zip" out of the idea zapper. Once Lena realized that Molly was giving her not more to do but suggestions to help her teach, she was more willing to listen to Molly's ideas. Sometimes therapists have to recognize that a teacher will not agree to a particular suggestion and suggest other strategies to reach the student's desired outcome.

Resource 6.2. Conflict Resolution Resources

As mandated by the Individuals With Disabilities Education Improvement Act of 2004, the organizations below provide many resources for teams in conflict regarding special education issues:

- Consortium for Appropriate Dispute Resolution in Special Education: www.directionservice.org/cadre/
- Hollier, F., Murray, K., & Cornelius, H. (2004). *Conflict resolution trainer's manual.* Chatswood, NSW, Australia: Conflict Resolution Network. Retrieved November 1, 2007, from www.crnhq.org/CR_Trainers_Manual
- International Institute of Conflict Prevention and Resolution: www.cpradr.org/
- WrightsLaw: Information on procedural safeguards and medication: www.wrightslaw.com/idea/law/section1415.pdf

Learn to Negotiate

Team members, no matter how cooperative, will not always agree with one another. Teams that work well freely admit that conflict is possible and use a specific method or decision-making process to address challenges to the team process as they arise. Conflict management and negotiation seminars have been widely taught in business and public schools (e.g., bullying programs, conflict management for at-risk kids, special education dispute resolution). This training typically focuses on teaching an entire staff, not just individuals or teams. Resource 6.2 identifies Web sites related to conflict management in schools.

Commitment to learn and practice negotiation skills takes time and patience requiring a systematic way to address conflict (Dettmer, Thurston, & Sellberg, 2005). Fisher, Ury, with Patton (1991) suggested seven elements to consider when negotiating with others to resolve a conflict.

Remember this. . . .
Teams that work well freely admit that conflict is possible and use a specific method or decision-making process to address challenges to the team process as they arise.

1. *Build and maintain relationships by separating the problem from the people.* Try to imagine a colleague's dissenting point of view. Why does he or she think like that? Do not blame a colleague or feel personally attacked so that emotions get in the way of a discussion. Instead, team members need to discuss and approach a conflict together and strive to recognize common ground and shared perceptions.

2. *Keep communication open.* Stay focused on maintaining an objective conversation with a dissenting team member and use active listening to convey understanding of this person's point of view. Try using third-space dialogue (described in Chapter 2, "Team Faces and Spaces") to understand another's perspective. Understanding another's perspective or opinion does not indicate agreement with it. Listen, share, and be honest about concerns without blaming the other team member.

3. *Share and respect one another's interests.* Ask the teammate to explain a certain position and whether personal interests may be influencing him or her. Focus on these interests, not personal positions. Share positions among team members and see whether mutual interests (student outcomes) can be found to discuss solutions.

4. *Brainstorm and give options for mutual gain.* Generate creative options by brainstorming solutions and looking for a win–win solution. Facilitate conversation around the four stages of brainstorming: Identify the problem, analyze why it's a problem, generate general ideas to fix the problem, and consider specific actions. Only after brainstorming is complete, begin to evaluate the ideas so premature decisions are not made.

5. *Agree on objective criteria or standards to evaluate decisions (legitimacy).* Before making intervention decisions, agree on objective criteria such as information from evidence-based practice, professional guidelines or standards, or previous legal or ethical decisions. Share decision making about objective criteria, and be open minded and reasonable with suggestions. Ask other team members why they chose the criteria and consider whether someone outside the team would think these are fair criteria.

6. *Find the best alternative to negotiated agreement.* Consider what will happen if no agreement is reached, and realize that a compromise is better than no agreement. Determine the bottom-line agreement that is acceptable to all team members.

7. *Make realistic and fair commitments to the team.* Don't agree to do something that is nearly impossible—for example, "The team will meet face to face with the aide and the teacher each week to assess whether suggestions are working and being carried out." Try instead, "As a team, commit to communicating with each other once a week to determine whether progress is being made. This communication may be done through meetings, a data collection chart, e-mail, or phone conversations."

Administrator Voices: Support, not judgment

As an administrator, if there is a problem that needs remediation, the team member and I develop a Plan of Improvement to affirm what is going right and to learn from each other to ensure student success. I listen to concerns but don't judge the team member. We review the objective essential components of the student's program, and I ask clarifying questions to discuss implementation and gauge the team member's comfort level with each component. I ask if he or she has other ideas to address these essentials and whether there is another team member that he or she would like to talk to or use as a mentor. We brainstorm alternatives and discuss how this would look in the classroom as well as how we will measure progress. I may share examples of how other teachers or therapists have addressed this issue, but I always enlist the team member's input into the problem-solving process. The team member, not me, identifies the problem, and this allows me to avoid direct conflict by being supportive.

—Rebecca Argabrite Grove, administrator, occupational therapist, and assistive technology specialist, Virginia

Collaborative partnerships are needed among school-based, private, and clinic-based occupational therapists. Students and families may be confused by the difference in recommendations from therapists in various settings (Hanft, Shepherd, & Read, in press; Tryon, 1997). When differences in opinions or conflict arise, use the principles of negotiation from Fisher et al. (1991) to understand parental and clinic and private therapists' perspectives. The goal is to communicate and work together for the student's success.

Tryon (1997), who is a clinic-based occupational therapist and mother of a child with a disability, reminded therapists to consider all the environments in which students perform everyday activities before recommending intervention and to allow parents time to understand and chose recommendations, particularly when parents are receiving occupational therapy from two different settings. Chapter 3 provides an example of how Wisconsin therapists educated parents about the differences between school and community therapy services. Chapter 7 discusses ways to address the "more is better" issue that often occurs when students are in both school- and clinic-based therapy.

Therapist Voices: Educate and value

As practitioners, we must educate parents and other professionals about our differing roles [school and clinic] and reinforce the value of each.

—Peggy Tryon, occupational therapist and parent (Tryon, 1997, p. 1)

Focus on Concerns, Not the Emotion in Negotiation

Fisher and Shapiro (2005) built on the knowledge learned from the Harvard Negotiation Project (Fisher & Ury, 1991; Stone, Patton, & Heen, 1999; Ury, 1993) to identify five core concerns that may generate emotions during negotiations: *appreciation, affiliation, autonomy, status,* and *role.* Core concerns can "be used as both a lens to understand the emotional experience of each party and as a level to stimulate positive emotions in yourself and in others" (p. 18). Addressing the core concerns during negotiation can help diffuse conflict. When they are ignored, negative emotions emerge and predispose team members to negativity, distrust, rigid thinking, and less willingness to work together. Use the core concerns as a "lens" while preparing, conducting, and evaluating a negotiation. The following sections are based on the work of Fisher and Shapiro (2005).

Appreciation

Everyone likes to be recognized for their thoughts, feelings, and actions. Sometimes all it takes is sharing a comment that recognizes the effort a team member has expended to implement an idea or a lesson. Asking team members for their point of view makes it easier to understand their position and perspective and allows team members to try on another team member's perspective. This approach can lead to greater appreciation of their responsibilities and tasks. For example, consider how a teacher might feel if an occupational therapist gave her three more things to do with her student, Zeke, when she is already overwhelmed with his academic and self-care needs and behavior problems.

Recognition of body language and voice intonation or emphasis helps one understand *metamessages* (i.e., the underlying meaning of words). For example, when asked by the occupational therapist to record how many times Zeke activates his switch, the teacher says, "I *could* collect this data if I had the time," as she grits her teeth or clenches her fist. Fisher and Shapiro (2005) suggested using reflective listening, finding merit in what the other person says, and acting like an impartial mediator while trying to appreciate the other person's point of view. This technique is similar to using third-space dialogue and anchored understanding (discussed in Chapter 2). It is important to allow a certain amount of time for discussion to hear other opinions and not blame another team member (Stone et al., 1999). Sometimes introducing a metaphor or metamessage may simplify the message. The occupational therapist could respond to the teacher who already feels overwhelmed by data collection, "I feel like we've hit a brick wall in deciding how to determine if Zeke is making progress. Do you have other ideas?" With this statement, the occupational therapist expresses understanding of the teacher's viewpoint and solicits her ideas to demonstrate appreciation. An example of how one occupational therapist expresses appreciation for her team members is provided below:

Administrator Voices: Token of appreciation

Throughout the year, I may send an e-mail or give the team a small token of appreciation with a note. During a stormy phase on one of my teams, I sent each team member a Tension Tamer tea bag with a note expressing my appreciation for everything each person does for the children. This act of appreciation went a long way in letting team members know I understand they are under a lot of stress as they are working on their team process.

> —Rebecca Argabrite Grove, special education coordinator,
> occupational therapist, and assistive technology specialist, Virginia

Affiliation

When in conflict, building on a team member's need for structural (e.g., agreed-on procedures or ways the negotiation will proceed) and personal connectedness is essential (Fisher & Shapiro, 2005). When members feel connected to a person or group process, they are willing to listen because someone has demonstrated concern about their well-being. Finding these personal links (e.g., where you grew up, common interests, family, values) between team members facilitates communication. Reducing the personal distance between team members, soliciting advice, and sharing opinions, yet giving team members time to react and decide what to say, aids in establishing connectiveness. When expecting a volatile situation or a difference of opinion between team members, talk to the team member about neutral topics and stay in close proximity to them (e.g., try to engage, not avoid, the team member; Fisher & Shapiro, 2005). For example, a mother demanded one-on-one services for her child, but the team recommended that the occupational therapist provide in-class hands-on and team supports. To facilitate affiliation with this parent, the teacher invited the mother to sit down and started a neutral conversation by asking about her new baby and sharing a positive anecdote about her child.

Although building personal connections and affiliation is essential, be careful that they do not manipulate or cloud one's judgment or decisions (Fisher & Shapiro, 2005). Sometimes a person may overidentify with another team member with whom he or she is in conflict, and he or she may try to use the friendship to influence decisions. Consider Lori, a teammate, who wants to provide services out of context and expects her friend, an occupational therapist, to support her position. The occupational therapist must not allow her friendship or past affiliation with Lori to influence her opinion of what is best for the student.

Autonomy

In schools as in families, administrators and parents expect differing levels of autonomy for decision making. Keep in mind that meaningful, and effective, decisions should result from information sharing, collaboration, and negotiation. Small decisions are usually made independently, and others are informed about them. For example, in a school, a parent, teacher, student, or occupational therapist may decide independently to try a different food type for snack or pencil grip during writing. If this change works, then other team members may be informed of the decision. Other decisions are made by a leader or small group in consultation with other members. For example, a parent, teacher, and occupational therapist may discuss the best way for Jake to participate in the class field trip to the museum. Input from all team members is needed to be sure this will be a successful trip.

Larger decisions, such as placement options, changes in IEPs, behavioral support plans, and so on must often be negotiated between members. Team members' ideas, perspectives, and contributions are needed, and supported, and a variety of choices identified before committing to them. By brainstorming together, possibilities may surface that allow all team members to make recommendations that no one may have thought of themselves. When individuals have a choice in making a decision, they are often more willing to work with other team members. For example, when negotiating with a reluctant teacher to provide hands-on services and team supports within a classroom, asking "I have two options to work with Suzy; which would be the best time to help her?" provides the teacher with much more autonomy than saying "This is when I can be here."

Status

Be aware of team members' status and demonstrate respect accordingly. In conflict situations, status may relate to a team member's education, skills, connections, past experiences, or emotional insights. Understanding and recognizing another's status may help negotiations go smoothly. With education and experience, team members can raise their status or level the playing field for all team members.

Remember this. . . . **By brainstorming together, possibilities may surface that allow all team members to make recommendations that no one may have thought of themselves.**

Collaboration in Action: Understanding parent perspectives

An occupational therapist, Brenda, works with Aklesia, whose mother, Zema, is a well-known lawyer. Before the IEP meeting, Brenda considers what to do to enhance her knowledge and status from the parent's perspective. For example, she could review the IDEA regulations related to Aklesia's educational plan, distribute specific sections of the regulations, or invite the special education coordinator to the meeting for support. Data about Aklesia's progress, research about proposed intervention, and specific examples of classroom observations will be useful as well, especially if well organized and presented.

In contrast, if Brenda meets with a family who has little knowledge of the IDEA, she may need to educate the parents about the law and is aware that they may now view her as an expert and defer to her, or other team members, in decisions. As Brenda provides information to the family, she encourages questions and decision making that are based on this family's values.

Team members should value parents' own knowledge and observations of their child and solicit their questions and opinions about education services and supports needed to reach desired outcomes. Affirming a parent's or teacher's status by asking about past experiences or knowledge often opens discussion as well.

Fulfilling Team Operational Roles

"Every role has a job label . . . and a corresponding set of activities that goes with it" (Fisher & Shapiro, 2005, p. 120). Most people have a variety of personal (e.g., the token male or female viewpoint, the social planner) and team operational roles (e.g., note taker, time keeper) that are fulfilling or unfulfilling. Sometimes teams add new, more fulfilling activities or roles to keep pace with new practices. Roles need to be personally meaningful, purposeful, and not pretentious. By acknowledging one another's roles, team members affirm the importance of each person in the collaborative process.

Conflict may surface when therapists move in and out of classrooms and only glimpse a snapshot of how a student, teacher, parent, or paraprofessional fulfill their collaborative and team operational roles and activities. For example,

Collaboration in Action: Considering the whole picture

Carol, an occupational therapist, helps two students learn to use tools during math group every Thursday after recess. During this time, Carol observes minimal enthusiasm from Grace, the classroom assistant, and sees that Grace uses the recommended tools (i.e., magnifier ruler, abacus number line) minimally with the students. Carol is concerned because both students need these tools for their arithmetic calculations.

As an itinerant therapist who comes to this classroom and school once a week, Carol does not know that Grace is anxious about three student altercations with sticks that occurred this month in the bus line under her watch. Grace is worried that her job is on the line and has decided not to use the ruler and abacus with both students to prevent any "sword duels" in the classroom. In addition, when Grace suggested different math activities to engage the students, the teacher never followed up on her ideas. At this point, Grace views her role as disciplinarian to prevent future incidents, and she does not feel valued or able to use the tools recommended by Carol.

What Happened Here?

Think about the scenario of Grace and Carol.

- Where did communication break down?

- What can Carol do to change her interaction with Grace?

Team members can grow irritated with each other even though they are working on common goals and no specific incident has occurred. When this happens, it is important to consider, "Is my role and this team member's role meaningful and purposeful?" Considering this question gives team members a time to reflect and consider what else they would like to do. Refer to Reflection 6.1 to consider what Carol can do to engage Grace in the teaming process.

Team members may need to try on temporary team operational roles to help the team process and diffuse the emotional content of a negotiation (Fisher & Shapiro, 2005; Thousand & Villa, 2000). Examples of temporary roles that may encourage collaboration include the

- *Joker:* Finds humor in team situations, eases tension, and makes others laugh;

- *Advocate:* Acts on behalf of team and supports team roles and operations;

- *Brainstormer:* Generates a variety of ideas and possibilities;

- *Standard setter:* States and applies agreed-on standards for team relationships and tasks; and

- *Peacemaker:* Defuses situations and facilitates compromises. (Fisher & Shapiro, 2005; Thousand & Villa, 2000)

Case Scenario: Managing Conflicts

In the scenario below, identify Fisher and Shapiro's (2005) five core concerns and consider how Lou Ann, a registered occupational therapist, and her colleagues might address them to resolve a team conflict. Use Worksheet 6.1A in the Appendix as a guide.

Collaboration in Action: Communicate to negotiate

Lou Ann noticed tension between herself and Micah, a certified occupational therapy assistant (COTA) who worked with Jacques, a fourth-grade student. Lou Ann thought that Micah only did the bare minimum with Jacques, and she wasn't sure that she could trust Micah to follow through using Jacques's new splint since he returned to school following hand surgery. Lou Ann considered Micah's point of view as a recent graduate of a COTA program. She wondered whether he had concerns about meeting Jacques's needs, was overwhelmed with data collection, or really wasn't confident with using splints.

Lou Ann began a negotiation with Micah by first trying to *affiliate* with him. "How's your day going, Micah? What did you do this weekend?" When Micah replied that he went to a high school art show, Lou Ann replied, "Oh, I went to that art show, too. Did you see the pen-and-ink picture of the little boy by the tree?" As they continued to talk, Lou Ann realized that Micah was quite observant and interested in painting himself. She *appreciated* and *affirmed* his knowledge about art.

After Lou Ann and Micah communicated on a neutral topic, Lou Ann suggested, "I'd like to talk about how we're working together with Jacques and I'd like to get your opinion. . . . I feel like we are banging heads (*appreciation of feelings, using a metaphor*) about how to manage this splint and data collection. You see him more than I do and know him better than me (*recognize status*). Can we brainstorm together how to do this so it's easy to get Jacques to wear his splint and recover from surgery?" (*respecting autonomy, choosing a fulfilling role*).

After further discussion, Micah stated, "I've never used a splint this complicated with a child before, and he cries whenever I try to put it on him." Lou Ann *acknowledged*, "This is a very difficult splint to use, and I should have shown you how to do this more than once." She watched Micah put the splint on Jacques and brainstormed some other techniques with him. She then modeled how to put on the splint while using a memory game with Jacques as a distraction technique.

After discussing the pros and cons of the technique, Micah placed the splint on Jacques and reflected, "That was easier. Thank you for showing Jacques and me how to do this less painfully! It is MY responsibility to be sure the splint schedule is not forgotten" (*autonomy*). Micah then made up his own chart for documenting how long Jacques wore his splint. He also suggested that Jacques could be in charge of a small timer on his lapboard to remind everyone when it was time to change his splint and showed Lou Ann his data chart (*autonomy*).

In this scenario, both Lou Ann and Micah realized that it is a team responsibility to address conflict and negotiate a solution. By addressing the conflict directly (i.e., appreciating, affiliating, and respecting each others' autonomy, status, and role in working with Jacques), Micah and Lou Ann negotiated a solution that worked for both of them and improved Jacques' performance, the most important outcome of all in resolving conflict among team members.

Remember this. . . .
Each team member should take responsibility for his or her contribution to the team's emotional temperature and initiate a Plan B before negative emotions get out of control (Fisher & Shapiro, 2005).

When Negative Emotions Are Strong and Disruptive

Occasionally, negative emotions become so strong that they disrupt a negotiation. Fisher and Shapiro (2005) suggested that prevention in this case is the most effective intervention: Each team member should take responsibility for his or her contribution to the team's emotional temperature and initiate a Plan B before negative emotions get out of control. When attempting to soothe or cool down one's emotions, consider the following techniques: Count backward, breathe deeply, pause, visualize a soothing place, take a break, change the subject, keep a relaxed position, and ignore comments that are upsetting. Prepare to consider an alternative plan if agreement cannot be reached and consider, "How important is this issue to me?"(Fisher & Shapiro, 2005, p. 151). Plan B for negotiating difficult situations could include changing faces (e.g., "Could we ask Judy [a neutral party] to join us and share her ideas, too?") or paces and places (e.g., "How about we take a break for 10 minutes and resume our discussion in the conference room instead of the hall?").

If all else fails and it feels necessary to react emotionally during a negotiation, first consider what will be achieved (Fisher & Shapiro, 2005):

- To ventilate and feel better?

- To inform others of their impact? For example, a change in team schedule will require the occupational therapist to switch schedules with five other teachers, who will not be happy with her.

- To possibly influence other team members in the negotiation?

- To improve the interaction by explaining the emotional reaction and then offering an apology? ("I was worried that Justin would fall, so I yelled across the room. I apologize if I embarrassed you.")

Consider how well you deflect conflict by answering Reflection 6.2.

Pulling It All Together: Team Process and Conflict Resolution

The following scenario describes how Pedro's core team—Carlotta (mother), Keegan (general educator), Bonita (special educator), Robert (physical therapist), and Bijul (occupational therapist)—handled a conflict that arose during their discussion about Pedro's transition plans for college. Bijul, an occupational therapist, assumed team operation roles as an advocate for Pedro as well as a diffuser of conflict. Note that the core concerns (Fisher & Shapiro, 2005) are italicized.

Reflection 6.2

How Well Do You Deflect Conflict?

When in a heated discussion, how do you address the core concerns (i.e., appreciation, affiliation, autonomy, status, fulfillment)? Consider a recent conflict situation you were involved in or observed, and complete Worksheet 6.1A to identify the strategies used and their effectiveness in diffusing the conflict.

Collaboration in Action: Team process and diffusing conflict

Pedro has just begun to lead his own IEP meeting and began by asking everyone to introduce themselves. Before he could bring up the first item on his list, his mother interrupted, "Now, let's get right to the point, Pedro needs more occupational therapy and physical therapy. He is unable to keep up with his class." Pedro became indignant and told his mother to shut up and tried to start the meeting again. Further words were exchanged, and soon they both were vying for other team members' attention. Keegan muttered under her breath, "We never should have allowed Pedro to do this." Other team members were also uncomfortable and doubted Pedro's ability to take charge of the meeting.

Setting the Tone

Before the meeting, Bijul agreed to assume a team operations role as Pedro's supporter and advocate. As they practiced, Bijul sat next to Pedro, nodded to him when it was time to start the meeting, and smiled when he introduced everyone (*affiliation*). When the conflict began, Bijul assumed a temporary role as peacemaker and humorist. Knowing that Pedro's brother, Charlie, was a boxer (*affiliation*), she exclaimed, "WHOA! Time out, like Charlie would say, everyone back to your corners."

Pedro and Carlotta both stopped and smiled a bit, so Bijul immediately took the opportunity to restate that Pedro was practicing how to run a meeting to learn to advocate for himself. Bijul complimented Carlotta on how she always has been an excellent advocate for Pedro (*affiliation* from previous meetings with Carlotta helped Bijul recognize the mother's *status* as a long-term advocate and decision maker for Pedro). Bijul reminded the team, "As we agreed beforehand (*autonomy*), it's Pedro's turn to advocate for himself." She then added, "As a mother, I know how hard it is to not to step in and to learn to take a back seat" (*affiliation*).

After Bonita reiterated the purpose of the meeting and the team's operating rules (e.g., follow the agenda, let everyone speak), everyone agreed to begin again. As team members modeled how to consult Pedro about decisions, Carlotta understood the process better. By addressing Carlotta's and Pedro's core concerns, Bijul diminished their conflict without any one losing face, and the team addressed their goal of helping Pedro learn self-advocacy skills.

Desired Outcome

Pedro's IEP meeting focuses on outcomes developed with him in a previous team meeting using a PATH (Planning Alternative Tomorrows With Hope; Pearpoint, O'Brien, & Forest, 1995). The PATH is a powerful person-centered tool used by teams to identify future dreams and goals of the student and family. After identifying the student's dream, team members determine the steps needed to meet team-identified goals. Pedro, a junior in high school, sustained a spinal cord injury in sixth grade.

During the PATH discussion, it became evident that Pedro's long-term goal was to own a computer business for people interested in science and technology. Before this, Pedro always thought he would work at a computer store, but with his recent academic success and support from his team, he decided to modify his transition goal from going to work to attending college.

As Pedro's team helped him identify his goals, they also developed a list of skills Pedro would need to care for himself at college. Because Pedro uses a wheelchair, his self-advocacy, self-care, mobility, and life-task skills were just as important to assess as his organizational and academic skills.

Issue Definition

After talking to Pedro and the team, Bonita and Bijul asked several key questions to prompt Pedro to think about his goals:

- What do you want to be able to do yourself?

- If you chose three things to get started, what would they be?

- If we could work with you at school, when and how should we work together?

Pedro was as concerned as the team about his ability to care for himself at college. While answering Bijul's and Bonita's questions, he revealed that his cousin would also be going to college and that they were planning to live together. Carlotta said this news was comforting to her because his cousin was already helping him get dressed in the morning before school. Although this type of assistance would be difficult for many adolescents to accept, Carlotta explained that in their family, helping each other was truly valued and expected of immediate and extended family members.

Like most teenage boys, Pedro was also worried about eating and how he would manage the dining hall and fix snacks. Carlotta expressed a concern about how he would get to and from classes when it took time to maneuver his wheelchair over curbs and onto the university bus.

Intervention Options

During the IEP discussion, possible interventions were identified. Pedro was adamant that he did not want to leave class to work on self-help skills (nor did he have the privacy he wanted in the classroom) because he wanted to keep his grades up for college applications. Therefore, out-of-context hands-on services and team supports during school were not an option. While the team *brainstormed* options, several ideas for team supports from the occupational therapist were discussed and evaluated:

- Pedro could work on self-care skills after school or during the summer with an aide. Bijul and Robert could help educate the aide about specific self-care and mobility strategies.

- Pedro could take a family and consumer sciences (home economics) class in his senior year, and Bijul could consult with the teacher about any adaptations he may need (team supports).

- Pedro and his family could work together to help him learn how to make simple snacks and practice meal preparation skills learned in home economics. They could also use the summer to work on money management and transportation skills (e.g., directing friends in how to transfer him, crossing streets independently, using public transportation) when Pedro goes out to restaurants and snack bars with his cousins and friends.

- A field trip to a local university was planned during school hours (and encouraged by Pedro's high school). Either Bijul or Robert would go with Pedro and Carlotta to assess the physical environment and determine what skills and modifications would be helpful to consider.

- A representative from the Department of Vocational Rehabilitation, an extended team member, was invited to attend future team meetings and contribute to Pedro's transition plan. She subsequently committed funds to provide occupational therapy services to Pedro after school and in the summer to prepare him for college.

- Bijul remembered hearing about the Disabilities, Opportunities, Internetworking, and Technology (DO–IT) program in Washington State for high school students with disabilities who were interested in science. After finding the Web site on the Internet, Bijul shared information on the program with the other team members. Later, Bonita asked the chemistry teacher to allow Pedro to apply to this program in lieu of another writing assignment, and she agreed. (When Pedro was accepted to DO–IT, Vocational Rehabilitation contributed funding for Pedro to attend this 4-week summer program before college.)

Reflection on Bijul's Collaboration With Her Team

Hands-On Services With Team Supports

Bijul initially worked with Pedro during home economics, using in-context strategies and adaptations to help him access kitchen equipment and food items during cooking activities (refer to Figure 1.3 in Chapter 1 regarding providing occupational therapy in the least restrictive environment). Bijul provided team supports to Bonita and Rachel, the home economics teacher, showing them how to change the location of kitchen items for easier access; use nonslip matting under dishes; purchase large-handled utensils and an adapted cutting board with an attached rocker knife; and use a wheeled cart to carry items back and forth from the countertops to the kitchen table or the appliances. After Bijul demonstrated how to use these items, the educators helped Pedro practice during each class and become independent.

After school once a week and for a few weeks during the summer, Pedro participated in intensive occupational therapy hands-on services and team supports to learn other essential activities of daily living (e.g., directing others to help him with personal skills) and instrumental activities of daily living skills, (e.g., transportation and mobility, money management, meal preparation). By helping the team learn about other resources available to Pedro, Bijul took a lead role in focusing the team's decision-making process on finding alternatives to promote Pedro's independence and expanded the team's knowledge about educating future students with similar issues.

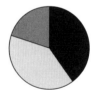

40% TS
40% HO
20% SS

System Supports

Through their discussions with Pedro and his family, the entire team became aware of the gap in services for students on a college track who also needed additional training to successfully transition to adult living. Bonita and Bijul brought this service gap to the attention of the administrator of transition services in their school district. They suggested that flexible work time be built into selected therapists' and special educators' schedules at least every 2 or 3 weeks so they could work with students after school on practical living skills. They presented convincing data about the number of students with disabilities who go to college but then drop out because of a lack of self-care or daily living skills. Through record review, they also demonstrated that almost 20 students with physical disabilities a year from their county drop out of higher education programs. The transition team administrator,

Resource 6.3. Transition Resources for Pedro

- DO–IT: Disabilities, Opportunities, Internetworking, and Technology has numerous resources for educators, students, and families. DO–IT Scholars is a program in which high school students live on campus and explore college life, including taking classes and directing personal self-care aides if needed: www.washington.edu/doit/
- Leading your own IEP meeting (downloadable manuals):
  - www.nichcy.org/pubs/stuguide/st1book.htm (workbook for the student)
  - www.nichcy.org/pubs/stuguide/ta2book.htm (technical assistance manual)
- Preparing for College: An Online Tutorial: www.washington.edu/doit/Brochures/Academics/cprep.html
- Planning Alternative Tomorrows With Hope (PATH): www.inclusion.com/path.html
- Vocational Rehabilitation State Offices: These resources are available through the Job Accommodation Network at West Virginia University: www.jan.wvu.edu/sbses/vocrehab.htm

convinced of the need to include life skills training, agreed to look for community grants to support an after-school program.

Summary

Teams often develop in predictable stages of forming, storming, norming, performing, and adjourning as they collaborate to work together to benefit students, develop rules of engagement, organize team meetings, facilitate communication, evaluate the effectiveness of their structure and operation, and address conflict. Examples of creative problem-solving strategies and negotiation strategies illustrated how school-based therapists can resolve conflict rather than be stymied by it.

Pedro's scenario demonstrates the value of using conflict management strategies, asking the right questions to understand everyone's point of view, and having a positive affiliation with team members. Pedro benefited from the knowledge and skills of a variety of team members who used their professional networks to develop and implement an effective transition plan for him. Pedro had many education issues that were most appropriately addressed by an occupational therapist providing team and system supports rather than solely by hands-on and team supports. This team's attention to its collaborative process helped an individual student develop life skills to attend college, educated team members about alternatives for intervention, and developed a systemwide program change that will benefit other students with disabilities. Some of the resources identified in this scenario are found in Resource 6.3.

Administrator Voices: Do the right thing!

Everyone in the long run has to decide what is more important: to hold on to conflict or get over it and do the right thing for the student.

—Jo Read, director of student services, Virginia

Acknowledgments

This chapter was produced in collaboration with Rebecca Argabrite Grove, Judith Schoonover, Jo Read, and our numerous team members over the years who have demonstrated the art of negotiation and getting over it!

Selected Resources

Fisher, R., & Shapiro, D. (2005). *Beyond reason: Using emotions as you negotiate.* New York: Penguin Books.

The authors identify five core concerns that may generate emotions during negotiations: appreciation, affiliation, autonomy and respect, status, and meaningful roles. Built on the knowledge learned from the Harvard Negotiation Project, these authors give explicit everyday life to worldwide examples of negotiation and how to address the core concerns to diffuse conflict. It is a quick read and user friendly. Downloadable forms for your team to use with the book are available at www.beyond-reason.net/teaching/index.html

Hanft, B., & Place, P. (1996). Conflict resolution. In *The consulting therapist* (pp. 125–139). Austin, TX: Pro-Ed.

> This chapter identifies the negotiation process and common conflicts that emerge for therapists and provides strategies to address how to work out conflicts. The use of examples in school settings are particularly helpful to the reader.

Program on Negotiation Clearinghouse at Harvard Law School.

> This resource center provides a variety of cases, articles, and worksheets based on the work of the Harvard Negotiation Project and the many colleagues who have taught about negotiation and alternative dispute resolution. www.pon.org/catalog/index.php

Ury, W. (2007). *The power of a positive no: How to say no and still get to yes.* New York: Random House.

> The author of the book *Getting to Yes* wrote this book to complete the picture of getting along in relationships. Using examples from everyday life and intercultural relationships, Ury gives readers examples of how to prepare, deliver, and follow through with a positive no instead of accommodating, attacking, or avoiding an issue.

References

American Occupational Therapy Association. (2002). Occupational therapy practice framework: Domain and process. *American Journal of Occupational Therapy, 56,* 609–639.

Dettmer, P., Thurston, L., & Sellberg, N. J. (2005). *Consultation, collaboration, and teamwork for students with special needs* (5th ed.). Needham Heights, MA: Allyn & Bacon.

Fisher, R., & Shapiro, D. (2005). *Beyond reason: Using emotions as you negotiate.* New York: Penguin Books.

Fisher, R., & Ury, W., with Patton, B. (Ed.). (1991). *Getting to yes: Negotiating agreement without giving in.* New York: Penguin Books

Giangreco, M. (1993). Using creative problem-solving methods to include students with severe disabilities in general education classroom activities. *Journal of Educational and Psychological Consultation, 4,* 113–135.

Giangreco, M. F., Cloninger, C. J., Dennis, R., & Edelman, S. W. (2002). Problem-solving methods to facilitate inclusive education. In J. S. Thousand, R. A. Villa, & A. I. Nevin (Eds.), *Creativity and collaborative learning: The practical guide to empowering students, teachers, and families* (2nd ed., pp. 111–134). Baltimore: Paul H. Brookes.

Hanft, B., Shepherd, J., & Read, J. (in press). Competence in numbers: Working on pediatric teams. In S. Lane & A. Bundy (Eds.), *Kids can be kids: Supporting the occupations and activities of childhood.* Philadelphia: F. A. Davis.

Holzmueller, R. L. (2005). Case report: Therapists I have known and (mostly) loved. *American Journal of Occupational Therapy, 59,* 580–587.

Individuals With Disabilities Education Improvement Act of 2004, Pub. L. 108–446, 20 U.S.C. § 1400 *et seq.* (2004).

Miller, D. L. (2003). The stages of group development: A retrospective study of dynamic team processes. *Canadian Journal of Administrative Sciences, 20*(2), 121–134. Retrieved January 14, 2007, from www.findarticles.com/p/articles/mi_qa3981/is_200306/ai_n9287378

Pearpoint, J., O'Brien, J., & Forest, M. (1995). *PATH: A workbook for planning positive possible futures: Planning alternative tomorrows with hope for schools, organizations, businesses, families.* Toronto: Inclusion Press.

Rainforth, B., & York-Barr, J. (1997). *Collaborative teams for students with severe disabilities: Integrating therapy and education* (2nd ed.). Baltimore: Paul H. Brookes.

Stone, D., Patton, B., & Heen, S. (1999). *Difficult conversations: How to discuss what matters most.* New York: Penguin Books.

Thousand, J., & Villa, R. (2000). Collaborative teaming: A powerful tool in school restructuring. In R. Villa & J. Thousand (Eds.), *Restructuring for caring and effective education* (pp. 254–291). Baltimore: Paul H. Brookes.

Tryon, P. (1997). Communication and collaboration with parents and between school and clinic base therapists. *Sensory Integration Special Interest Section Quarterly, 20*(4), 1–2.

Tuckman, B. (1965). Developmental sequence in small groups. *Psychological Bulletin, 63,* 384–399.

Tuckman, B. W., & Jensen, M. A. C. (1977). Stages of small group development revisited. *Group and Organizational Studies, 2,* 419–427.

Ury, W. (1993). *Getting past no: Negotiating your way from confrontation to cooperation.* New York: Bantam Books.

Wheelan, S., & Hochberger, J. (1996). Assessing the functional level of rehabilitation teams and facilitating development. *Rehabilitation Nursing, 21*(2), 75–81.

Williams, M., & Shellenberger, S. (1996). *How does your engine run?* Albuquerque, NM: TherapyWorks.

Williams, M., & Shellenberger, S. (2001). *Take five! Staying alert at home and school.* Albuquerque, NM: TherapyWorks.

Williams, M., & Shellenberger, S. (2006). *Test drive: Introducing the ALERT program through song.* Albuquerque, NM: TherapyWorks.

CHAPTER 7

Reframing Perspectives About Collaboration

Barbara Hanft, MA, OTR, FAOTA, and Jayne Shepherd, MS, OTR, FAOTA

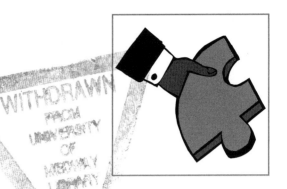

*S*chools are led by teams, not individuals. To accomplish change in a system requires collaboration with team members, including teachers, parents, and administrators.

—Case-Smith, 1998, p. 13

This chapter focuses on how occupational therapists and education personnel can initiate and sustain changes in interactions to expand their collaborative practices. Part 1, "Encouraging Team Members to Collaborate," discusses how to encourage individual team members to collaborate with occupational therapists in all school places and spaces. Part 2, "Initiating Change Systemwide," identifies the steps involved in making collaboration a key component in occupational therapy supports and services throughout a school system.

After reading this material, readers will be able to

- Select strategies for encouraging school personnel and families to collaborate with occupational therapists;

- Identify information and assistance to provide to team members at various stages of a change process;

- Identify the essential components of an action plan to expand collaborative occupational therapy services in the schools; and

- Recognize the factors that influence how receptive team members are to collaborative practices and use them in daily interactions with teachers, families, and students.

Key Topics

- Engaging reluctant collaborators
- Family perspectives
- Change process in schools
- Initiating systemwide collaboration

Part 1: Encouraging Team Members to Collaborate

Collaboration in Action: Connecting with reluctant team members

Joan Bryant has taught seventh-grade history for more than 25 years and says she "is tired of new policies and procedures when what I've been doing has worked just fine." She thinks collaboration is yet another trend and doesn't think having therapists in her classroom while she is teaching will be helpful. "OTs have worked with my students in their therapy room, and it's always worked fine. I don't want anyone touching my computers and changing my lessons."

Maria, a special educator, co-teaches with Elena, an early childhood educator, in their kindergarten for 18 "regular" students and 4 "special-needs" students. Both teachers are determined that all of their students will progress through the district curriculum in preparation for first grade. Their energies are focused on ensuring that their students "stay on track" and "demonstrate Level 10 classroom behavior." Maria and Elena are worried that "OTs take away valuable teaching time whether they work with our kids in class or their therapy room."

What will influence teachers like Joan, Maria, and Elena to collaborate with occupational therapists in their classrooms? Will they change their minds about collaborating with therapists once they experience the benefits of integrated therapy and teamwork for their students? What must happen before these teachers will try a different approach to working with related service providers such as occupational therapists? Rather than hoping for the best, occupational therapists and their team members should first consider their readiness for collaboration before attempting to influence one another's perceptions and expectations regarding the benefits of working together (see Chapter 3 for further discussion about readiness for collaboration).

To influence teachers like Joan, Maria, and Elena who doubt that in-class services and supports can be helpful, occupational therapists and their team members must demonstrate a genuine interest in finding a win–win solution for all parties to work together. A win–win strategy, one of the key principles of effective negotiation (Fisher, Ury, & Patton, 1991), focuses teachers, educators, and families on the benefits students and adults gain from collaboration (see "Learn to Negotiate" in Chapter 6). An educator or family member who believes that an occupational therapist can help them promote a student's learning and socialization in school will be more interested in team collaboration than the teacher or parent who thinks that his or her daily responsibilities and to-do list will only grow longer as a result of collaborating with an occupational therapist.

Family Voices: Benefits of occupational therapy

One of my hardest hang-ups was when my son had go through the lunch line with other children and carry a tray to the table. Jake has a birth defect and could not turn his hands sideways, so carrying a tray was totally out of the question for him. First, the OT helped me understand that no other kindergarten child would be expected to carry a full tray and not to spill it sometimes. Not even the fifth graders can do that! This helped me not to worry over every little thing and helped me not to transfer my fears to my son. Then she set to work to teach him how to carry a tray. She made a game out of it. He got to be the helper who passed out things to the other children from a tray. This gave him a real reason to be doing the task and made him feel special. He practiced at home and at school and was doing fine in no time.

The main thing was that the OT listened to my fears and concerns. When that worry was out of the way, we could begin working on other school-oriented goals. She heard what was important to our family and helped me to find a concrete way to resolve my concerns. It was good to be heard at the table and given a voice just like everyone else there. I knew that we would work together to meet all the goals listed that year.

—Melanie Cashion, parent of fourth-grade student, North Carolina

The following strategies—listen, observe, educate, and translate—focus on understanding the perspectives of reluctant team members regarding collaboration as a precursor for initiating, and then sustaining, win–win partnerships that will enhance the education of all students (Giangreco, Cloninger, Dennis, & Edelman, 2000; Hanft & Place, 1996). Keep in mind that there are many reasons why a team member may be reluctant to collaborate with an occupational therapist, especially in the classroom. As stated succinctly by one therapist,

Therapist Voices: Reluctant partners

I think sometimes educators are shy or unsure, or don't feel they can spare the time because of their dedication to what they need to accomplish as opposed to disinterest; then of course there are some who simply do not think about anything other than what they have to do.

Remember this. . . .
Listen, observe, educate, and *translate* are strategies to help occupational therapists understand team members' perspectives on collaboration.

Listening to Reframe Perspectives

Clearly communicating what occupational therapy is and how it can promote student learning and socialization may not be enough to convince a reluctant team member to collaborate. Therapists must also demonstrate that they recognize the classroom, school, and parenting responsibilities of families and educators and respect their knowledge and experience. In particular, the perspectives of core team members (i.e., educators, paraprofessionals, family members, and other related services providers) should be solicited because they spend the most time with and best understand a particular student. Listen to what those team members say about their roles and responsibilities as well as about what a student needs to learn and do to participate successfully in school. Worksheet 2.4A, introduced in Chapter 2 and included in the Appendix, includes sections for recording what team members say, in their own words, about a student's strengths, interests, challenges, and desired education outcomes.

As initial conversations with a teacher or parent unfold and teaching and parenting challenges are identified, descriptions of occupational therapy can be individualized to illustrate how hands-on services and team supports address a specific student's learning and socialization goals. An occupational therapist might suggest to a teacher, "I can help you figure out how to make it easier for Amil to participate in his reading group." To a parent, she could explain, "Amil tires quickly when he has to sit still and look at a page with lots of print. I could help you set up a home work plan that builds in time for movement breaks and helps him keep track of where he is on the page." The goal of initial conversations with reluctant team members is to help them understand how occupational therapy complements and supports their education or parenting perspectives. Therapists must also convey to families and school personnel how occupational therapy can promote student learning and participation in school. When suggestions are offered to team members, solicit their feedback by asking "How will this work for you in your classroom or at home?" If therapists' suggestions are not practical or are irrelevant, they are likely to be disregarded (McWilliam & Scott, 2001). Soliciting information and perspectives from team members before offering a strategy conveys a desire to individualize suggestions to the implementer's context.

Concerns About Previous Attempts to Collaborate

During initial conversations, teachers and parents may express concerns about their previous experiences with occupational therapists and other school personnel. If that happens, invite the teacher or parent to describe what did not work and listen for opportunities to discuss how to implement a more effective collaboration. In the following scenario, Mina, an occupational therapist, would like to work with Carly in Joan's classroom. Mina believes pairing hands-on services with team supports is essential and is interested in hearing about Joan's expectations of "helpful help" from therapists.

Collaboration in Action: Initial steps toward collaboration

Mina introduces herself to Joan and then asks, "Have you ever worked with an occupational therapist before?" When Joan replies unenthusiastically that she has, Mina adds, "How did that OT help you teach your students? (If Joan indicates that she has never worked with an occupational therapist before, Mina could take the opportunity to clearly and briefly describe school-based occupational therapy, emphasizing the three collaborative roles: hands-on service with team supports, team supports, and system supports.)

Joan describes how the previous occupational therapist worked on her own therapy tasks in the classroom, disrupting Joan's schedule and distracting her class so much that she asked the occupational therapist to see her students someplace else. Mina listens respectfully and suggests, "Let's see if we can work out a more positive experience this time with Carly. I'd like to work with you on one of Carly's IEP goals and help you find a comfortable position for Carly to use her computer so she can finish her assignments. What are your two most challenging parts of the day helping Carly finish her assignments?"

In this vignette, Mina invites Joan's comments and then listens to what she says about her less-than-positive interactions with the previous occupational therapist. Mina listens for an opening to express that she wants to help Joan structure classroom lessons to address Carly's individualized education program (IEP) goals in ways that will benefit all the students. Mina avoids discussing the details of Joan's previous interaction with an occupational therapist by inviting her to focus on how the two of them can collaborate to help a current student, Carly, find comfortable positions to use her hands and eyes effectively in classroom lessons and activities. Mina's question, "What are your two most challenging parts of the day helping Carly get set up to work on the computer?" invites Joan to describe her teaching routines and schedule rather than recite a list of what Carly cannot do. This approach opens up possibilities about when and how Mina could provide team support that is helpful to Joan.

Mina could also ask, "Have you ever had a student like Carly in your classroom?" to understand what Joan already knows about students who have muscle weakness and limited mobility because of spina bifida as well as learn about strategies she has tried with other students with similar educational needs as Carly. Knowing how to build on a teacher's current knowledge and skills, a key principle of adult learning, is a vital component of the art of collaboration (see Chapter 3 for additional information about adult learning).

Observing to Reframe Perspectives

Remember this. . . .
One benefit of collaboration in education settings is to help education team members teach and interact with students effectively so that they achieve their outcomes.

Observation, as a strategy for changing attitudes about collaboration, is closely aligned with listening. While talking with a teacher or parent, make careful mental notes about a teacher's classroom etiquette (i.e., his or her rules, schedules, and routines) and a family's culture to understand how they expect itinerant therapists and other personnel to behave and interact in their school space or home. Chapter 2 discusses classroom culture and suggests brief questions that quickly convey a desire to fit into a teacher's environment while observing students and working with them.

In the following vignette, an occupational therapist paired an observation of her students' functional hand skills with an introduction to occupational therapy for the teacher. Notice how the occupational therapist built upon a classroom lesson to benefit the teacher, the students, and herself.

Therapist Voices: Tailoring a description about occupational therapy

The opportunity for me to observe and participate in regular class activities is immensely valuable for identifying and solving individual student issues related to development and classroom success. After a group of 14 first graders listened to a story about a Christmas mouse who wrapped himself in a quilt, they decided to make a paper quilt. I offered to show the children how to fold paper to make mice. With patterns, materials, glue sticks, and scissors assembled ahead, I outlined the steps on the chalkboard, and the teacher and I worked together to help them through each step. The project was a big success, and I made some valuable observations about all the students to share with the teacher (e.g., tool use; fine motor planning; attention, distractibility, and sensory overload; and social interaction).

—Dottie Marsh, occupational therapist, Maryland

Educating Team Members to Reframe Perspectives

It is important that key stakeholders in a school district (e.g., parents, educators, administrators, supervisors, related services providers) share a common understanding of collaboration and have similar expectations about what it takes to make it work (Graham & Wright, 1999; Nochajski, 2001). As illustrated in Resource 1.2 in Chapter 1, the education literature uses many complementary terms to describe collaboration (e.g., *collaborative teaming, collaborative consultation, co-teaching*). All team

Reflection
7.1

A Common Definition of
Collaboration

Does your team or school district have a formal definition of collaboration? If not, how would you, and other team members, describe it? If yes, compare and contrast your definition with the one presented in Chapter 1: "Collaboration is an interactive team process that focuses education, family, and student partners on addressing the academic and nonacademic performance of all students in a school setting."

Remember this. . . .
All team members must share a common understanding of collaboration and what it takes to make it work.

members should be introduced to collaboration (e.g., what it is, how it works, what the benefits for all stakeholders are) through discussion groups, newsletters, and in-services (see Reflection 7.1).

Before initiating or expanding collaborative practices among educators, families, and related services providers, it is critical to secure support from key administrators such as building principals, special education directors, and teacher supervisors. An effective strategy for securing administrative support for collaborative practice is to share success stories and evidence about the benefits of collaboration (see Table 1.3 in Chapter 1). Success stories about occupational therapy collaboration should be data based (e.g., use progress monitoring to track the effectiveness of a specified intervention for a particular student rather than communicate solely through anecdotes; Clark & Miller, 1996). The vignette about Charlie in Chapter 4 is an example of a data-based success story that demonstrates how an occupational therapist collaborated with a general education teacher to improve a student's written assignments. Competent occupational therapists "make informed decisions about [occupational therapy] service provision using available research-based evidence, professional judgment, incorporating the client's (e.g., student, teacher, parent) values and preferences, and effectiveness data collected systematically and evaluated against targeted student outcomes" (Swinth, Spencer, & Jackson, 2007, p. 13).

When introducing occupational therapy services and supports, it is helpful to present successful examples of how hands-on services, team supports, and system supports benefited students and education teams. Emphasize that hands-on services for students should always be paired with team supports and describe how occupational therapists' contributions to systemwide school programs and initiatives can help students access the general curriculum. (In Chapter 4, system supports are illustrated through a description of an occupational therapist's participation on an early intervening services response-to-intervention team; other examples are provided in Chapter 1.) Success stories can also be disseminated via school newsletters, informal meetings, and lunch discussions and more formally through in-services for school personnel, information sessions for families, and scheduled team meetings. Be sure to include stories from students who have benefited from occupational therapy, such as fourth-grader Jake, who in Chapter 1 describes how his classmates no longer make fun of him since his occupational therapist helped him ask his physical education teacher to loosen his bow tie so he could participate successfully with his peers.

Stories from teachers can highlight how they and their students benefited when an occupational therapist blended hands-on services and team supports in their classrooms. For example, one study reported on the experience of a group of general educators during their first year of including children with severe motor delays in their second-grade classrooms (Giangreco, St. Denis, Cloninger, Edelman, & Schattman, 1993). The teachers expressed many pointed sentiments about helpful help and valued therapists who shared the teachers' framework and goals, actually worked in the classroom as a partner, and validated the teachers' perspectives and contributions.

The vignette below illustrates how Ancolien, an occupational therapist, collaborates with a speech–language pathologist (Shelby) and a general educator (Britt) to ensure that Colin, one of Britt's students, interacts with his classmates and demonstrates what he knows. Colin is a bright second-grade student with spastic quadriplegia who communicates via his computer and alternative augmentative communication (AAC) device. His mother, Nikki, shares important information about how he communicates at home. Ancolien provides helpful help to Britt in several ways (see Reflection 7.2).

Remember this. . . .
Success stories from students, teachers, and families about occupational therapists' collaboration are effective communication tools.

Collaboration in Action: Interdisciplinary team supports

Sharing Britt's framework and goals. Colin is extremely motivated to learn but must have adaptations to communicate because his expressive language is significantly delayed. Britt, Ancolien, and Shelby work together with Colin and his mother to figure out how he can express his knowledge to Britt and interact with his peers during social activities.

Working in the classroom on a regular basis. Ancolien meets with Britt before introducing any new equipment or techniques to try with Colin. Before the AAC device was ordered, Colin's core team—Ancolien, Colin's mother, Shelby, and Britt—pooled their expertise to try a variety of low-tech and AAC devices with Colin. Britt described assignments and communication needs; Colin and his mother shared their personal preferences for the size and attractiveness of the AAC device; Shelby considered pragmatics and language development to assess how each device would grow with Colin, and Ancolien problem solved with the team regarding the different ways Colin could access the device, carry it, and use it at home and in school places and spaces. Ancolien was particularly concerned with helping Colin keep up with the pace of the classroom and interface the device with his other technology (e.g., computer, wheelchair, electronic aids for daily living). The team shared information, listened to one another, and collectively decided on a device. When his AAC device arrived, Ancolien, Shelby, and Britt identified what symbols and phrases Colin needed to participate in class and figured out how to set up the ACC device, charge it, and attach it securely to his wheelchair so it would not be dropped.

Validating Britt's contributions and perspectives. Ancolien and Shelby responded to Britt's suggestion that Colin's classmates also needed to learn his symbols and showed his classmates how to work his machine so they could help him toggle between screens when they talked to one another. Ancolien also asked Britt, "How else can I help you encourage the kids to interact with Colin?" Britt replied that she was looking for games the children could play on their own with Colin during free time to increase the opportunities for Colin to practice his accuracy in using his new communication device.

Working as a partner on Colin's team. As part of her team supports for Britt, Ancolien developed a game to quiz classmates about Colin's symbols and initiated "quiz shows," in which classmates used Colin's AAC device to talk with him. With every piece of equipment or adaptation she suggested for Colin, Ancolien first asked Britt, "How will this work in your classroom?" Sometimes Ancolien e-mailed her idea to Britt to try out before her scheduled visit to the class, and sometimes she asked Britt if she could try it first to work out the kinks, and then conferred with Britt later to hear her reaction. Ancolien always helped Britt explain the AAC devices to Colin and modeled how to use any equipment and materials for Britt and Colin's classmates during the activities and routines when he needed to use them.

Reflection 7.2

"Helpful" Help

Consider one student and the *helpful* help you provide team members. How do you

- Share the framework and goals of teachers, parents, paraeducators, other therapists, and so on?
- Work in the classroom on a regular basis?
- Validate team members' contributions and perspectives? and
- Work as a partner on the student's team?

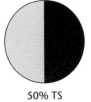

50% TS
50% HO

Translating to Find Common Ground

In the context of encouraging team members to collaborate with one another, *translating* refers to adapting all strategies and suggestions to fit comfortably in a specific school place or space (Hanft & Place, 1996). The teachers in the study cited above (Giangreco et al., 1993) also shared their comments about the "worst of times." They identified three categories of "help" from related services providers and special educators that required significant translation to actually be useful in their classrooms.

The first category addressed goals not identified or shared by teachers or that was not referenced to their classroom programs. Separate frameworks and disciplinary goals often resulted in the use of pull-out intervention from therapists and educators who used specialized techniques and equipment to help a student acquire defined skills. These skills were often unconnected to a student's school experience or used only when prompted.

The second category of misdirected team support relate to disrupting the classroom routine. Some teachers felt that the presence of special educators and therapists disrupted their classrooms more than learning to teach a student with a significant disability. One of the biggest disruptions reported by the teachers was "traffic coming through the classroom" and "the number of people who came in and watched" or talked in the back of the room while the classroom teacher tried to present a lesson (Giangreco et al., 1993, p. 367).

The third category was overly technical and specialized suggestions and strategies. Recommendations that required specialized training to implement often created confusion, particularly when the occupational therapist or special educator was not available for follow-up support in the classroom. When ongoing team supports were not provided, the recommended intervention was ultimately viewed as irrelevant by the general educators and classroom assistants. For example, a specialized feeding program suggested by an occupational therapist was so foreign to the lunch experience that it was never implemented.

Teacher Voices: Suggestions must fit the lunch context

And the way they were going to do it, it sounded like they were going to rig up this really cumbersome thing and nail it to the cafeteria table. We might as well put a sign over her [the student] and say, "Look we're practicing over here, you guys go right ahead and eat." It would be like a freak show. (Giangreco et al., 1993, p. 368)

The overly technical feeding program described above needed to be translated into a comfortable routine that school personnel could reasonably implement during lunch with classmates in the cafeteria. Recommendations for an eating program that addressed only this student's physical factors would have isolated the student from her peers in a key social context. This therapist overlooked an important opportunity to solicit input from the student and her teacher, classroom aide, and parent, a collaboration misstep that could have been avoided if the therapist had considered her team support role before recommending any intervention. Asking "How will this work for you and your student?" could have opened up many possibilities for adapting routines, materials, and the physical and social environment before implementing an out-of-context intervention (see Figure 1.3 in Chapter 1). Specifically, the therapist could have

- Talked with the student about her interests and abilities and what she would like to be able to do during lunch;

- Invited the student's mother to share her experiences and knowledge related to her daughter's mealtime routine;

- Prompted the paraprofessional who helps the student eat to describe what is working and identify challenges; and

- Solicited from team members what helpful help might look like to ensure an effective and meaningful eating experience for the student.

Summary

When challenges to collaboration arise, they create an opportunity for all team members to consider how to refine their interaction and translate their expertise so suggestions are meaningful and relate to each team member's role and responsibilities (see Reflection 7.3 and Chapter 6). In the lunch room example above, the occupational therapist needed to translate her recommendations so that they would complement, not contradict, the teacher's goal for encouraging her student's socialization during lunch. In many challenging situations, occupational therapists must artfully encourage reluctant team members to consider collaboration, as expressed below:

Using Reframing Strategies

- How could you use the strategies *listen, observe, educate,* and *translate* to influence a reluctant teacher in your work setting to view collaboration more favorably?

Therapist Voices: Encouraging collaboration in the classroom

When a teacher wanted me to take a student out of the classroom rather than work in the context, I replied, "I understand that your reading group would go smoother without Jackie, but IDEA says I should try working with him in the least restrictive environment first." When a teacher wanted to leave the classroom after I arrived, I let it go the first time and tried to reengage him on his return by saying, "Mr. Cermak, look how Johnnie formed his letters!" or "We had a question for you, Mr. Cermak; what can we do about fitting the worksheet your students are using with the computer screen?"

—Judith Schoonover, occupational therapist and
assistive technology specialist, Virginia

Reframing Perspectives: Family Concerns

Collaboration in Action: Transferring to a new school district

Sandi and Jon Watson have just moved to a new school district and have enrolled their children Samantha and Alex in high school and Jason in eighth grade. Mrs. Watson explains, "Jason has autism spectrum disorder and received sensory integration therapy twice per week with the OT in his previous school. But our new special ed coordinator told us that the therapists don't provide OT in a therapy room here and work with the majority of students within school activities." The Watsons are really worried that Jason will not get the therapy he needs and are considering appealing the district's plan for implementing Jason's IEP.

Where to start? Before attempting to dispel a family's assumption about what they think will help their child, talk with parents and listen to their past experiences in securing specific services for family members and interacting with occupational therapists and other medical and education professionals. If parents' first introduction to occupational therapy was in a hospital setting or private clinic, they are very likely to expect that school-based services will also be provided as a one-on-one session with specialized equipment and activities. Perhaps a grandfather or aunt received occupational therapy in a rehabilitation program. Daily therapy in a hospital or rehabilitation center is expected practice for these settings and is covered by health insurers. Maybe a young cousin was in a local early intervention program. Infants and toddlers with disabilities who qualify for early intervention programs under the Individuals With Disabilities Education Improvement Act of 2004 (IDEA) receive occupational therapy and other services in "natural environments" (i.e., the community and home settings in which other children their age typically spend their time (34 CFR 303 § 303.12[b])). Families transitioning from early intervention to public school are accustomed to home-based services and supports and may feel cut off from familiar therapists and teachers.

Family Voices: Help me help my child

My experience is that family members often long for a partner or a model in learning ways to help their child, but they often lose the contact and the direct ability to observe a model and develop strong partnerships when the child goes to [school]. Instead, parents receive, if anything, verbal directions via a phone call or written notes that, although possibly helpful, usually never foster the growing feeling of competence family members have when they have a direct model of helping and direct interaction with the professional. (Gretz, 1999, p. 3)

Myths About School-Based Services and Supports

In addition to their experiences with occupational therapy in hospitals and private clinics, parents also hold some common assumptions about the desirability of individualized therapy for their children. It is helpful to recognize how some myths (e.g., "more is better," "hands-on is real therapy") are very appealing to parents who want the best for their children and may be reinforced by referral sources outside the education system (Case-Smith & Nastro, 1993; Giangreco, Edelman, MacFarland, & Luiselli, 1997; Thress-Suchy, Roantee, Pfeffer, Reese, & Jennings, 1999). When families seek school-based therapy, they may be admonished by a physician to "request one-on-one therapy five times a week, but don't accept less than twice per week" (Edward Feinberg, personal communication, April 17, 2007).

Table 7.1 identifies common misassumptions about meeting children's educational needs by providing hands-on therapy and team supports in the context of typical school lessons and activities. Consider compiling discussion points to give families another perspective about hands-on services and team supports.

Remember this. . . .
Parents may believe "more is better" because they want a partner or model to show them how to help their child in school and home.

Table 7.1. Myths About Collaborative Occupational Therapy Supports and Services

Perspective	Myths About Collaboration and Teamwork
Administrator	• Teachers can incorporate therapy goals with just a little input from therapists. • Therapists can double and triple their caseloads.
Therapist	• I'll ask the teacher to do what I would have done in therapy. • It's all talk, and I won't work with kids myself anymore.
Teacher	• This is a back-door approach to making teachers into therapists. • Another "fad du jour" from administrators who are removed from classroom teaching.
Family	• Another strategy by the school district to abdicate their legal responsibility to my child. • The school districts will save money by not hiring as many therapists.

From Feinberg, E. (2003). *Collaboration and consultation in the schools.* Unpublished workshop presentation, Albuquerque, NM. Copyright © by author. Used with permission.

Administrator Voices: Addressing "hands-on is better"

Listen to what families tell us they want, and then piggyback your explanation of OT to their comments. "I'm so glad you've brought this up—let me explain how we can meet your child's educational needs." One family wanted a sensory diet for their child, so the occupational therapist observed in class and then explained to the mother, "You'd be amazed how many sensory strategies are already incorporated in your child's day. He doesn't need OT in a separate place, but I will work with his teacher to help your child be successful in his classroom."

Explain that we do not provide separate therapy in school; rather, we support a student in school. What are a child's priorities for learning and "doing" in class, on the playground, in art, in the band after school? When a parent asks for occupational therapy before the team agrees on goals, reassure the parent by explaining, "I'm going to withhold my final recommendation until I hear about your son's education program. Can you tell me about what you want him to learn and do in school (or about his IEP goals, if they are already are identified)?" Parents often think, "I'm afraid he won't get what he needs." So ask parents what they think their child needs to learn (not get), and explain how you can address these goals.

—Jean Polichino, occupational therapist and
administrator of school programs, Texas

Therapist Voices: Addressing "hands-on is better"

For example, when confronted with the situation of a parent persisting in a request that the school practitioner see her child three times a week for pull-out services, one reaction might be to become upset and say, "That's impossible. There is no way I could do that, and I don't think your child needs that type of service." Another, more constructive, approach might be to say, I understand that you really want to help your daughter by having her receive as much service as possible. Can you tell me some of the things you would like to see her accomplish this year?" In this approach, the practitioner joins the parent in problem solving while acknowledging the parent's feelings.

—Tryon, occupational therapist and parent, Massachusetts
(Tryon, 1997, p. 2)

When occupational therapists provide team supports so that all team members understand how to engage students in therapeutic activities throughout the day rather than once a week, then more is indeed better (Shepherd, 1999).

Communicating With Families About Collaborative Occupational Therapy

Help families understand the benefits of blending hands-on services, when needed, with team and system supports in typical school spaces and places by using the four strategies discussed previously (i.e., listen, observe, educate, and translate). Open the door to discussion without passing judgment about how, or where, therapy was provided in other settings. Begin a conversation with families such as the Watsons by asking, "What would you like Jason to learn and do in school?" and listen closely to their answer. The Watsons responded that they wanted Jason to have sensory integration therapy; however, that is an intervention, not an education outcome reflecting what Jason should learn in school. Occupational therapists must help families understand that the goal of related services in the schools is to achieve a desired academic or functional outcome for a particular student to facilitate participation in the general curriculum, not deliver a set number of therapy sessions. "Sometimes families are caught up in the mindset that more is better and don't really focus on a specific goal or purpose for therapy, or how the therapy is going to improve daily life" (McWilliam & Scott, 2001, p. 5).

When prompted again, the Watsons describe how they want Jason to pay attention to his teacher and schoolwork and not get so overstimulated. The occupational therapist now must consider how to *translate* school-based practice for the Watsons to focus on their desired outcomes for Jason. The therapist explains how she could work with Jason in his classroom to achieve his goals and describes how Jason could benefit from hands-on services with team supports in school contexts and activities, as follows (see also Reflection 7.4):

Reflection 7.4

Encouraging Families to Consider Collaborative Occupational Therapy

Think about a family who has asked for individual occupational therapy in an occupational therapy space. How would you explain the benefits of teacher–therapist–family collaboration? Consider the points discussed in this section.

- *Jason will learn skills and behaviors in the spaces and places in which he will need to use them.* "I can help Jason use sensory strategies to calm down and pay attention when he has problems focusing on the task at hand, as they come up in the classroom, lunchroom, hallways, and so on. I may work with Jason in a quiet spot in the classroom when he is really overstimulated, but separating him from his typical routines will only be used as a last resort."

- *Jason will have opportunities for practicing emerging skills and behaviors in the context of a familiar environment with familiar people and materials, a prerequisite for mastery of any new skill* (Schmidt & Lee, 2005). "Jason needs numerous opportunities every day—not once per week—to benefit from sensory strategies to help him pay attention to specific people and activities. If I'm the only person who helps him use them, he'll miss out on numerous critical learning opportunities. That's also why we need to consider how I can help you use sensory strategies at home, too."

- *Jason will participate in social relationships, classroom lessons, and school activities instead of being pulled out of the classroom.* "Movement and sensory breaks can be scheduled throughout the day to help Jason stay on task and interact with other children in his classroom. Taking him out of class eliminates the time I can help him with schoolwork and join activities with the other kids."

- *Therapists and teachers can address learning challenges together, as they arise.* "If I am walking with the class to the cafeteria when Jason gets overloaded by too much noise, I can help his teacher figure out immediately what will help calm him down."

- *Jason's teachers can see what an occupational therapist does to help him focus in school places and paces and continue the same strategies.* "Rather than trying to describe what kind of sensory input helps Jason calm down and pay attention, I can demonstrate what to do, and when. His teachers and I can share our observations and together come up with a more specific plan that fits their classroom routine and teaching."

- *Observing Jason's abilities, interests, and performance within a specific context (physical, social, cultural, temporal, etc.) helps individualize occupational therapy intervention for him.* "When I see how Jason reacts to the space and environment in the gymnasium, I can help the physical education teacher prompt his participation by building on his great ball-handling skills and interest in keeping time and recording scores."

Part 2: Initiating Change Systemwide

Administrator Voices: System change

We need to make sure that the "work of OT" gets done every day, all day, for each student—not just once a week. The place to start with changing [occupational therapy] practice is at the building level, and administrative support is a must.

> —Jean Polichino, occupational therapist and administrator of school programs, Texas

When a group of therapists would like to expand or refine how they provide their occupational therapy services and supports across a school district, five key considerations guide the change process:

1. Understand the *impact* of changing occupational therapy practice on potential stakeholders.
2. Identify *outcomes* desired by key stakeholders.
3. Scan the environment to identify *resources and challenges* to achieving the desired outcomes.
4. Develop an *action plan* to guide changes in occupational therapy practice
5. Evaluate *progress* toward reaching desired outcomes.

Each consideration is explored below with regard to encouraging colleagues, families, and school administrators to collaborate with occupational therapists to blend hands-on services, as needed, with team and system supports in education settings.

Resource 7.1 provides tips from two education change agents that apply to any initiative to reframe school-based practice.

Understand the Impact of Change on School Personnel, Students, and Families

Before taking action to initiate a districtwide change in occupational therapy practice, consider how to "go slow to go fast"—that is, take the time to understand the perspectives of all stakeholders or potential users of a new practice in a particular school system. Any change in occupational therapy roles and services may run into stiff resistance from stakeholders.

Teacher Voices: Keep stakeholders informed

It is critical that all parties to be affected by a change in service delivery understand the need for and the nature of the changes being implemented. Directly presenting the strengths and weaknesses of present modes of service delivery to students while examining the driving and restraining forces that influence a change in current practice provides the foundation on which changes are built. (Korinek, McLaughlin, & Gable, 1994, p. 38)

Key stakeholders of collaborative occupational therapy services in school settings include

- *Families:* parents and legal guardians of all students;
- *Students:* children with and without disabilities;
- *Related service providers:* occupational and physical therapists, speech–language pathologists, psychologists, social workers, nurses, and guidance counselors;
- *Education personnel:* special, general, and early childhood educators and paraprofessionals;
- *Administrators:* school superintendents, principals and assistant principals, supervisors, coordinators, and directors of education, special education and related services; and
- *Community partners:* local businesses owners and staff from private and public mental health and vocational rehabilitation agencies.

Resource 7.1. Lessons Learned About Initiating a Collaborative Handwriting Program
- Be aware that dreams are not realized overnight.
- Find kindred souls and "dream and scheme" together.
- Be flexible and open-minded.
- Be steadfast; modify but do not give up when faced with adversity.
- Keep dreaming; there always are new heights to climb (Schoenfeld & Mesquitit, 2002).

Two models of system change, Diffusion of Innovations (Rogers, 2000) and the Concerns-Based Adoption Model (CBAM; Hall & Hord, 2006), can assist occupational therapists, occupational therapy assistants, and other school stakeholders in understanding and engaging in collaborative teaming. Both models can help an individual or team deal with the personal and professional concerns associated with changing how education and related services are provided in school settings.

Diffusion of Innovations

Everett Rogers (2000) identified five factors that influence how quickly new ideas and practices are accepted by multicultural groups around the world. Rogers referred to a new idea or practice as an "innovation" and uses the term *diffusion* to describe the dissemination of those new ideas and practices to the people who will potentially use them. When deciding whether to adopt a collaborative practice or policy, stakeholders need information that will help them understand the practice and consider how it will affect their daily interactions and work responsibilities. Five key characteristics influence how new practices are accepted by individuals and groups.

Remember this. . . .
Before taking action to initiate a districtwide change in occupational therapy practice, consider whom to include and how to "go slow to go fast."

1. *Relative Advantage: "Show me the benefits."* Team members want to know if the new practice will be better than the one currently in use or the one "I'm-used-to-and-don't-want-to-give-up." The greater the benefits of the proposed practice or policy as perceived by team members, the more likely they are to use it.
2. *Complexity: "Give it to me real simple."* Will the proposed practice or policy be hard to understand and then to use? The easier it is for team members to understand the proposed practice or policy, the more likely they are to use it.
3. *Compatibility: "Help me see how it relates to what I know and believe."* Is the proposed practice or policy consistent with team members' values, experiences, and needs? The more the new practice fits in with their values and past experiences, the more likely team members are to use it.
4. *"Trialability": "How about a test drive first?"* Can I try out this new practice or policy before we begin full implementation? The more frequently team members can give a proposed practice or policy a trial run, the more likely they are to use it later.
5. *Observability: "I want a look-see."* Can team members watch someone else using the proposed practice or policy and see what happens when they do? When team members observe someone (especially someone like themselves whom they respect) implement a proposed practice or policy, they are more likely to try it themselves. Resource 7.2 identifies media resources that illustrate hands-on services with team supports in school and community contexts.

When a change in occupational therapy intervention is first proposed, the perceptions of school personnel and families about the new practice or policy are more important in convincing them to accept the change than what experts report or school administrators say about it. Each person wants to hear (or see) what people like themselves say about a collaborative practice or policy to understand its impact on their daily interactions and professional lives.

Concerns-Based Adoption Model

CBAM describes the impact of introducing a new practice in an education setting and is a useful guide for

Resource 7.2. Videos Illustrating Collaboration in Early Childhood and High School
Integrating Therapies Into Classroom Routines (McWilliam, 2002) and *Just Being Kids* (Edelman, 2001) illustrate collaborative occupational therapy, physical therapy, and speech–language therapy services and supports in preschool classrooms and early intervention settings. *I'm Tyler* (www.imtyler.org) offers a peek into the life of a typical high school student who happens to have cerebral palsy but also has a team who believes what he can do is more important than what he cannot do.

navigating through seven stages of a change process: awareness, informational, personal, management, consequences, collaborative, and refocusing (Hall & Hord, 2006). CBAM reminds leaders of a change effort to pay attention to the needs and desires of team members for specific kinds of information, assistance, and emotional support at various points when introducing or refining collaborative occupational therapy services. The stages of concern are not rigid and may be cycled through more than once.

Awareness (Stage 0)

Initially, educators, occupational therapists and families hear or read about school-based collaboration and may wonder how it works. Although most people have heard the word *collaboration* and understand that it entails some form of working together, they may be unsure what collaboration among therapists, educators, and families actually looks like in the classroom and in other school contexts (Graham & Wright, 1999). Team members may not even be sure about what questions to ask. Strategies for individuals and groups entering the awareness stage should promote a general understanding of collaboration, what it looks like and where additional resources can be found.

Informational (Stage 1)

School personnel and families may understand what collaboration is but need more information about how collaborative practices work. This information gathering most typically occurs by talking with colleagues and friends or posing questions on an e-mail list (e.g., "What have you heard about the district's plan to initiate more therapy services in the classroom?") or requesting information from someone who engages in collaborative practices (e.g., "What does the OT do when she works with Sonya in the classroom?"). Team members may also search for print or online resources. Individuals who already engage in a collaborative team process will need more detailed information to answer their questions about the proposed change, its benefits, and how it differs from current practice. It is important to establish a common understanding and examine various perspectives to allow participants to share their personal views and clarify the need for change to answer such questions as "Why is there a need to change our current approaches to service delivery?" or "Why consider more collaborative approaches to service delivery at this time?" (Korinek et al., 1994, p. 38).

Some team members may not show much interest in the proposed collaborative practice or program or may actively resist it, thinking that "the way we are" has worked just fine. Exposure to a new practice, without pressure for immediate adoption, helps resistors consider the proposed change. Two strategies described previously in this chapter, listening and translating, are particularly important to implement with resistors. Listen to their comments, consider their concerns, and translate for them how students and families as well as school staff could benefit from the proposed collaborative practice or policy.

Personal (Stage 2)

In this stage, team members now personalize what they have heard about proposed collaborative practices to their own school situations. They focus on learning what is expected of them and consider how they will have to change their current behavior, schedules, and practices to implement a new policy or practice regarding collaboration. Parents may wonder, "Will my child get the occupational therapy he or she really needs?" Teachers might ask, "What will it mean to have OTs working with students in my classroom?" Occupational therapists and their colleagues may speculate, "Will my students make progress?" Other questions focus on how much time will be required to learn the new practice and the effort it will take to change one's professional behavior.

Resistors may actively question the proposed practice and raise numerous concerns, many of which may be quite valid (e.g., "What if I don't know what to do?" "Who's going to help me figure this out?"). By raising concerns and asking questions, resistors can help identify critical information to share with all stakeholders (Hall & Hord, 2006). Keep in mind that resistance can be a rational or irrational concern or fear related to a proposed change or one that has just been initiated (Carner & Alpert, 1995).

Teacher Voices: Concerns about change

Another example of fear related to the change itself may be the philosophy or value system associated with the change. If you are a [therapist] who believes strongly in the value of therapy offered in separate settings, then the plan to have you work with students primarily in classes may cause you to be resistant. Alternatively, if you believe that integrative therapy should be the standard in your field, you are likely to be resistant to the plan in which you will provide only [therapy] in a separate clinical setting. (Friend & Cook, 2007, p. 307)

Issues about confidentiality and competency may also surface in the personal stage. Educators and occupational therapists, concerned about working closely with colleagues in the same school places and spaces, may wonder (but be afraid to ask), "Will Carmen talk to other team members about what she sees me doing in her class with her students?" and "If we are supposed to share responsibility for implementing Stacy's IEP, will I be held accountable for what her aide is supposed to do?" Families of children with disabilities typically have more concerns about staff competency than about confidentiality because they already know their child is being served by a team of professionals and have consented to an IEP. Parents may also worry that classroom collaboration is really a way to decrease therapy for their children (review other myths and assumptions various school stakeholder groups may entertain privately about collaboration in Table 7.1).

Management (Stage 3)

Team members focus in Stage 3 on developing and mastering the skills needed to implement collaborative practices. At this point, occupational therapists may wonder, "What if I don't know anything about math and that's what is going on when I go to work with Sam?" A parent may fret, "Sam is reluctant to work with his occupational therapist when other students are watching." Or a teacher worries, "Where will I ever find the time to plan and talk to Sam's occupational therapist?" Learning new practices takes time and energy, but as team members' skills increase, the new behaviors and interaction become more routine and team members grow more comfortable and confident with collaborative practices.

Even when the benefits of collaboration for students, teams, and the school system are fully explained and accepted, management issues arise related to the logistics of scheduling, finding time to jointly plan and assess intervention, and learning to negotiate team conflicts (Chapter 6 addresses negotiation and problem solving). Finding time to collaborate is a major challenge and requires creativity and flexibility from therapists, educators, and administrators and supervisors (Dettmer, Thurston, & Dyck, 2005; Idol & West, 1987). Table 5.5 in Chapter 5 identifies strategies used by therapists and educators across the country to find time to collaborate.

Another management issue relates to how competent an occupational therapist feels about his or her ability to provide team supports (e.g., "How will I manage classroom behavior problems?") or participate in schoolwide initiatives (e.g., "I've never been on a task force, and I don't know how to write guidelines, let alone transfer files by e-mail!"). Team members need concrete answers to their questions, and it is helpful for them to talk with colleagues about how they negotiate these challenges to effective collaboration or to attend an in-service highlighting management issues.

Consequence (Stage 4)

When team members have gained interpersonal and communication skills to collaborate competently, they can devote more attention to achieving desired results for students, their teams, and the school system. Once therapists and educators understand the basics of collaboration and its benefits, they can develop an in-depth appreciation of collaboration and why it is worth their personal attention and professional effort. In this stage, they also consider the consequences of not providing team and system supports for themselves and other school stakeholders:

- Students lose opportunities to generalize emerging skills.
- Occupational therapists do not benefit from other perspectives.
- Teachers limit assistance to facilitate student performance in their classrooms.
- Parents miss valuable support for in-home strategies.
- Teams lack support for addressing difficult or complex student behavior.

Collaboration (Stage 5)

At this stage, team members understand what they need to do to successfully change their personal and professional behavior and seek the advice of others to continue learning about specific topics related to collaboration (e.g., in-context services, supports to improve student outcomes). They may request assistance in individualizing hands-on services and team supports to help a particular student participate in school spaces and places (e.g., "Do you have any ideas about how can I help Jana introduce games at recess that Milo can play in his wheelchair?"). Many people will try a new practice while holding on to their traditional ways of providing services. Team members still need support to work through the challenges that arise ("It's harder to find time to share ideas than I thought!") and benefit from focused information to answer their questions as well as on-site coaching, mentoring, and consultation. It is one thing to attend a professional development workshop about new practices such as team collaboration and quite another to implement these new ideas after returning to work (Cutspec, 2004).

Refocusing (Stage 6)

Refocusing is the final stage in the change process; it occurs when occupational therapists and their teammates begin to address their own doubts and share insights about how to make collaboration work effectively for others as well. As challenges arise, they are critiqued objectively as opportunities for reassessment and refinement rather than as a justification to abandon the collaborative practice. Refocusing occurs after a core group of occupational therapists, educators, and families have experienced success with the proposed collaborative practice and become role models for other practitioners. Their experiences highlight the benefits of collaboration for themselves, their colleagues, and the students and families who are the heart of educational teams.

Summary of CBAM Stages

CBAM's stages of concern describe human learning and development along a continuum on which a person's focus or concern shifts in predictable ways. The first three stages—awareness, informational, and personal—focus on individual concerns about change (e.g., "What is this all about, and how will I be affected?"). In the middle stage, management, the person shifts to a task-oriented focus: "How does collaboration work, and how can I use collaborative practices efficiently?" When the majority of self-centered and task concerns are resolved, the last three stages—consequences, collaborative, and refocusing—emphasize the impact of collaborative practices on students, therapists, teachers, and the school system. For example, teams can review student progress: "Our students are really improving their tool use since the OT has spent more time in the classroom" and "How else can OTs assist teachers in the classroom?" (Sweeney, 2003).

Table 7.2 organizes change strategies in a matrix using two categories: characteristics influencing how individuals adopt new practices (Rogers, 2000) and the stages of concern for individuals contemplating, and engaging in, a change process (Hall & Hord, 2006).

Identify Outcomes Desired by Key Stakeholders

Occupational therapy leaders should articulate with key stakeholders what they hope to achieve by implementing collaborative practices. The goal is for stakeholders to draft a collective vision statement describing the outcomes for providing collaborative occupational therapy supports and services. Ultimately, occupational therapy intervention should assist education personnel and families in promoting the academic achievement and functional performance of students with disabilities so that they can participate successfully in school lessons and activities with their peers.

Teacher Voices: A shared vision for collaboration

A first step in moving toward a changed and improved future is the development of a shared dream or vision of what will be—that is, a vision of the future that increases student outcomes. . . . Many change efforts fail because the participants do not share mental images or pictures of what classroom and/or

Table 7.2. Strategies for Influencing Others to Collaborate in School Settings Using the Concerns-Based Adoption Model (CBAM; Hall & Hord, 2006) and Characteristics of Innovations (Rogers, 2000)

	Characteristics of Innovations				
	Relative Advantage	Complexity	Compatibility	Trialability	Observability
CBAM Stage 0: Awareness					
Share basic information (e.g., what collaboration is and benefits) through staff meetings, brief articles, fact sheets, and newsletters.	✔	✔			
Post notices about presentations emphasizing collaboration in schools (e.g., cooperative learning, co-teaching, consultation).			✔		
CBAM Stage 1: Informational					
Draft a 5-minute talk or PowerPoint presentation about collaboration based on Figure 1.1 in Chapter 1.		✔	✔		
Describe how other teams or schools use collaborative practices to help students learn and participate in the general curriculum.	✔				✔
Present collaboration as a set of team tools to make informed decisions about student outcomes and intervention.	✔		✔		
Recruit families, educators, administrators, therapists, and students, as appropriate, to share their experiences with occupational therapy collaboration.		✔			✔
Use videos to illustrate collaborative teaming (see Resource Box 7.2).		✔			✔
Distribute a Frequently Asked Questions sheet regarding occupational therapy supports to promote student performance (e.g., organizing work, using a locker, handwriting tips).	✔		✔		
CBAM Stage 2: Personal					
Describe collaboration as an opportunity to use one's professional knowledge and skills differently (not to abandon them).			✔		
Encourage colleagues to consider refining their current practice to increase collaboration (see Chapter 5).	✔		✔		
Share success stories and lessons learned about initiating collaboration with teammates (i.e., observe, listen, educate, and translate) to build on existing relationships.		✔			✔
Distribute examples of teams collaborating for student learning (e.g., transition to work and independent living; Shepherd, 2004).	✔				✔
Share an administrator's comments about collaboration myths to spark discussion (see Table 7.1).		✔	✔		
CBAM Stage 3: Management					
Schedule visits to classrooms to observe how occupational therapists, families, and teachers collaborate effectively to address student needs.					✔
Identify strategies for addressing the challenge of finding time to talk, plan, and work together (see Chapter 5).		✔			
Discuss how to use collaborative strategies to meet work responsibilities (e.g., individualized education program meetings, assessment, prereferral, response to intervention).	✔	✔			
Model how occupational therapists and teachers can plan and co-lead groups.		✔			✔
Pair presentations from experts with respected clinicians, educators, and students to address time, resources, schedules, and so on.		✔	✔		
CBAM Stage 4: Consequence					
When "test driving" a collaborative practice, collect ongoing data to document outcomes and refine intervention (see vignette about tracking Charlie's progress in Chapter 4).				✔	
Schedule a discussion (in person or online) to revisit the benefits of collaboration outlined in Chapter 1 after a pilot test.	✔			✔	
Interview supportive educators about helpful team supports from occupational therapists and what students and teams would have missed without them.	✔		✔		
CBAM Stage 5: Collaboration					
Encourage occupational therapy colleagues to collaborate with just one teacher or family and then facilitate a discussion about what they learned.		✔		✔	
Set timelines to try the proposed collaborative practice, and then hold a face-to-face or online debriefing to discuss what is going right and what needs adjusting.		✔		✔	
Keep a journal or file about what works and why, as well as dead ends encountered. Talk regularly with team members about what to do about challenges.		✔	✔		

Note. Stage 6 is not included.

school practice will look like when an identified change is implemented to a high quality. Picturing the change in operation provides the target for beginning the change journey. (Hall & Hord, 2006, p. 190)

Seek input and support from the people who have a stake in educating students, particularly those with disabilities, in a specific school district. Begin a discussion with stakeholders by prompting them to draft a description of collaboration in education settings that they can all support. Families and school personnel often have very different ideas about what collaboration looks like and what it can achieve (Graham & Wright, 1999). Educators and therapists often describe the specific team supports (e.g., co-teaching, consulting, coordination) with which they are familiar or have observed others engaging in. Although these are prime examples of one collaborative role (i.e., team supports), the critical element of collaboration as an ongoing, interactive team process is often overlooked. In one school survey investigating collaboration between educators and therapists, all 51 interdisciplinary respondents reported that, although they had daily informal discussions with team members, they never met periodically to plan intervention (Nochajski, 2001). Fewer than 4% of the respondents in this study reported that they engaged in a problem-solving process together, and only 16% felt collaboration increased family involvement in planning and decision making (see Chapter 3 for a discussion of team decision making). Collaboration can take place in more than one way, all of which should focus on how stakeholders can work together to promote student achievement and performance, the competency of team members, and school productivity and efficiency.

One approach to facilitating an informed discussion among stakeholders about collaborative occupational therapy is to objectively review how therapists currently use their knowledge and skills to provide team and system supports as well as hands-on services. Worksheet 3.4A in the Appendix can help occupational therapists identify their hands-on services and team supports for a sampling of students. Space is also provided on the worksheet to identify the system supports provided to a school district or districts.

After reviewing how current school-based therapy services are offered in a school district, discussions with stakeholders can then focus on drafting a succinct and brief statement articulating the broad program outcomes to which collaborative occupational therapy services and supports could contribute. This statement highlights the ultimate "vision" supported by all stakeholders.

Therapist Voices: Articulating a vision

This vision must be believable and related to the mission of the school district. All who are concerned with a school district or a school must come together and articulate a goal or vision of what a transformed school or district will look like. . . . For example, a focus on student learning might be articulated. (Chandler, 2005, p. 2)

Vision statements regarding the impact of collaboration among occupational therapists and education personnel at state and local levels were drafted by occupational therapists and school administrators for a national advocacy project sponsored by the American Occupational Therapy Association (AOTA) to support effective school-based services (Case-Smith, 1998; Hanft, 1995). Examples of those vision statements are as follows:

- *Delaware:* To develop and implement a coordinated, collaborative personnel that meets the needs of families and youths and includes the following components: collaboration; coordinated flow of delivery of services; systems change; preservice and continuing education to accommodate role changes; and development of qualified, transdisciplinary teams.

- *Indiana:* Educational needs for students will be met in the most productive way through collaboration of comprehensively trained service providers.

- *New Jersey:* To provide a comprehensive educational experience that will meet the changing needs of the children and families and provide them with the skills necessary to become productive, contributing members of society to the fullest extent of their individual capabilities.

To be effective agents of change, therapists, educators, and families are also guided by personal visions, or scenarios of the future for a student or group of students, that are shaped by their professional and personal experiences, as well as state and federal education laws. Case-Smith (1998) described how one occupational therapist's vision for full inclusion for her high school students guides her hands-on services and team and system supports:

Therapist Voices: A vision guides intervention

Part of Diane's effectiveness relates to the vision that she holds for her students. She believes that they will become full participants in the community and helps them see how this is possible. She helps them to understand the barriers and to identify the resources. She creates opportunities that enable students to participate in their community and promotes the community's acceptance of those individuals. (p. 18)

Remember this. . . .
Draft a vision statement with all stakeholders to guide team collaboration.

Families articulate their vision for their children when they, and other members of the education team, engage in a collaborative decision-making process associated with team assessments such as Making Actions Plans (MAPS; Falvey, Forest, Pearpoint, & Rosenbury, 2004). These vision statements are generated for individual students, and they remind all school personnel of the importance of focusing education and related services on ensuring that students participate in typical school activities and lessons with peers. A team's vision for a student using the MAPS process is illustrated in Susannah's story at the end of Chapter 5, and Chapter 2 includes a family's vision for their daughter.

Scan the Environment to Identify Challenges and Resources

After a vision or outcome statement for collaboration is specified, the next step is to scan the school environment to identify current issues and trends that could affect any proposed changes in occupational therapy supports and services. This "wide-angle" picture helps leaders analyze the challenges and resources that could limit or enhance a group's chances of reaching their vision (Bryson, 1995; Newberry, 1992). An environmental scan provides a broad view of a school system and lays the groundwork for developing goals and strategies for action.

Therapist Voices: Identifying system issues

To create change, the occupational therapy practitioner must know how his or her school system works. . . . Schools operate according to a systems model in which all of the parts are interdependent and thus an interdisciplinary team of professionals who bring different perspectives to each situation is needed. Students, occupational therapy practitioners, and educators have reciprocal relationships; however, these relationships are complicated by many variables that enter into the system and influence the students' learning and the professional's work. (Case-Smith, 1998, p. 10)

Key categories for scanning current trends that could influence collaborative occupational therapy supports and services in education settings include the following areas:

- *Stakeholder beliefs:* What are the attitudes and beliefs of each stakeholder group regarding school-based occupational therapy? (Key stakeholders identified previously include student, families, educators, related service providers, other school personnel, administrators, and community agencies.)

- *Political and economic considerations:* Which current or proposed laws and regulations and administrative policies may affect school-based occupational therapy and its financing?

- *Professional development:* What current and anticipated changes in theory, research, and practice may affect school-based occupational therapy and other school personnel? What standards for professional licensing and certification may apply?

- *School trends and demographics:* How many related services and education staff work in a school district? What is their discipline and experience? How many students are currently served, and what are the projections for the next 5 to 10 years? What is the typical workload for occupational therapists and other related services providers?

Additional categories that may be helpful to analyze for related trends and issues include community climate (e.g., community acceptance and support of recent immigrants) and employment opportunities for occupational therapists and educators within a specific community (e.g., competition with private clinics and hospitals for therapists). Table 7.3 summarizes an environmental scan compiled by occupational therapists and school administrators attending the Promoting Partnership summit sponsored by AOTA (Hanft, 1995). A blank copy of the environmental scan (Worksheet 7.1A) is included in the Appendix.

Table 7.3. Environmental Scan: Issues Influencing Occupational Therapists' Collaborative Role in "Any School District"

Stakeholders	Stakeholder Beliefs	Political and Economic Trends	Professional Development	School Trends and Demographics
Key stakeholders invested in school-based OT?	*Beliefs and attitudes regarding school-based OT?*	*Federal, state, and local laws and regulations and administrative policy affecting OT services and financing?*	*Current and anticipated changes in OT theory, research, and practice?*	*Staff training and experience? Changes in student population? Occupational therapists workload?*
• *Administrators:* Educators with administrator credentials • *Educators:* Shortage of general and special educators, paraprofessionals • *Families:* Race and ethnicity, religious beliefs, and socioeconomic status varies by school and influences expectations regarding educating a student with a disability (e.g., 170 languages spoken within district) • *Students:* ages, numbers, medical and/or learning conditions • *OT practitioners:* Uneven distribution of occupational therapists across state and between rural and urban districts • *Community partners:* corporate executives, chamber of commerce, social services, mental health/ vocational rehabilitation agencies, and independent living centers	• *Administrators:* Frustrated by OT salaries and manpower shortages; unsure how to use OTs; view professional organization as "gatekeeper"; oppose unfunded government mandate (IDEA) • *Families:* Unfamiliar with education model; often believe the more hands on the better; strong reactions (pro and con) to inclusion • *Teachers:* Want more support to implement inclusion; may view OT in classroom as a "fad"; time limited for collaboration • *Therapists:* Itinerant services present challenge to teamwork; high caseloads limit consultation; some view hands-on therapy as more efficient	• IDEA: Related service provisions bundle OT to special education; federal funds flow to districts through state department of education; early intervening services; response to intervention • Rehabilitation Act Amendment of 1986 Section 504 ensures accommodations for students, but no funds are provided • NCLB demands annual yearly progress for all student groups, including those in special education • Families use litigation and due process safeguards to secure OT services • Medicaid for medically necessary services only • Contract therapists may answer to health or private agency rather than school district	• Demand for evidence-based practice reinforces data-based decision making for assessment and intervention • Limitations in Levels 3 and 4 research studies; OT studies generally focus on case and descriptive studies • Inconsistent preparation for school-based practice • Limited onsite supervision and mentoring opportunities • Occupational therapists have little knowledge of education trends (e.g., high-stakes testing, co-teaching, response to intervention) • Percentage of occupational therapists who are members of state or national professional associations (AOTA, Council for Exceptional Children)	• Standards and certification for teachers and paraprofessionals as mandated in NCLB • One in 150 children born in 2007 has autism spectrum disorder (Centers for Disease Control and Prevention, 2007) • Extended school year upheld for specific students • Related services must be provided per individualized education program

Note. OT = occupational therapy; IDEA = Individuals With Disabilities Education Improvement Act of 2004; NCLB = No Child Left Behind Act of 2001.

Analyze Resources and Challenges

Once issues and trends are identified, the resources and challenges that will support or hinder a group's ability to achieve its outcomes regarding collaborative therapy services can be summarized. *Resources* are the opportunities, people, funding, and school capabilities available both within and outside a school system. Some examples of internal resources include support from building principals and special education coordinators for classroom collaboration or funding from the state Department of Education for training on school-based collaboration. Examples of external supports include Web sites with articles about collaboration or funds available through state occupational therapy associations for workshops and developing informational brochures.

Challenges to an initiative to refine occupational therapy practice in a district can also arise from internal and external sources. Internal challenges may surface if insufficient effort is dedicated to securing and maintaining stakeholder support as well as failing to monitor and revise a plan of action for achieving goals. Internal challenges

Table 7.4. Examples of Resources and Challenges Affecting School-Based Occupational Therapy Practice

Internal (Within School System)	External (Outside School System)
Resources (opportunities, people, funding, etc., that will help achieve outcomes)	
• Individuals (occupational therapists, educators, supervisors, principals, etc.) with expertise regarding school-based practice and collaboration • Support for collaboration from administrators • Educators and families who want to collaborate with occupational therapist • Funds for external consultant, professional development	• Print or online articles, success stories, research studies • Availability of consultant, coach, or mentor to guide change process • Workshops and conference presentations regarding school-based collaboration • IDEA least restrictive environment mandate creates an opportunity for collaboration within classroom • IDEA 2004 provision for early intervening services creates opportunity for occupational therapist participation on education teams
Challenges that may hinder collaboration	
• Lack of leadership for change in practice • Resistance from occupational therapists and educators not addressed • Key stakeholders groups not identified and contacted for support • Ultimate outcomes (vision) not embraced by stakeholders • Goals either too narrow or broad • Action plan lacks specificity about who will do what by when • No plan for monitoring progress and evaluating outcomes	• Increased demand for occupational therapists to increase hands-on services and supports services to serve special populations • Higher salaries for occupational therapists in medical and rehabilitation settings and other school districts result in unfilled job positions • Medicaid will fund only hands-on services • Families resist any change from hands-on service only

Note. IDEA = Individuals With Disabilities Education Improvement Act of 2004.

can also arise from occupational therapists and other education team members who resist changes in how services and supports are provided in the schools. A common external challenge comes from private therapists and physicians who urge families to specify how often hands-on services should be provided for a student. It is extremely important to anticipate, and address, reactions from all stakeholders at various stages of a change process, as discussed previously in this chapter. Table 7.4 summarizes the internal and external resources and challenges typically encountered when moving to more collaborative school-based practices.

The final two steps in the change process, developing an action plan and monitoring progress, are illustrated below in a vignette about a group of occupational therapists and educators who plan to expand their collaborative teaming efforts to educate students with disabilities in general education classrooms.

Remember this. . . .
Conduct an environmental scan to identify current issues and trends that could affect proposed changes in occupational therapy supports and services.

Develop an Action Plan

An action plan identifies the specific goals and action steps that will help a group achieve their valued outcome. This vision is the "big picture" for collaborative services and describes what a school-based planning group hopes to ultimately achieve with regard to student achievement and participation in the schools. Whereas a vision statement describes an outcome that a school district values highly, an action plan with goals and action steps identifies how to go about achieving stakeholders' vision for collaboration. The following vignette illustrates how one group of educators and teachers worked with administrators and families to develop an action plan to support their vision for collaborative teaming in their school.

Collaboration in Action: Crafting a vision for collaboration

After reading several articles about the benefits of teamwork and collaboration, Leslie, an occupational therapist, and Oma, a third-grade educator, decided it was time to learn more about blending hands-on services with team supports in Oma's classroom. Students typically received hands-on services in the occupational therapy room, once per week, throughout the school district. Therapists and teachers exchanged greetings as the occupational therapists picked up students from class and shared information about student progress and intervention strategies at monthly staff meetings.

Over the summer, Leslie and Oma and three colleagues attended a workshop about collaborative teaming in education settings and spent several weeks afterward discussing what they might try. With input from other colleagues, families, therapy supervisors, and building principals, they drafted a vision statement to guide their efforts: "We will support all students' participation in typical school activities and lessons through collaborative teaming in the classroom and other education contexts."

On behalf of their colleagues, Leslie and Oma also met several times with their respective supervisors and the director of special education to gain support for piloting hands-on occupational therapy services with team supports in three classrooms when school started. These administrators encouraged Oma and Leslie to talk with interested families about providing OT services and supports with their children in the classroom and to be sure to follow the frequency and duration times already listed on the students' IEPs. Leslie and Oma were also encouraged to set up another meeting for final approval after drafting an action plan with their colleagues to specify their goals and action steps.

***Remember this*. . . .**
An action plan with goals, action steps, facilitators, criteria for success, and timelines identifies how to achieve a team's vision for collaborative services.

Oma and Leslie, and their colleagues, wisely decided to implement a change in their practice by working first with teachers and families who welcomed their collaboration in the classroom. They did not expect to change where and how occupational therapy services and supports were provided in their school district without first developing, with their supervisor's support, a vision statement describing their desired outcome and an action plan to guide their efforts.

Identify and Prioritize Goals

In a brainstorming session, key stakeholders should generate a list of goals to help them work toward their group's desired outcome, or vision. During this discussion, an impact–likelihood analysis can be conducted to help prioritize the identified goals. Worksheet 7.2A in the Appendix is a useful tool for identifying goals that could have a high impact and are likely to be accomplished because of adequate resources, support of stakeholders, time availability, administrative support, etc. Worksheet 7.2A is divided into four quadrants to help identify and categorize goals as follows:

1. High impact and unlikely to accomplish (Quadrant A)
2. High impact and likely to accomplish (Quadrant B)
3. Low impact and unlikely to accomplish (Quadrant C)
4. Low impact and likely to accomplish (Quadrant D)

Stakeholders rate each goal identified in their brainstorming session using a scale ranging from 1 to 5 (1 is the lowest rating, and 5 the highest). Each person gives each goal two ratings: one for the impact the goal will have in advancing the group's vision and the other for how likely it can be accomplished. All ratings for each goal are then plotted on a grid illustrating the impact of the goal and the likelihood that it can be accomplished within a specific timeframe. Figure 7.1 illustrates how Leslie's and Oma's group used Worksheet 7.2A to rate goals generated during their brain storming session.

The benefit of completing an impact–likelihood analysis is that it provides a visual illustration of how various stakeholders perceive identified goals so that a planning group can prioritize those goals. Goals that fall into Quadrant B reflect a group's belief that those goals will have the most impact in moving a group toward its vision for collaboration and are most likely to be accomplished. Quadrant C goals have low impact and are unlikely to be accomplished. Clearly, a planning group should be

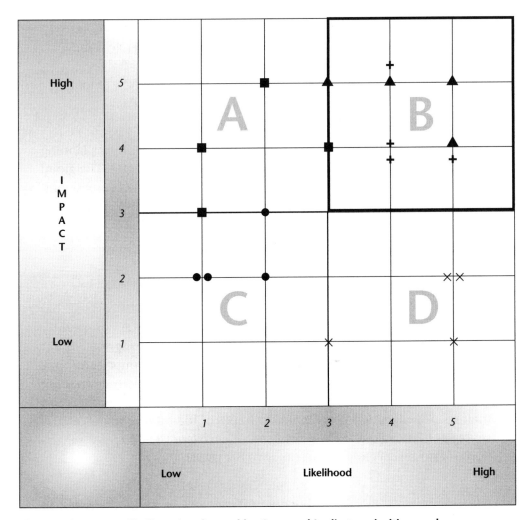

Figure 7.1. Impact–likelihood scale used by Oma and Leslie to prioritize goals.

Key: A: high impact and unlikely to accomplish; B: high impact and likely to accomplish;
C: low impact and unlikely to accomplish; D: low impact and likely to accomplish.

▲ Goal 1: Prepare two teams for pilot test of collaborative services.
+ Goal 2: Increase in-class occupational therapy with team supports in two classrooms.
● Goal 3: Present in-service on benefits of collaborative occupational therapy services and supports.
✕ Goal 4: Disseminate article about occupational therapist–teacher collaboration on school Web site.
■ Goal 5: Develop collaborative goals for students' IEPs.

cautious about tackling any goals that fall into Quadrant C of the grid. Quadrant A goals have high impact but are unlikely to be accomplished; those goals should be discussed further to determine what factors would have to change, or they should be changed to improve the likelihood that they can be achieved. Quadrant D goals have a low impact but are likely to be accomplished, and they may give a group a boost of confidence that they can work together to complete them.

Collaboration in Action: Prioritizing goals

Oma and Leslie facilitated a discussion with parents, supervisors, and their colleagues and identified five possible goals to work on for the next year to move them toward their vision of collaborative teaming in their classrooms:

1. Prepare two teams for a pilot test of collaborative services (see Resource 7.3)
2. Increase in-class, hands-on OT with team supports in two classrooms
3. Present an in-service on the benefits of collaborative OT services and supports
4. Disseminate an article about OT–teacher collaboration on the school Web site
5. Develop collaborative goals for students' IEPs.

Leslie posted one big grid on a flip chart so that everyone in the planning group could plot their rating for all five goals on the same grid. The group identified two goals in Quadrant B that they were likely to accomplish and that could have a high impact on helping them achieve their vision for collaborative teaming:

• *Goal 1:* Prepare teams for a pilot test of collaborative services

• *Goal 2:* Increase hands-on OT with team supports in the classroom.

As Oma and Leslie facilitated the group's discussion, they discovered that Goal 5, "develop collaborative goals for students' IEPs," was consistently rated as high impact but unlikely to be accomplished during the current school year. Rather than discard a goal the group felt was important, they decided to continue exploring the challenges associated with developing collaborative IEP goals. They planned to discuss Goal 5 with supervisors and their special education coordinator in hopes of identifying resources and strategies that could make it possible to achieve (see Chapter 5 for suggestions regarding developing collaborative IEP goals).

Resource 7.3. Piloting Collaborative Practices

Selecting pilot sites to test and refine a collaborative program or practice before widespread implementation reinforces team members' need for "trialability," one of five characteristics that promote adoption of new practices (Rogers, 2000; see also Table 7.2). Select sites by staff interest, previous success with collaboration, and administrative support (Korinek et al., 1994).

Goal 3, "present an in-service on the benefits of collaborative OT services and supports," fell in Quadrant C and was neither high impact nor likely to be accomplished, so the group set it aside. Goal 4, "disseminate an article about OT–teacher collaboration on the school Web site," was also rated as low impact but likely to be accomplished (Quadrant D). An occupational therapist and a teacher volunteered to write a short article and share their success thus far with in-class collaboration.

The impact–likelihood worksheet completed by Oma and Leslie with their education team is displayed in Figure 7.1 (for simplification, only four team members' ratings are shown). As illustrated, Goals 1 and 2 in Quadrant B were identified as the group's priorities. Goals 3 and 4, in Quadrants C and D, were rated as low impact; however, Goal 4 was also rated as likely to be accomplished, and the group voted to keep it because volunteers were willing to write the article.

Specify Action Steps With Timelines and Responsibilities

An action plan also specifies the steps necessary to accomplish each goal, including timelines and responsible group members. Action steps spell out who will do what and by when. Assigning responsibility for carrying out action steps can be a challenge unless all members of a planning group take a broad view about who can do what. It is helpful to consider the various roles different stakeholders may assume as implementing, supporting, and guiding partners (Hanft & Read, 2001). Although partners will play different roles in carrying out a group's action plan, they all must support the group's vision for promoting student success in the schools through collaborative teaming. Ultimately, as goals are achieved a group will move closer and closer to realizing its vision.

One definition of *partner* as "a player on the same side or team as another" (*Random House,* 2006) provides a useful metaphor for how implementing, supporting, and guiding partners can achieve common goals that will move them toward fulfilling their desired outcome, or vision.

> Consider a baseball team. The number of players on the team far outnumbers who can be on the field at one time. Regardless of how many players are on the field, however, each member plays a role to support the team's effort. Players on the bench observe the other team and reflect those observations to their teammates when they take the field. Every team member shows his or her support for each individual as they take their turn at bat. While each team has identified leaders, not every player plays at the same time. Some players rarely leave the bench, but the whole team is committed to their collective success. The entire team shares in the glory of winning and the sting of defeat. (Read & Hanft, 1999, p. 4)

Implementing partners are the people who will actually carry out the action steps identified by a planning group such as Oma, Leslie, their supervisors, and colleagues. Implementing partners are the players (e.g., therapists, teachers, paraprofessionals) who are actually on the field during the game, educating and interacting with students in various school places and spaces on a routine basis. *Guiding partners* have regulatory, funding, or statutory authority and therefore can significantly influence the implementation of a group's action plan. Guiding partners may promulgate and administer regulations, set standards for professional credentials, or administer school funds and control helpful resources. They do not actually implement a group's action plan, but they contribute substantially to the shape it takes. In baseball, the coach or manager is a guiding partner. They are not on the field playing, but they significantly influence how the players play the game. In a school setting, guiding partners at the local level include therapy and education supervisors, building principals, or the director of special education. More distant guiding partners include members of education committees in state and federal legislatures and state licensure boards.

Supporting partners offer information, political support, or positive public relations, but they do not participate in the day-to-day work of implementing or supervising a group's action plan. Continuing the baseball metaphor, supporting partners would include a team's fans and sponsors. In an education setting, the most important supporting partners are families of children with and without disabilities. Supporting partners also include a school parent–teacher association, professional organizations such as a state occupational therapy association or a local chapter of the Council for Exceptional Children, and community agencies that collaborate with the schools (e.g., social services or mental health agencies).

Collaboration in Action: Partner roles

Oma and Leslie talked with their colleagues about partner roles and decided the six therapists, teachers, and class assistants were the obvious implementers of their plan to integrate hands-on services and team supports in their classroom. However, they realized that they needed to keep their local guiding partners (e.g., their supervisors, building principals) informed of their action plan and what happened as they implemented it in their classrooms. The families of children receiving occupational therapy services and the families of the other students were their key supporting partners. Leslie and Oma decided to use their monthly class newsletters as one way to keep families informed about the different ways in which occupational therapists were collaborating with teachers to help students in the classroom and other school settings. They planned to use their newsletters to continue the themes presented in the Web site article their colleagues had agreed to write about occupational therapist–teacher collaboration in the classroom (Goal 4 identified during their brainstorming session).

Remember this. . . .
Stakeholders in a change process can assume different roles as implementing, supporting, and guiding partners.

Develop Accountability Measures to Monitor Progress

Another important component of developing an action plan is to draft accountability indicators (i.e., measurable criteria) to assess the group's progress toward each goal. These indicators are critical guides for assessing whether goals are achieved and how a group moves toward its desired outcome, or vision, for promoting successful student performance and participation in school lessons and activities. Figure 7.2 is a draft of the action plan developed by Oma and Leslie with their planning group of teachers, supervisors, and families; a blank copy of the action plan is included in the Appendix (Worksheet 7.3A). The group's action plan identifies their two priority goals and the action steps, responsible parties, criteria for success, and timelines.

Evaluate the Effectiveness of Reaching Stated Outcomes

Action plans should be considered a draft document that will need to be modified at regular intervals to account for what is and is not working. "Planning is both essential and dangerous. If the organization does not plan well, change efforts can go off

Goals and Action Steps	Facilitated by	Criteria for Success	Completed by
Goal 1: Prepare two teams for pilot test of collaborative OT services (each with 1 occupational therapist, 1 teacher, 1 aide, 3 students/families)	Oma	**Teams schedule in-class OT and identify strategies and supports to implement students' IEPs.**	**September of school year '07–'08**
Action Steps 1.1. Schedule visits to a local school district to observe occupational therapists/teachers collaborating in typical school contexts.	Teacher	At least one school visit completed by each team (parents encouraged to attend also).	Spring of school year '06–'07
1.2. Review video (e.g., McWilliam, 2002), print (e.g., Swinth et al., 2002), and online (e.g., Swinth, 2004) resources regarding collaboration.	Occupational therapists	Teachers, aides, and occupational therapists identify strategies and activities to use in class	Summer '07 in-service
1.3. Identify how to address each student's IEP goals with in-context OT supports and services	Occupational therapists	Each team reviews curriculum and IEP goals for 3 students; schedules in-class OT.	By September '07
Goal 2: Provide in-class OT services and supports in two classrooms		**Occupational therapist, teachers, and aides work together to promote students participation in school assignments, activities, and interactions.**	10 in-context visits per grading period per student during '07–'08
Action steps: 2.1. Implement strategies and supports to address specific goals from students' IEPs.	Teachers/aides	Collaboration notebook for each class is up to date (e.g., communication with parents, "Keep-it-up" forms, IEP progress reports).	Ongoing
2.2. Exchange feedback by e-mail, phone, and in-person; reassess activities in monthly team meeting.	Occupational therapists	"Keep-it-up" feedback notes completed by occupational therapist after each visit; team meetings held monthly (with parents, as possible).	Weekly notes Monthly meetings
2.3. Teams engage in peer coaching to observe one another implementing strategies and activities with students.	Education supervisor	Teams engage in self-reflection and provide verbal feedback for each another within 3 days of observation.	Two sessions per team each semester

Completed by:

Dates reviewed:

Figure 7.2. Oma's and Leslie's action plan (for two goals in Year 1).

Note. OT = occupational therapy; IEP = individualized education program.

half-cocked. 'Let's try this and see what happens' is not bad as a condiment but should not be a staple" (Egan, 1988, p. 10). Conversely, excessive planning can stifle a group's flexibility in responding to changes in internal and external resources and challenges.

Progress toward achieving goals identified in an action plan like the one Oma and Leslie drafted for implementing collaborative practices must be periodically assessed, just as student progress is monitored for IEP reviews. This assessment is an opportunity to revisit the group's vision and review how far it has come in reaching its valued outcomes. What do all partners (implementing, guiding, and supporting) think about the goals and action steps achieved thus far? Have any partners changed their perspective on collaboration? If so, why has their perspective changed, and what do they now think? Progress reviews can be accomplished through verbal discussion at meetings, by means of short surveys, and by conducting focus groups. The need to conduct periodic reviews also raises an opportunity to keep local guiding partners (e.g., supervisors, building principals) informed of successes and challenges. It also presents an opportunity to link with distant guiding partners (e.g., university faculty in occupational therapy and education departments) who might provide guidance regarding program evaluation of and resources on effective collaborative practices.

Administrator Voices: Stable yet flexible planning

Planning is not a one-time event. Like a holiday trip, destinations sometimes change, and frequently, unexpected additions may be made for increased effectiveness and/or satisfaction. Thus, while a plan is essential for understanding where the change journey is moving, it should never be cast in concrete. (Hall & Hord, 2006, p. 191)

Remember this. . . .
Expect to revise an action plan, and always keep your vision in mind.

Expect to revise an action plan and revisit the partnership roles assumed by various stakeholders. Implementing partners typically carry out the action steps and assume the lion's share of the work. To forestall burnout and promote creative problem solving, consider the following:

- Can responsibilities be shared by recruiting additional implementers?

- What resources can supporting partners contribute (e.g., success stories from families about occupational therapy services and supports)?

- Are guiding partners, especially local school administrators and supervisors, still on board?

- Have satisfactory communication links been maintained to keep them informed about key outcomes of the in-class collaboration among occupational therapists, educators, and families?

Conclusion

This chapter has reviewed strategies for reframing the perspectives of individual team members and school systems about the benefits of collaboration for students, families, therapists, and educators. Typically, occupational therapists are more familiar and comfortable with individual change at the student level than with system-level change; at either level, it is a multifaceted process (Chandler, 2005). When planning for a system change in providing occupational therapy services and supports in school places and spaces, consider how to do the following:

1. Solicit the input of key school stakeholders (i.e., teachers, families, therapists, students, administrators) to craft a vision for collaborative occupational therapy services and supports.
2. Scan the environment with stakeholders to review the impact of the proposed changes on stakeholders as well as identify resources and challenges to achieving the identified outcomes.
3. Identify goals and conduct an impact–likelihood analysis.
4. Develop an action plan linking goals with action steps, people responsible, criteria for success, and timelines.
5. Assess progress toward reaching the stated vision for team collaboration.

It is not enough to have good intentions to successfully blend hands-on services, when needed, with team and system supports in an interactive team process. Therapists and their team members must also consider how to plan and implement a change process to include the input and support from all stakeholder groups if occupational therapy practice in school settings is to become truly collaborative.

The ultimate benefit for all stakeholders? Consider the possibilities expressed in this final vignette:

Therapist Voices: Collaborating for student success

In my local school district, our essential early education (EEE) team is working to address a new influx of preschoolers on the autism spectrum in a collaborative, planful way. I have assumed a role in a statewide training program with a speech–language pathologist and special educator who bring energy and a desire to learn to our seasoned team. One thing we've developed is an engaging way to train our paraeducators, who were typically unfamiliar with these kids. We scheduled 2-hour seminars at one of the staff's houses, so staff could bring their own kids and let them play while we presented some basic topics (e.g., using a picture exchange communication system, designing schedules and work systems to fit different preschools). This worked really well, and the paraeducators began to understand what the therapists and special educators had to offer in terms of expertise and program design. The ideas exchanged were very specific to just our students and our settings, and we built a collegial bond as we sat, talked, brainstormed, and shared meals.

The net effect was that program ideas that usually take months of cajoling and pushing for one small change were now requested, and people felt empowered to talk together, plan, and work on designs. Our paraeducators didn't feel like they were stuck with materials they didn't understand. Now they noticed how terrifically kids were doing and felt they had a part in that success.

Given that my OT role in the EEE program has always been a bit stretched, due to funding issues and just not enough time, it has been a great way to mix and match OT skills and build capacity in the school. It allows me to support the school system by helping with program design and training. This is also economical for the school district, as my expertise can be stretched much farther, and the results of my team consults are visible and can be duplicated in other places and with other students.

The energy in our office now is remarkable, and instead of complaints about how things are not going well, there are requests for more materials, new ideas, how to document changes, etc. For me, it is the epitome of OT contributions to program design and training, and the results and spin-off effects have been just wonderful. OTs now have a highly visible role as collaborators, designing classrooms, materials, and accommodations for preschool activities for a special group of children.

—Chris Knippenberg, occupational therapist, Vermont

Acknowledgments

This chapter was produced in collaboration with Melanie Cashion, Judie Davis, Ed Feinberg, Christine Knippenberg, Dottie Marsh, Jean Polichino, Jo Read, and

Judith Schoonover. Thanks to all for their perspectives on changing practice in the schools.

Selected Resources

Bober, P. (2002). Moving toward evidence-based practice in schools: Wisconsin's model. *School System Special Interest Section, 9*(4), 1–6.

> This article is authored by the occupational therapist who works as an Education Consultant in Wisconsin's state education agency. Bober describes a planned statewide systems change process for school-based occupational therapists and highlights the environmental scan of issues and trends that influenced a reconsideration of how services are provided to students with disabilities in the public schools.

Case-Smith, J. (1998). Thinking out of the box. In J. Case-Smith (Ed.), *Occupational therapy: Making a difference in school system practice* (Unit 2, AOTA Self-Paced Clinical Course). Bethesda, MD: American Occupational Therapy Association.

> This lesson describes how occupational therapists can fulfill the IDEA mandates of least restrictive environment and free appropriate education for all children by making significant contributions as members of an education team and working as change agents in the school setting. Detailed case studies illustrate how occupational therapists across the country provide system supports (e.g., writing state guidelines, enlisting administrator support for expanding team supports, reframing teacher–family attitudes toward collaboration, translating a personal vision for student achievement into a team vision for collaborative services).

Friend, M., & Cook, L. (2007). *Interactions: Collaboration skills for school professionals* (5th ed.). Boston: Allyn & Bacon.

> This book provides tools, principles, and guidelines for teachers and therapists to collaborate with other school professionals and for parents to educate students with special needs within typical school settings. Two special features, "A Basis in Research" and "Putting Ideas Into Practice," are included in all chapters. Chapter 11, "Difficult Interactions," discusses the causes of personal resistance to change and how to respond effectively. Other chapters address the fundamentals of collaboration, problem solving, teaming, consultation, co-teaching, paraeducators, and interpersonal communication.

Hall, G., & Hord, S. (2006). *Implementing change: Patterns, principles, and potholes* (2nd ed.). Boston: Pearson Education.

> An in-depth analysis of the patterns, themes, and principles connected with the process of changing practice in education settings, including classic perspectives for understanding change (systems thinking, diffusion of innovations, and organization development), the Concerns-Based Adoption Model to examine the personal reaction to change, and tools and recommendations for leading change.

References

Bryson, J. (1995). *Strategic planning for public and nonprofit organizations.* San Francisco: Jossey-Bass.

Carner, L., & Alpert, J. (1995). Some guidelines for consultants revisited. *Journal of Educational and Psychological Consultation, 6,* 47–57.

Case-Smith, J. (1998). Thinking out of the box. In J. Case-Smith (Ed.), *Occupational therapy: Making a difference in school system practice* (Unit 2, AOTA Self-Paced Clinical Course). Bethesda, MD: American Occupational Therapy Association.

Case-Smith, J., & Nastro, M. (1993). The effect of occupational therapy intervention on mothers of children with cerebral palsy. *American Journal of Occupational Therapy, 47,* 811–817.

Centers for Disease Control and Prevention. (2007). *Prevalence of the autism spectrum disorders in multiple areas of the United States, surveillance years 2000 and 2002.* Retrieved January 7, 2008, from www.cdc.gov/od/oc/media/pressrel/2007/f070208.htm

Chandler, B. (2005). Anything changed around here lately? The change process in public education. *School System Special Interest Section Quarterly, 12,* 1–4.

Clark, G. F., & Miller, L. E. (1996). Providing effective occupational therapy services: Data-based decision making in school-based practice. *American Journal of Occupational Therapy, 50,* 701–708.

Cutspec, P. (2004). Origins of evidence-based approaches to best practice. *Centerscope, 1,* 2. Retrieved September 1, 2005, from www.researchtopractice.info/centerscopes/centerscope_vol2_no1.pdf

Dettmer, P., Thurston, L., & Sellberg, N. J. (2005). *Consultation, collaboration, and teamwork for students with special needs* (5th ed.). Needham Heights, MA: Allyn & Bacon.

Edelman, L. (2001). *Just being kids* (video). Denver: University of Colorado Health Sciences Center.

Egan, G. (1988). *Change-agent skills B: Managing innovation and change.* San Diego, CA: University Associates.

Falvey, M., Forest, M., Pearpoint, J., & Rosenbury, R. (2004). *All my life's a circle: Using the tools: circles, MAPS & PATHS.* Toronto: Inclusion Press.

Feinberg, E. (2003). *Collaboration and consultation in the schools.* Unpublished workshop presentation, Albuquerque, NM.

Fisher, R., Ury, W., & Patton, B. (1991). *Getting to yes: Negotiating agreement without giving in.* New York: Penguin Books.

Friend, M., & Cook, L. (2007). *Interactions: Collaboration skills for school professionals* (5th ed.). Boston: Allyn & Bacon.

Giangreco, M. F., Cloninger, C. J., Dennis, R. G., & Edelman, S. W. (2000). Problem-solving methods to facilitate inclusive education. In R. Villa & J. Thousand (Eds.), *Restructuring for caring and effective education* (pp. 254–291). Baltimore: Paul H. Brookes.

Giangreco, M., Edelman, S., MacFarland, S., & Luiselli, T. (1997). Attitudes about educational and related service provision for students with deaf-blindness and multiple disabilities. *Exceptional Children, 63,* 329–342.

Giangreco, M., St. Denis, R., Cloninger, C., Edelman, S., & Schattman, R. (1993). "I've counted Jon": Transformational experiences of teachers educating students with disabilities. *Exceptional Children, 59,* 359–371.

Graham, J., & Wright, J. (1999). What does "interprofessional collaboration" mean to professionals working with disabilities? *British Journal of Special Education, 26,* 37–41.

Gretz, S. (1999). Commentary: Parents. *School System Special Interest Section Quarterly, 6*(3), 2–3.

Hall, G., & Hord, S. (2006). *Implementing change: Patterns, principles, and potholes* (2nd ed.). Boston: Pearson Education.

Hanft, B. (1995). *Promoting partnerships* (final report). Bethesda, MD: American Occupational Therapy Association.

Hanft, B., & Place, P. (1996). *The consulting therapist.* Austin, TX: Pro-Ed.

Hanft, B., & Read, J. (2001). Collaborative partnerships. In K. Murray & J. Stockhouse (Eds.), *Professional development leadership academy.* Alexandria, VA: National Association of State Directors of Special Education.

Idol, L., & West, J. (1987). Consultation in special education (Part II): Training and practice. *Journal of Learning Disabilities, 20*(8), 474–494.

Individuals With Disabilities Education Improvement Act of 2004, Pub. L. 108–446, 20 U.S.C. § 1400 *et seq.* (2004).

Korinek, L., McLaughlin, V., & Gable, R. (1994). A planning guide for collaborative service delivery. *Preventing School Failure, 38*(4), 37–40.

McWilliam, R. (2002). *Integrating therapies into classroom routines.* Nashville, TN: Vanderbilt University, Center for Child Development and Outreach Services.

McWilliam, R., & Scott, S. (2001, November). *Integrating therapy into the classroom.* Retrieved December 21, 2006, from www.fpg.unc.edu/~inclusion/IT.pdf

Newberry, A. (1992). *Strategic planning in education.* Vancouver, BC: EduServ.

Nochajski, S. (2001). Collaboration between team members in inclusive educational settings. *Occupational Therapy in Health Care, 15*(3/4), 101–112.

No Child Left Behind Act of 2001, Pub. L. 107–110, 115 Stat. 1425 (2002).

Random House Unabridged Dictionary. (2006). Retrieved April 1, 2007, from http://dictionary.reference.com/browse/partner

Read, J., & Hanft, B. (1999). IDEA '97: Professional development and collaborative partnerships. *NASDSE Liaison Bulletin, 29*(4), 1–7.

Rehabilitation Act Amendments of 1986, Pub. L. 99–506.

Rogers, E. (2000). *Diffusion of innovation* (5th ed.). New York: Free Press.

Schmidt, R., & Lee, T. (2005). *Motor control and learning: A behavioral emphasis* (4th ed.). Champaign, IL: Human Kinetics.

Schoenfeld, H., & Mesquitit, P. (2002). A collaborative partnership: Creating developmentally appropriate teaching practices for pre-K and kindergarten. *School System Special Interest Section Quarterly, 9*(1), 1–4.

Shepherd, J. (1999). Commentary: Practitioners. *School System Special Interest Section Quarterly, 12*(4), 1–3.

Shepherd, J. (2004). Addressing transition and school-to-work in school settings. In Y. Swinth (Ed.), *Occupational therapy in school-based practice: Contemporary issues and trends* (Lesson 1, AOTA Online Course). Bethesda, MD: American Occupational Therapy Association.

Sweeney, B. (2003). *The CBAM: A model of the people development process.* Retrieved June 20, 2007, from www.mentoring-association.org/membersonly/CBAM.html

Swinth, Y. (Ed.). (2004). *Occupational therapy in school-based practice: Contemporary issues and trends* (AOTA Online Course). Bethesda, MD: American Occupational Therapy Association.

Swinth, Y., Hanft, B., DiMatties, M., Handley-Moore, D., Hanson, P., Schoonover, J., et al. (2002, September 16). School-based practice: Moving beyond 1:1 service delivery. *OT Practice,* pp. 12–16.

Swinth, Y., Spencer, K. C., & Jackson, L. L. (2007). *Occupational therapy: Effective school-based practice within a policy context* (COPSSE Document No. OP–3). Gainesville: University of Florida, Center on Personnel Studies in Special Education.

Thress-Suchy, L., Roantee, E., Pfeffer, N., Reese, K., & Jennings, T. (1999). Mothers', fathers' and teachers' perceptions of direct and consultative occupational therapy services. *School System Special Interest Section Quarterly, 6*(3), 1–2.

Tryon, P. (1997). Communication and collaboration with parents and between school- and clinic-based therapists. *Sensory Integration Special Interest Section Quarterly, 29*(4), 1–2.

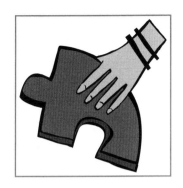

Appendix:
Exhibits and Worksheets

Exhibit or Worksheet	Purpose	Discussed in Chapter
Exhibit 1.1A	Individuals With Disabilities Education Improvement Act of 2004 Definitions of *Free Appropriate Public Education, Least Restrictive Environment,* and *Individualized Education Program* Requirements	1, 5
Exhibit 1.2A	Providing Team Supports via a Report of an Assistive Technology Evaluation	1, 2
Exhibit 2.1A	Collaborative Teaming Assessments Commonly Used in Pediatrics	2, 4
Worksheet 2.1A	How Student- or Family-Oriented Is Your School Team?	2
Worksheet 2.2A	Observation of the School Environment	2
Worksheet 2.3A	Reflection on Team Support Role	2
Worksheet 2.4A	Faces, Spaces, and Paces	2, 4, 5, 7
Worksheet 3.1A	Interpersonal Communication Skills Checklist	3
Worksheet 3.2A	Reflections on Team Collaboration	3
Worksheet 3.3A	Collaborative Team Meeting Worksheet	3
Worksheet 3.4A	School Workload: Collaborative Roles Review	3, 7
Worksheet 6.1A	Resolving Team Conflict by Addressing Core Concerns	6
Worksheet 7.1A	Environmental Scan: Issues Influencing Occupational Therapists' Collaborative Role in the Schools	7
Worksheet 7.2A	Impact–Likelihood Scale: Assessing an Action Plan for Collaboration	7
Worksheet 7.3A	Action Plan for Collaboration	7
Exhibit A	Vignettes Illustrating Hands-On and Team Supports	

Exhibit 1.1A. Individuals With Disabilities Education Improvement Act of 2004
Definitions of *Free Appropriate Public Education, Least Restrictive Environment,*
and *Individualized Education Program* **Requirements**

Free Appropriate Public Education (FAPE)

(34 CFR § 300.17)

Free appropriate public education or FAPE means special education and related services that—

    (a) are provided at public expense, under public supervision and direction, and without charge;

    (b) meet the standards of the SEA, including the requirements of this part;

    (c) include an appropriate preschool, elementary school, or secondary education in the State involved; and

    (d) are provided in conformity with an individualized education program (IEP) that meet the requirements of §§300.320-300.324

Authority: 20 U.S.C. 1401(9)

Least Restrictive Environment (LRE)

(34 CFR § 300.114)

(2) Each public agency must ensure that—

    (i) To the maximum extent appropriate, children with disabilities, including children in public or private institutions or other care facilities, are educated with children who are nondisabled; and

    (ii) Special classes, separate schooling, or other removal of children with disabilities from the regular educational environment occurs only if the nature or severity of the disability is such that education in regular classes with the use of supplementary aids and services cannot be achieved satisfactorily.

Authority: 20 U.S.C. 1412(a)(5)

Individualized Education Program (IEP)

(34 CFR §300.20)

(a) General. As used in this part, the term individualized education program or IEP means a written statement for each child with a disability that is developed, reviewed, and revised in a meeting in accordance with Sec. 300.320 through 300.324, and that must include—

(1) A statement of the child's present levels of academic achievement and functional performance, including—

    (i) How the child's disability affects the child's involvement and progress in the general education curriculum (i.e., the same curriculum as for nondisabled children); or

    (ii) For preschool children, as appropriate, how the disability affects the child's participation in appropriate activities;

(2)(i) A statement of measurable annual goals, including academic and functional goals designed to—

        (A) Meet the child's needs that result from the child's disability to enable the child to be involved in and make progress in the general education curriculum; and

        (B) Meet each of the child's other educational needs that result from the child's disability;

    (ii) For children with disabilities who take alternate assessments aligned to alternate achievement standards, a description of benchmarks or short-term objectives;

(3) A description of—

    (i) How the child's progress toward meeting the annual goals described in paragraph (2) of this section will be measured; and

    (ii) When periodic reports on the progress the child is making toward meeting the annual goals (such as through the use of quarterly or other periodic reports, concurrent with the issuance of report cards) will be provided;

(4) A statement of the special education and related services and supplementary aids and services, based on peer-reviewed research to the extent practicable, to be provided to the child, or on behalf of the child, and a statement of the program modifications or supports for school personnel that will be provided to enable the child—

    (i) To advance appropriately toward attaining the annual goals;

    (ii) To be involved in and make progress in the general education curriculum in accordance with paragraph (a)(1) of this section, and to participate in extracurricular and other nonacademic activities; and

    (iii) To be educated and participate with other children with disabilities and nondisabled children in the activities described in this section;

(5) An explanation of the extent, if any, to which the child will not participate with nondisabled children in the regular class and in the activities described in paragraph (a)(4) of this section;

(6)(i) A statement of any individual appropriate accommodations that are necessary to measure the academic achievement and functional performance of the child on State and districtwide assessments consistent with section 612(a)(16) of the Act; and

(ii) If the IEP Team determines that the child must take an alternate assessment instead of a particular regular State or districtwide assessment of student achievement, a statement of why—

(A) The child cannot participate in the regular assessment; and

(B) The particular alternate assessment selected is appropriate for the child; and

(7) The projected date for the beginning of the services and modifications described in paragraph (a)(4) of this section, and the anticipated frequency, location, and duration of those services and modifications.

Authority: 20 U.S.C. 1414(d)(1)(A)(i)

Exhibit 1.2A. Providing Team Supports via a Report of an Assistive Technology Evaluation

---

Your Public School
Department of Special Education
Classroom Assistive Technology Evaluation

Teacher's Name: ___Tony Teacher___   **School:** ___Community of Learners Middle School___
Program Type: ___"School Within a School"___   **Date of Evaluation:** ___11/30/06___
Reason for Referral: ___AT support to increase/improve student-generated written expression.___

Dear Tony,

Chris and I really enjoyed our visit to your classroom for the assistive technology classroom evaluation you requested. On the day of our visit, there were four students present, and one (substitute) Teaching Assistant. A fifth student arrived just as we were leaving. Whenever we come out and do classroom evaluations, we end up learning new ideas that we can spread around the county. The visit to your classroom was no exception. Although your classroom is small, you have used your space creatively. We were especially impressed with your pocket chart that not only displayed examples of the lesson you were teaching (*prefixes*) but doubled as an organizer for student work as well. We observed that student work was arranged in the pocket chart labeled with student names, which contained each student's notebook and journal. We noted that you had two networked computers, one printer, an overhead projector, and a wall-mounted TV and VCR. Audiotapes and videos of core literature were on bookshelves.

Student input and interaction is clearly part of your teaching style. Student work was posted and evident around the room. You asked your students for input ("What do you think *judge* means?") and gently guided their thought process with compliments and clarification ("Nice use of *example*, but what do you think the word means?). You accepted and revised all answers in a positive manner.

Tony, you introduced us to your students as individuals who assist you in increasing your competence in using technology and mentioned that your students were likely more "tech-savvy" than you felt. You were hoping that one of the outcomes of our visit was to. . . . During our visit, we had a chance to brainstorm with you about some other strategies that might benefit your students, and after our visit Chris and I further discussed various strategies and ideas for possible implementation within your classroom based on the activities viewed during our visit.

Please feel free to use any of these solutions at your discretion, but don't feel like you need to do them all at once. Please select the recommendations you would like to implement first, and then I can help you get those in place. Any specialized equipment or training will be provided. After these are working, you can pick the next few recommendations and we can move from there.

Recommendations: [Specific ideas, where to purchase, Web sites, etc., are suggested in the actual report]

Thanks again, Tony, for letting us come and visit your class. When you get this e-mail, if you have any questions about what is described or suggested, let me know and we can go over them together. We are always available to brainstorm solutions to any concerns you might be having.

Judith Schoonover, MEd, OTR/L, ATP
Assistive Technology Trainer
Your Public School

Exhibit 2.1A. Collaborative Teaming Assessments Commonly Used in Pediatrics

Name	Age Range	Comments
Canadian Occupational Therapy Performance Measure, 4th ed. (COPM; Law et al., 2005)	8 years to adult	*Purpose:* Interview designed by occupational therapists for use with clients with a variety of disabilities and across all developmental stages to detect the client's self-perception of occupational performance over time. It promotes client–occupational therapist collaboration, which can then be shared with the entire team.
Choosing Outcomes and Accommodations for Children, 2nd ed. (COACH; Giangreco, Cloninger, & Iverson, 1998)	3 to 21 years old with moderate, severe, or profound disabilities	*Purpose:* A decision-making process to assist a team to identify collaborative individualized education program (IEP) goals for students with moderate to severe or profound disabilities that can be integrated within the routines of the day. With modifications, components of the COACH may be used with students who are older or who have mild disabilities.
Child Occupation Self Assessment (COSA; Keller, Kafkes, Basu, Federico, & Kielhofner, 2005)	Elementary through high school	*Purpose:* A client-centered assessment tool that allows a child to share perceptions about competence and values. This information could help teams select appropriate goals, and the interview could be conducted by various members of the team.
Making Actions Plans (MAPS; Falvey, Forest, Pearpoint, & Rosenbury, 2004)	All ages	*Purpose:* A person-centered process that helps collaborative teams identify a student's current level of functioning, identify goals, and determine how the team will work together. It is used in schools and community settings.
Planning Alternative Tomorrows With Hope (PATH; Pearpoint, O'Brien, & Forest, 1993)	All ages	*Purpose:* A tool to facilitate a team's collective decision making regarding long- and short-term planning for a student's education program.
School Function Assessment (SFA; Coster, Deeney, Haltiwanger, & Haley, 1998)	Elementary	*Purpose:* A client-centered interview to determine the student–environment fit for students with physical disabilities. Based on the Model of Human Occupation (Kielhofner, 2007), a student describes how he or she is doing in school environments (e.g., classroom, playground, field trips) and interpersonal relationships. Teams would then develop a plan to make necessary accommodations, based on the student-identified needs.
School Setting Interview (SSI; Hemmingson, Egilson, Hoffman, & Kielhofner, 2005)	Elementary through high school	*Purpose:* A semistructured interview that assists a team to make collective decisions when planning interventions and modifications.
Sensory Profile (Dunn, 1999)	3 to 10 years	*Purpose:* A questionnaire that identifies a caregiver's responses to sensory events in a child's daily life. Teams can use this information to develop collaborative IEP goals, make accommodations, and target intervention for specific school contexts.
Adolescent/Adult Sensory Profile (Brown & Dunn, 2002)	11 years or older	*Purpose:* A self-questionnaire that identifies a person's responses to sensory events in everyday life. Teams can use this information to develop collaborative IEP goals, make accommodations, and target intervention for specific school contexts.
Sensory Profile School Companion (Dunn, 2006)	3 to 11 years	*Purpose:* A teacher questionnaire that identifies a student's responses to sensory events in the educational setting. Teams can use this information to develop collaborative IEP goals, make accommodations, and target intervention for specific school contexts.
Vermont Independent Services Team Approach (Giangreco, 1996)	Elementary through high school	*Purpose:* A cross-disciplinary process for a team's collective decision making about related services. This process supports collaborative problem-solving and prioritizing services for a student's IEP.

Note. Developed in 2007 by Gloria Frolek Clark. Information was obtained from Web sites or test manuals.

References

Brown, C., & Dunn, W. (2002). *Adolescent/adult sensory profile.* San Antonio, TX: Psychological Corporation.

Coster, W., Deeney, T., Haltiwanger, J., & Haley, S. (1998). *School function assessment (SFA).* San Antonio, TX: Psychological Corporation.

Dunn, W. (1999). *Sensory profile.* San Antonio, TX: Psychological Corporation

Dunn, W. (2006). *Sensory profile school companion.* San Antonio, TX: Psychological Corporation.

Falvey, M., Forest, M., Pearpoint, J., & Rosenbury, R. (2004). *All my life's a circle: Using the tools: Circles, MAPS, and PATHS.* Toronto: Inclusion Press.

Giangreco, M. (1996). *Vermont Independent Services Team Approach (VISTA)*. Baltimore: Paul H. Brookes.

Giangreco, M., Cloninger, C., & Iverson, M. (1998). *Choosing outcomes and accommodations for children* (2nd ed.). Baltimore: Paul H. Brookes.

Hemmingson, H., Egilson, S., Hoffman, O., & Kielhofner, G. (2005). *School Setting Interview* (Version 3.0). Chicago: MOHO Clearinghouse.

Keller, J., Kafkes, A., Basu, S., Federico, J., & Kielhofner, G. (2005). *Child Occupational Self Assessment* (Version 2.1). Chicago: MOHO Clearinghouse.

Kielhofner, G. (2007). *Model of Human Occupation: Theory and application* (4th ed.). Baltimore: Lippincott Williams & Wilkins.

Law, M., Baptiste, S., Carswell, A., McColl, M., Polatajko, H., & Pollock, N. (2005). *Canadian Occupational Therapy Performance Measure* (4th ed.). Ottawa: Canadian Association of Occupational Therapists.

Pearpoint, J., O'Brien, J., & Forest, M. (1993). *PATH (Planning alternative tomorrows with hope): A workbook for planning positive futures*. Toronto: Inclusion Press.

Worksheet 2.1A. How Student- or Family-Oriented Is Your School Team?

Read the following items, and in the column for students or parents, check if you do that item to give students or parents input to your team. ✔+ yes, most of the time ✔− sometimes 0 no or rarely		
Do you . . .	**Students**	**Parents**
1. Ask the student/parent what he or she likes to do when at home or at school?		
2. Ask what is working well for this student at home as well as at school?		
3. Allow them to voice their opinion about their own strengths and needs?		
4. Help students/parents voice their opinions even if you disagree with them?		
5. Acknowledge their opinions and preferences?		
6. Give students/parents the opportunity to lead groups (e.g., class, IEP meeting, teacher meeting, extracurricular activities)?		
7. Use identified concerns to help guide goals and objectives?		
8. Identify and use interests and preferences to guide activities and accommodations?		
9. Give options or choices for goals and activities?		
10. Give options for communication between staff and family (e.g., phone calls, e-mail, communication notebook, videos)?		
Regarding IEP meetings, do you . . .		
11. Include the student as well as the family in the IEP meeting?		
12. Give choices about who will come to their IEP meeting (e.g., parents, siblings, friends, specific teachers)?		
13. Give options for IEP and other meetings (who, when, where, what to discuss)?		
14. Assist in getting prepared for meeting ahead of time (e.g., what to bring to the meeting, a transition checklist, or welcome them bringing a friend)?		
15. Help the student and family feel welcomed and valued in the IEP meeting (e.g., refer to them; ask their opinion)?		
16. Give students/parents the opportunity to lead groups (e.g., class, IEP meeting, teacher meeting, extracurricular activities)?		
17. Help students/parents voice their opinions even if you disagree with them?		
18. Acknowledge their opinions and preferences?		
Regarding the team process, do you . . .		
19. Ask the student and family individually, "What can our team do better?"		
20. Reevaluate team's comfort level with student-centered practices and communication with family?		
COMMENTS:		

Note. IEP = individualized education program.

Worksheet 2.2A. Observation of the School Environment

Student: _____　Grade: _____　Date/time: _____

"Place/space": _____　Activity: _____

Context	Description of Characteristics		
Cultural *Customs, ethnicity, beliefs, values, school climate, teaching practices, behavior standards.*	School atmosphere/expectations: Classroom atmosphere/expectations: Relationships between students, parents, school staff and administrators: Acceptance of diversity in students?　☐ Yes　　☐ No		
Social *Peer/adult interaction* *Expectations for roles and routines*	What is the class size? Impressions? When are there opportunities for socialization with peers? Are there others with disabilities?　☐ Yes　　☐ No Expected social norms and routines (e.g., classroom rules, jobs/chores)		
Temporal *Duration, time of day, sequencing, age appropriate*	☐ Adequate ☐ Inadequate	Materials and routines are age appropriate.	
	☐ Adequate ☐ Inadequate	Sequencing and timing of activities:	
		☐ Adequate ☐ Inadequate	Classroom schedule (structured/unstructured)
		☐ Adequate ☐ Inadequate	Variety of activities with quiet and active times
		☐ Adequate ☐ Inadequate	Movement opportunities
		☐ Adequate ☐ Inadequate	Duration of activities
	Comments:		
	Routines		
	☐ Adequate ☐ Inadequate	Beginning the day/class	
	☐ Adequate ☐ Inadequate	Academics (e.g., time of day, placement of homework, objects brought to reading group, review of materials)	
	☐ Adequate ☐ Inadequate	Time management, organizational strategies	
	☐ Adequate ☐ Inadequate	Self-care (e.g., bathroom, cafeteria, handwashing, putting on coats)	

Worksheet 2.2A. Observation of the School Environment *(continued)*

Context	Description of Characteristics		
Virtual *Computers, whiteboards, electronic devices using airways*	☐ Adequate ☐ Inadequate	Going to and from classes or different areas of the school	
	☐ Adequate ☐ Inadequate	Transitioning between activities; ending the day/class	
	Comments:		
	Check whether the following are adequate and describe if needed:		
	☐ Adequate ☐ Inadequate	Computers are used	
		☐ Adequate ☐ Inadequate	Frequency?
		☐ Adequate ☐ Inadequate	Internet capabilities?
	☐ Adequate ☐ Inadequate	Personal digital assistants (e.g., Palm Pilot, BlackBerry)	
	☐ Adequate ☐ Inadequate	Electronic schedulers, memory devices	
	☐ Adequate ☐ Inadequate	Augmentative communication devices, electronic aids for daily living	
	☐ Adequate ☐ Inadequate	Computer projection systems, virtual blackboards, etc.	
	Comments:		
Physical *Accessibility of building, objects, tools, devices, terrain, plants, animals*	*Check if the following are adequate and describe if needed below:*		
	Accessibility and availability		
	☐ Adequate ☐ Inadequate	Classroom materials (e.g., books, writing tools, papers)	
	Context	Furniture height and size	
	☐ Adequate ☐ Inadequate	Computer or assistive technology setup and adjustability	
	☐ Adequate ☐ Inadequate	Personal belongings	
	☐ Adequate ☐ Inadequate	Bathrooms/sinks	
	☐ Adequate ☐ Inadequate	Other areas of the school	
	Comments:		

(continued)

Worksheet 2.2A. Observation of the School Environment *(continued)*

Context	Description of Characteristics		
Physical *Space dimensions*	**Space Dimensions**		
	☐ Adequate ☐ Inadequate	Size for number of people and objects	
	☐ Adequate ☐ Inadequate	Organization/arrangement of furniture and space (diagram)	
	☐ Adequate ☐ Inadequate	Traffic pathways are defined	
	☐ Adequate ☐ Inadequate	Intent of space is clear (e.g., academics, social/play area, self-care, independent/cooperative, quiet/active areas)	
	Comments:		
	Sensory Characteristics of Materials or Environment		
Sensory characteristics	☐ Adequate ☐ Inadequate	**Tactile/kinesthetic (materials, furniture, carpet):**	
		☐ Adequate ☐ Inadequate	Textures
		☐ Adequate ☐ Inadequate	Proximity to others
		☐ Adequate ☐ Inadequate	Other features
	☐ Adequate ☐ Inadequate	**Auditory:**	
		☐ Adequate ☐ Inadequate	Noise level in or outside classroom
		☐ Adequate ☐ Inadequate	Acoustic features
	☐ Adequate ☐ Inadequate	**Visual:**	
		☐ Adequate ☐ Inadequate	Light source (any glare?)
		☐ Adequate ☐ Inadequate	Color
		☐ Adequate ☐ Inadequate	Chalkboard, computer, projection systems, written materials
		☐ Adequate ☐ Inadequate	Bulletin boards, visual schedules, decorations
		☐ Adequate ☐ Inadequate	Other features
	☐ Adequate ☐ Inadequate	**Movement opportunities**	
	☐ Adequate ☐ Inadequate	**Temperature/humidity/ventilation**	
	Comments:		

Recommendations to discuss with teacher and other team members (ways to increase or decrease accessibility, distractions, socialization, or the "fit" between the student, the demands of the activity, and the environment):

Worksheet 2.3A. Reflection on Team Support Role

Student: _____

Team member(s) supported: _____

Are my suggestions working for this team?	Yes	No	Examples
1. Do activities and strategies address educational goals?			
2. Do they "fit" within a school context?			
3. Do they "fit" with the needs of ALL students in the classroom?			
4. Are they practical and doable by a specific team member?			
5. Do they "fit" with a team member's role and instruction–interaction style?			
6. Is there evidence that they will make a difference?			
7. How follow-up will be provided:			
8. How activities and strategies might be modified to promote student's participation in school:			
9. How data will be collected to measure progress:			

Worksheet 2.4A. Faces, Spaces, and Paces

Student: _____   Grade: _____   Date: _____

1. FACES (core team members):

2. Listen to key team members and record their words below.	
Student's Strengths and Interests	**Student's Challenges**
Desired Educational Outcomes	

3. PLACES and SPACES student was observed in the school environment: a. b. c.	
What's working for this student in this environment?	What challenges are present in this environment?

4. PACES: Describe how the student meets role expectations and keeps up with the pace of school life (e.g., schedule, study habits, homework, time use, hygiene and health habits).	
What is expected of this student?	How do the student's routines and habits influence his or her performance?

5. Collaborative Roles (suggestions for IEP/team meetings)	Who will do what?
☐ Hands-on/team supports	
☐ Team supports	
☐ System supports	

6. COMMENTS	

Worksheet 3.1A. Interpersonal Communication Skills Checklist

Skills	Specific Tasks	Needs to Improve	OK	My Strength
Interpersonal and Communication	1. I communicate with others in everyday language.			
	2. I support team members giving positive and descriptive feedback about what they are doing.			
	3. I communicate positively verbally and with body language (e.g., eye contact, body stance, gestures).			
	4. I ask others their opinion and acknowledge their expertise.			
	5. I listen to others and reiterate what I hear.			
	6. I state my appreciation of team members' thoughts, feelings or actions.			
	7. I communicate trust to fellow team members by displaying empathy, positive regard, and credibility.			
	8. I recognize my own biases and emotions when dealing with team issues.			
	9. I address and manage conflict skillfully.			
Collaborative Problem Solving and Decision Making	10. I understand the roles and talents of team members.			
	11. I am optimistic that problems can be solved.			
	12. I offer multiple suggestions for the team to choose a plan of action.			
	13. I brainstorm ideas with the team or administrators to improve team and system supports.			
	14. I listen to others' suggestions prior to making judgments and work with my team to evaluate their benefits for students.			
	15. I blend roles when appropriate to benefit the student.			
	16. I coach others to try new techniques or ideas.			
	17. I commit to the team decision even if I disagreed during the decision-making process.			
	18. I encourage the team to use data to make decisions.			
	19. I employ strategies for coping with challenging team behaviors.			
Professional Development	20. I evaluate my effectiveness in achieving student outcomes and providing team and system supports.			
	21. I share information with team members that is relevant and practical to them.			
	22. I ask for, accept, and incorporate suggestions to improve my practice.			
	23. I seek professional development within and outside my profession (e.g., workshop, in-service, journals).			
	24. I help coach or mentor new therapists or team members to be a collaborative partner.			

Worksheet 3.2A. Reflections on Team Collaboration

Check how frequently your team demonstrates the following characteristics of collaboration during meetings and other interactions. Discuss together, or complete individually and share comments.

Collaborative Characteristics	Example	Definitely	Sometimes	Rarely
Team Functions				
Voluntary membership	"We want to be part of this team."			
Equality among team members	"Your opinion as a COTA (or whomever) is considered as equally as my opinion."			
Shared purpose	"We share the common goal to get this child to be as independent as possible."			
Mutual values	"We believe in inclusion."			
Defined roles and responsibilities	"My job is to schedule IEP meetings with parents and document that I did this."			
Shared responsibility for decision making	"As a team, we reviewed our options and decided to try this technique."			
Joint accountability for outcomes	"This year, we did not reach Mark's goal of learning to ride the bus. What happened?"			
Shared resources	"I added some new toys to the fidget basket for you to use during reading."			
Value collaboration	"Let's talk about how we can help Horatio and his classmates play together at recess."			
Trust team members	"I believe that Jill thought this was the best solution."			
Sense of community	"Our team works together to help high school students learn work skills."			
Communication				
Guidelines govern roles and communication	"We all have input before we take a vote or make a decision."			
Flexible process	"I will take notes for you now and next time I will leave you an e-mail message."			
Opinions and contributions are respected	"Great idea! How do you think it will work for Josie?"			
Concerns and conflicts addressed and resolved	"Can we talk about what happened yesterday in my classroom with Mary Jo?"			
Lifelong learning is expected	"Let's learn how to do this together. I have an article to share."			
Process Skills				
Agenda accomplished	"We followed the agenda and met our goals."			
Contributions to the team process stated	"I will show Mrs. Davalos the data we have been keeping."			
Reflect on team process and interactions	"We really listened to Duncan and used his ideas and preferences for possible jobs."			
Develop team and individual goals	"Next week, can we keep to our time schedule by using a 2-minute warning?"			

Note. COTA = certified occupational therapy assistant; IEP = individualized education program.

Worksheet 3.3A. Collaborative Team Meeting Worksheet

Collaborative Team Meeting Worksheet		
Date: _____		
Members present: 1.	Members absent: 1.	Others who need to know
Roles	**This Meeting**	**Next Meeting**
• Facilitator	_____	_____
• Recorder	_____	_____
• Timekeeper	_____	_____
• Processor or observer	_____	_____
• Jargon buster	_____	_____
• Other: _____	_____	_____
Agenda		
Items	**Time Limit**	**Synopsis of Discussion**
1. _____	_____	_____
2. _____	_____	_____
3. _____	_____	_____
4. _____	_____	_____
5. _____	_____	_____
Action Plan		
Action Items	**Person Responsible**	**By When?**
_____	_____	_____
_____	_____	_____
_____	_____	_____
_____	_____	_____
_____	_____	_____
Agenda for Next Meeting		
Date: _____	Expected agenda items	
Time: _____	1. _____	4. _____
Location: _____	2. _____	5. _____
_____	3. _____	6. _____
How Did We Work as a Team Today?		
What worked well?	What needs improvement?	How will we improve?

From Snell, M. E., & Janney, R. (2005). Collaborative team meeting worksheet. In M. E. Snell & R. Janney (Eds.), *Collaborative teaming* (2nd ed., Appendix, p. 50). Baltimore: Brookes. Copyright © 2005 by Brookes. Adapted with permission.

Worksheet 3.4A. School Workload: Collaborative Roles Review

_____ (Name)   ☐ OTR   ☐ COTA   _____ Date

| Sample of Students (Initials, Grade) | Hands-On Role *(must include team support)* | | Team Support Role |
	In Context: Where/How Often	Out of Context: Where/How Often	Whom I Collaborate With and How Often
1.			
2.			
3.			
4.			
5.			
6.			

System supports I provide *(check those that apply):*

☐ Coordinate/supervise OT   ☐ Handwriting curriculum   ☐ In-services: _____   ☐ School policies or procedures

☐ Playground design   ☐ Positive behavior support team   ☐ Prereferral screening   ☐ Program evaluation

☐ Aide training   ☐ Assistive technology team   ☐ Other task force or committee   ☐ After-school activities

☐ _____   ☐ _____   ☐ _____   ☐ _____

Note. OTR = registered occupational therapist; COTA = certified occupational therapy assistant; OT = occupational therapy.

Worksheet 6.1A. Resolving Team Conflict by Addressing Core Concerns

Core Concerns and Reflections	I Did This	I Need to Consider This
1. Appreciation: Of others' thoughts, feelings and actions		
• Do I communicate understanding?		
• Do I understand others' points of view?		
• Do I share my point of view?		
2. Affiliation: Build a feeling of connectedness		
• Do I look for professional links between others and myself?		
• Do I look for personal links between others and myself?		
• Do I treat the person as a colleague?		
3. Respect autonomy: Support decision-making process and choices		
• Are we here to inform others about decisions, collaborate with others, or to negotiate?		
• Do we brainstorm recommendations together?		
• Do we consider all stakeholders and/or decision makers?		
4. Recognize status: Understand how the status or knowledge of team members affects interactions		
• Do I recognize the status of others and show respect but not give it more weight in negotiation?		
• Do I acknowledge status in others and in myself?		
• Do I educate myself about other's knowledge?		
5. Choose a fulfilling team operational role: meaningful, purposeful, and not pretentious		
• Do I acknowledge the purpose of this interaction?		
• Did I clarify my and other person's roles during this interaction?		
• Did I choose a temporary operational role that encourages collaboration (e.g., joker, brainstormer, or advocate)?		

Note. Based on the work of Fisher, R., & Shapiro, D. (2005). *Beyond reason: Using emotions as you negotiate.* New York: Penguin.

Worksheet 7.1A. Environmental Scan: Issues Influencing Occupational Therapists' Collaborative Role in the Schools

Stakeholders	Stakeholder Beliefs	Political and Economic Trends	Professional Development	School Trends and Demographics
Key stakeholders invested in school-based occupational therapy?	Beliefs and attitudes regarding school-based occupational therapy?	Federal, state, and local laws and regulations and administrative policy affecting occupational therapy services and financing?	Current and anticipated changes in occupational therapy theory, research, and practice?	Staff training and experience? Changes in student population (general and special education)? Occupational therapists' workload?
Issues:	Issues:	Issues:	Issues:	Issues:
Resources:	Resources:	Resources:	Resources:	Resources:
Challenges:	Challenges:	Challenges:	Challenges:	Challenges:

Worksheet 7.2A. Impact–Likelihood Scale: Assessing an Action Plan for Collaboration

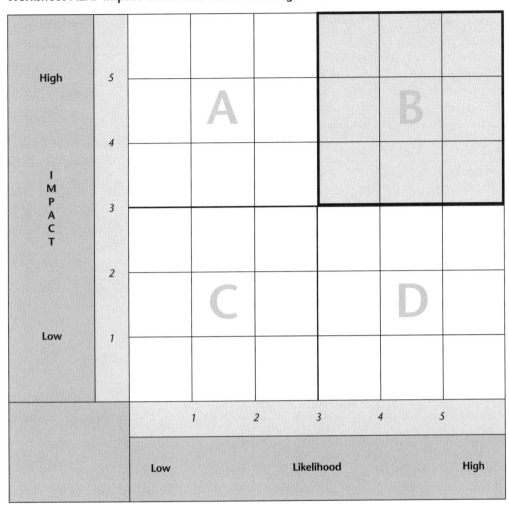

Key: A: High impact and **unlikely** to accomplish   **B: High** impact and **likely** to accomplish
        C: Low impact and **unlikely** to accomplish   **D: Low** impact and **likely** to accomplish

GOALS:

Worksheet 7.3A. Action Plan for Collaboration

Goals and Action Steps	Facilitated by	Criteria for Success	Completed by
Goal # ___			
Action Steps 1			
2			
3			
4			

Exhibit A. Vignettes Illustrating Hands-On and Team Supports

Page	Collaborators	% of Occupational Therapy Time in HO and TS	Focus of Collaboration
		Chapter 1: 2 . . . 4 . . . 6 . . . 8 . . . How Do You Collaborate?	
10	**Julio,** preschool student Derrick, occupational therapist Marianne, Julio's teacher	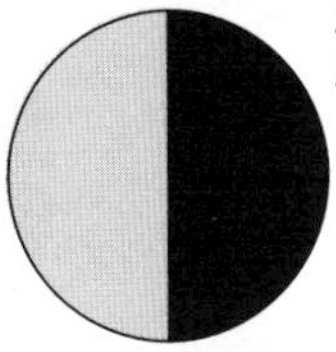 50% TS 50% HO	Eating lunch within 20 min.
11	**Adamo,** student, second grade Linda, occupational therapist Mr. Sylvester, custodian	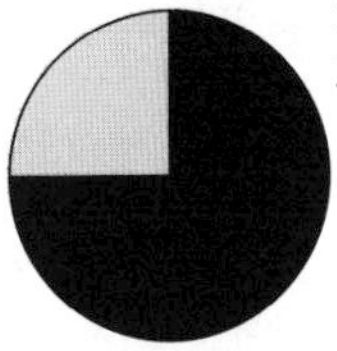 75% TS 25% HO	Using appropriate social skills throughout the school
		Chapter 2: Team Faces and Spaces	
37	**Jonell,** student, kindergarten Jonell's parents Heidi, occupational therapist Jonell's teacher Anita, speech–language pathologist Nutritionist Cafeteria staff Custodian Administrator	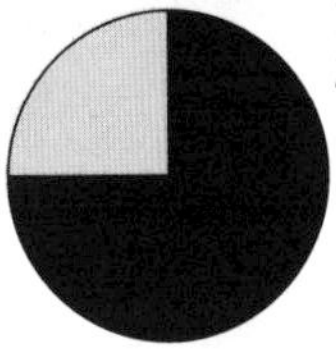 75% TS 25% HO	Carry cafeteria tray to the table
		Chapter 3: Teamwork Versus the Lone Ranger	
83–84	**Preschool Class for Children With Autism** Matt, occupational therapist Preschool teacher Speech–language pathologist Assistive technology team	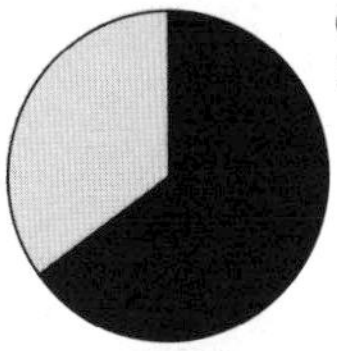 65% TS 35% HO	Support students in school routines and activities using assistive technology
85	**Gretchen,** student, 10th grade Judy, occupational therapist Teachers: special education, physical education, life skills, art, music, social studies Paraprofessional Speech–language pathologist Physical therapist Job coach	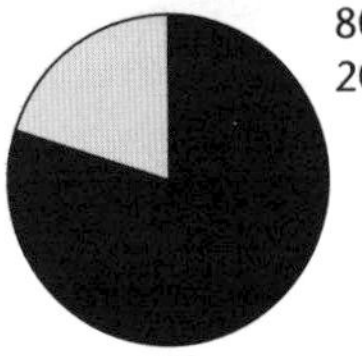 80% TS 20% HO	Wants to participate with her peers in physical education, art, music, leisure activities, social studies, life skills class, and have a job in the community.

(continued)

Exhibit A. Vignettes Illustrating Hands-On and Team Supports (continued)

Page	Collaborators	% of Occupational Therapy Time in HO and TS	Focus of Collaboration
		Chapter 4: Getting Into a Collaborative School Routine	
109	**Marina,** student, third grade June, registered occupational therapist Lisba, general educator Eva, school nurse	40% TS 60% HO	Assessment for reading and writing fluently post–head injury
110–111	**Amos,** student, first grade Alex, occupational therapist Lyla, general educator Michael, special educator	80% TS 20% HO	Assessment and documentation of activities of daily living and behavior
113	**Jamald,** student, third grade Wynn, occupational therapist Sabrina, mother Bonita, general educator	85% TS 15% HO	After assessment, drinking to stay hydrated
114	**Daniel,** student, first grade Doreen, occupational therapist Mrs. Willow, general educator	10% TS 90% HO	Tool usage: developing cutting and writing skills
114–115	**Galiana,** student, first grade Maureen, occupational therapist Virginia, general educator	80% TS 20% HO	Tool usage: developing cutting and writing skills
116	**Huang,** student, 11th grade Remy, occupational therapist Will, vocational educator Mr. D'Angelo, onsite work supervisor	50% TS 50% HO	Assessment of community work—washing dishes at local pizzeria
121–124	**Charlie,** student, first grade Rhonda, occupational therapist Anne, general educator Brock, paraprofessional	70% TS 30% HO	6 weeks of response to intervention with progress monitoring for handwriting legibility
126–128	**Kekoa,** student, middle school Cheryl, occupational therapist Charlotte, general educator Jonathan, paraprofessional	65% TS 35% HO	Community prevocational training for student with autism

Exhibit A. Vignettes Illustrating Hands-On and Team Supports *(continued)*

Page	Collaborators	% of Occupational Therapy Time in HO and TS	Focus of Collaboration
		Chapter 4: Getting Into a Collaborative School Routine *(continued)*	
129–131	**Sakina,** preschooler Occupational therapy assistant Parents Special educator Paraprofessional	50% TS 50% HO	Developing self-feeding and handwashing skills within a preschool routine
132–134	**Leo,** high school student Leon and Angelica, parents Jada, special educator Barney, general educator Raab, occupational therapist Zeke, paraprofessional Chestina, speech–language pathologist	50% TS 50% HO	Learning personal hygiene and social and job skills for a student with moderate to severe disabilities
		Chapter 5: Collaboration in Action: The Nitty Gritty	
157–165	**Susannah,** student, second to fourth grade Mina, occupational therapist Sarah and Ryan Hudson, parents Felicia, paraprofessional Arleathia, special educator Rebekah, third-grade general educator	20% TS 80% HO 80% TS 20% HO	Developing social skills and anger management to move to full inclusion; facilitate Making Action Plans (MAPS; Pearpoint, Forest, & O'Brien, 1996) process for team decision making
		Chapter 6: Conflict Happens: Negotiate, Collaborate, and Get Over It	
173–174	**Elaina,** student, second grade Christy, occupational therapist Shawn, special educator Mildred, paraprofessional Lakshmi, school psychologist	70% TS 30% HO	Team problem solving to determine how to help Elaina transition between activities and address handwashing, dressing, and tool usage skills
175–176	**Carmine,** student, third grade Molly, occupational therapy assistant Lena, general educator Niaz, special educator Jacqueleen, art teacher	60% TS 20% HO 20% SS	Providing sensory strategies to use in general education classrooms
184–188	**Pedro,** 12th grade Bijul, occupational therapist Carlotta, mother Keegan, general educator Bonita, special educator Robert, physical therapist	40% TS 40% HO 20% SS	Team supports to develop self-advocacy and instrumental activities of daily living in preparation for college

(continued)

Exhibit A. Vignettes Illustrating Hands-On and Team Supports *(continued)*

Page	Collaborators	% of Occupational Therapy Time in HO and TS	Focus of Collaboration
		Chapter 7: Reframing Perspectives About Collaboration	
197	**Colin,** student, second grade Ancolien, occupational therapist Nikki, mother Britt, general educator Shelby, speech–language pathologist	50% TS 50% HO	Assessing adaptive equipment to promote communication and social interaction in the classroom and at home

Note. TS = team supports; HO = hands-on and team supports; SS = system supports.
Reference. Pearpoint, J., Forest, M., & O'Brien, J. (1996). MAPS, Circle of Friends, and PATH: Powerful tools to help build caring communities. In S. Stainback & W. Stainback (Eds.), *Inclusion: A guide for educators* (pp. 67–86). Baltimore: Paul H. Brookes.

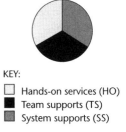

KEY:
☐ Hands-on services (HO)
■ Team supports (TS)
▨ System supports (SS)

Subject Index

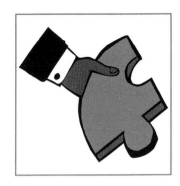

3:1 transition model, 152–153

A

AAC (alternative augmentative communication) device (collaboration in action), 196–197

accessibility
    defined, 54–55
    in physical environment, 53, 54–56

accountability indicators, as part of action plan, 220

action plans
    accountability indicators, 220
    Action plan for collaboration (worksheet), 246
    brainstorming, 216
    creating (collaboration in action), 215–216
    defined, 215
    developing, 215–222
    as draft, 220
    evaluating effectiveness of, 220–222
    identifying and prioritizing goals, 216–219
    impact-likelihood analysis, 217–218
    Impact-likelihood scale: assessing an action plan for collaboration (worksheet), 245
    timelines and responsibilities, 219–220
    vs. vision statement, 215

action steps, defined, 219

activities of daily living (ADLs), as occupation area, 105

adjourning, as teaming stage, 170, 171–172

ADLs. See activities of daily living

administrators
    administrative support (therapist voices), 149
    brainstorming (administrator voices), 178
    clarifying questions (administrator voices), 178
    collaboration, initiating with (therapist voices), 86
    conflict resolution (administrator voices), 188
    determining how OT will fit into school, 43
    early collaboration, importance of (administrator voices), 124–125
    as essential to team collaboration, 74, 165, 196
    as faces on team, 36
    family goals (administrator voices), 201
    flexible services and supports and, 148–153
    hands-on services, misassumptions about (administrator voices), 201
    mentoring, importance of (administrator voices), 99–100
    as mentors, 95
    negotiation, appreciation during (administrator voices), 179
    planning, as ongoing process (administrator voices), 222
    problem-solving (administrator voices), 178
    school culture and teamwork (administrator voices), 57
    student goals (administrator voices), 201
    system change (administrator voices), 203
    team, importance of (administrator voices), 76

adult learning, using principles of in collaboration, 80–82

advocate, as temporary role during negotiation, 182

affiliation, as concern during negotiation, 180

Alert Program, 158, 176

alternative augmentative communication (AAC) device (collaboration in action), 196–197

alternative programs
    recognition of importance of, 14

American Occupational Therapy Association (AOTA)
    Guidelines for Supervision, Roles, and Responsibilities During the Delivery of Occupational Therapy Services, 50
    professional standards in public education, 107
    Promoting Partnership summit, 213
    vision statement of OT services at state and local levels, 212–213
    See also Occupational Therapy Practice Framework: Domain and Process

anchored understanding
    defined, 47
    as used in negotiation, 179

AOTA. See American Occupational Therapy Association

appreciation, as concern during negotiation, 179

Asperger syndrome, 157

assessments
    Child Occupation Self Assessment (COSA), 40, 41
    collaboration during, 112–113
    COSA (Child Occupation Self Assessment), 40, 41
    importance of teamwork in creating, 76–77
    measurable IEP goal, developing, 112–113
    student-centered, 40–41

Citation Index

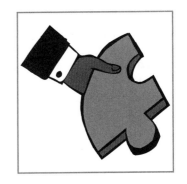